S0-AFC-695

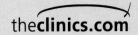
theclinics.com

MAGNETIC RESONANCE IMAGING CLINICS

OF NORTH AMERICA

Body MR Imaging: 1.5T versus 3T

Guest Editor

ELMAR M. MERKLE, MD

August 2007 • Volume 15 • Number 3

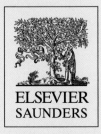

ELSEVIER
SAUNDERS

An imprint of Elsevier, Inc
PHILADELPHIA LONDON TORONTO MONTREAL SYDNEY TOKYO

W.B. SAUNDERS COMPANY
A Divison of Elsevier Inc.

Elsevier Inc. ● 1600 John F. Kennedy Boulevard ● Suite 1800 ●
Philadelphia, Pennsylvania 19103-2899

http://www.mri.theclinics.com

MRI CLINICS OF NORTH AMERICA Volume 15, Number 3
August 2007 ISSN 1064-9689, ISBN 13: 978-1-4160-5088-9, ISBN 10: 1-4160-5088-4

Editor: Lisa Richman

Copyright © 2007 by Elsevier Inc. All rights reserved. No part of this publication may be reproduced or transmitted in any form or by any means, electronic or mechanical, including photocopy, recording, or any information retrieval system, without permission from the Publisher.

Single photocopies of single articles may be made for personal use as allowed by national copyright laws. Permission of the publisher and payment of a fee is required for all other photocopying, including multiple or systematic copying, copying for advertising or promotional purposes, resale, and all forms of document delivery. Special rates are available for educational institutions that wish to make photocopies for non-profit educational classroom use. Permission may be sought directly from Elsevier's Global Rights Department in Oxford, UK: phone 215-239-3804 or +44 (0)1865 843830, fax +44 (0)1865 853333, e-mail: healthpermissions@elsevier.com. Requests may also be completed online via the Elsevier homepage (http://www.elsevier.com/permissions). In the USA, users may clear permissions and make payments through the Copyright Clearance Center, Inc., 222 Rosewood Drive, "Danvers, MA 01923, USA; phone: (978) 750-8400, fax: (978) 750-4744, and in the UK through the Copyright Licensing Agency Rapid Clearance Service (CLARCS), 90 Tottenham Court Road, London W1P 0LP, UK; phone: (+44) 171 436 5931; fax: (+44) 171 436 3986. Other countries may have a local reprographic rights agency for payments.

Reprints: For copies of 100 or more, of articles in this publication, please contact the Commercial Reprints Department, Elsevier Inc., 360 Park Avenue South, New York, New York 10010-1710. Tel. (212) 633-3813, Fax: (212) 462-1935, email: reprints@elsevier.com.

The ideas and opinions expressed in *Magnetic Resonance Imaging Clinics of North America* do not necessarily reflect those of the Publisher. The Publisher does not assume any responsibility for any injury and/or damage to persons or property arising out of or related to any use of the material contained in this periodical. The reader is advised to check the appropriate medical literature and the product information currently provided by the manufacturer of each drug to be administered to verify the dosage, the method and duration of administration, or contraindications. It is the responsibility of the treating physician or other health care professional, relying on independent experience and knowledge of the patient, to determine drug dosages and the best treatment for the patient. Mention of any product in this issue should not be construed as endorsement by the contributors, editors, or the Publisher of the product or manufacturers' claims.

Magnetic Resonance Imaging Clinics of North America (ISSN 1064-9689) is published quarterly by Elsevier Inc., 360 Park Avenue South, New York, NY 10010-1710. Months of issue are February, May, August, and November. Business and Editorial Offices: 1600 John F. Kennedy Blvd., Suite 1800, Philadelphia, PA 19103-2899. Customer Service Office: 6277 Sea Harbor Drive, Orlando, FL 32887-4800. Periodicals postage paid at New York, NY and additional mailing offices. Subscription prices are $226.00 per year (US individuals), $336.00 per year (US institutions), $110.00 per year (US students), $253.00 per year (Canadian individuals), $413.00 per year (Canadian institutions), $149.00 per year (Canadian students), $308.00 per year (international individuals), $413.00 per year (international institutions), and $149.00 per year (international students). International air speed delivery is included in all *Clinics* subscription prices. All prices are subject to change without notice. **POSTMASTER:** Send address changes to *Magnetic Resonance Imaging Clinics*, Elsevier Periodicals Customer Service, 6277 Sea Harbor Drive, Orlando, FL 32887-4800. **Customer Service: 1-800-654-2452 (US). From outside of the US, call 1-407-345-4000.**

Magnetic Resonance Imaging Clinics of North America is covered in the *RSNA Index of Imaging Literature*, *Index Medicus*, *MEDLINE*, and *EMBASE/Excerpta Medica*.

Printed in the United States of America.

BODY MR IMAGING: 1.5T VERSUS 3T

GUEST EDITOR

ELMAR M. MERKLE, MD
Professor of Radiology, Department of Radiology;
and Director of Body MR Imaging; and Medical
Director, Center for Advanced MR Development,
Duke University Medical Center, Durham,
North Carolina

CONTRIBUTORS

ERSAN ALTUN, MD
Department of Radiology, University of North
Carolina at Chapel Hill, Chapel Hill, North
Carolina

ULRIKE I. ATTENBERGER, MD
Institute of Clinical Radiology, University
of Munich–Grosshadern Campus, Munich,
Germany

SUSANNE BOOTH, MRCOG
Specialist Registrar in Obstetrics and Gynaecology;
and Lecturer in MR Imaging, Centre for MR
Investigations, Hull Royal Infirmary, United
Kingdom

DAVID D. CHILDS, MD
Assistant Professor, Department of Radiology,
Wake Forest University School of Medicine,
Winston-Salem, North Carolina

DANIEL M. CORNFELD, MD
Assistant Professor of Diagnostic Radiology,
Department of Diagnostic Radiology, Yale
University School of Medicine, New Haven,
Connecticut

BRIAN M. DALE, PhD
Siemens Medical Solutions, Cary, North Carolina

ROBERT R. EDELMAN, MD
Chairman, Department of Radiology, Evanston
Northwestern Healthcare; Professor of Radiology,
Feinberg School of Medicine, Northwest
University, Evanston, Illinois

MICHAEL FENCHEL, MD
Resident, Eberhard Karls University, Tubingen,
Germany

J. PAUL FINN, MD
Professor of Radiology and Medicine;
and Chief, Diagnostic and Cardiovascular
Imaging, Department of Radiological Sciences,
David Geffen School of Medicine, University
of California Los Angeles, Los Angeles, California

JOHANNES M. FROEHLICH, PhD
MR Research Group, Cantonal Hospital,
Winterthur, Switzerland

ELIZABETH M. HECHT, MD
Assistant Professor, Department of Radiology,
New York University School of Medicine,
New York, New York

VASCO HERÉDIA, MD
Department of Radiology, University of North
Carolina at Chapel Hill, Chapel Hill, North
Carolina

CHRISTIANE K. KUHL, MD
Professor of Radiology, Oncologic Imaging and
Intervention, Department of Radiology, University
of Bonn, Bonn, Germany

HARALD KRAMER, MD
Institute of Clinical Radiology, University
of Munich–Grosshadern Campus, Munich,
Germany

THOMAS C. LAUENSTEIN, MD
Assistant Professor of Radiology, Department
of Radiology, The Emory Clinic, Atlanta, Georgia

RAY F. LEE, PhD
Assistant Professor, Department of Radiology,
New York University School of Medicine, New York,
New York

JOHN R. LEYENDECKER, MD
Associate Professor, Department of Radiology,
Wake Forest University School of Medicine,
Winston-Salem, North Carolina

DIEGO R. MARTIN, MD, PhD
Professor of Radiology, Department of Radiology,
The Emory Clinic, Atlanta, Georgia

ELMAR M. MERKLE, MD
Professor of Radiology, Department of Radiology;
and Director of Body MR Imaging; and Medical
Director, Center for Advanced MR Development,
Duke University Medical Center, Durham, North
Carolina

HENRIK J. MICHAELY, MD
Institute of Clinical Radiology, University
Hospital Mannheim, Medical Faculty
Mannheim-University of Heidelberg,
Mannheim; Institute of Clinical Radiology,
University of Munich–Grosshadern Campus,
Munich, Germany

KAMBIZ NAEL, MD
Resident; and Research Fellow, Department
of Radiological Sciences, David Geffen School
of Medicine, University of California,
Los Angeles, Los Angeles, California

MICHAEL A. PATAK, MD
Institute of Diagnostic Interventional and
Pediatric Radiology, Inselspital, University
Hospital, Bern, Switzerland

MIGUEL RAMALHO, MD
Department of Radiology, University of North
Carolina at Chapel Hill, Chapel Hill, North
Carolina

MAXIMILIAN F. REISER, MD
Institute of Clinical Radiology, University
of Munich–Grosshadern Campus, Munich,
Germany

BETTINA SAAR, MD
Institut für Diagnostische, Interventionelle, und
Pädiatrische Radiologie der Universität Bern,
Inselspital, Bern, Switzerland

ROYA SALEH, MD
Department of Radiological Sciences, David
Geffen School of Medicine, University
of California, Los Angeles, Los Angeles, California

RICHARD SEMELKA, MD
Department of Radiology, University of North
Carolina at Chapel Hill, Chapel Hill, North
Carolina

SEBASTIAN T. SCHINDERA, MD
Interventional and Pediatric Radiology, University
Hospital of Bern, Institute for Diagnostic,
Inselspital Bern, Bern, Switzerland

STEFAN O. SCHOENBERG, MD
Institute of Clinical Radiology, University
Hospital Mannheim, Medical Faculty
Mannheim-University of Heidelberg,
Mannheim; Institute of Clinical Radiology,
University of Munich–Grosshadern Campus,
Munich, Germany

DANIEL K. SODICKSON, MD, PhD
Associate Professor, Department of Radiology,
New York University School of Medicine;
Director, Center for Biomedical Imaging, New
York University Medical Center, New York,
New York

BRIAN J. SOHER, PhD
Research Assistant Professor of Radiology, Center
for Advanced MR Development, Duke University
Medical Center, Durham, North Carolina

BACHIR TAOULI, MD
Assistant Professor, Department of Radiology, New
York University School of Medicine, New York,
New York

LINDSAY TURNBULL, FRCR, MD
Professor of Radiology; and Scientific Director
of the Centre for MR Investigations, Centre for MR
Investigations, Hull Royal Infirmary, United
Kingdom

JEFFREY C. WEINREB, MD
Professor of Diagnostic Radiology, Department
of Diagnostic Radiology, Yale University School
of Medicine, New Haven, Connecticut

CONSTANTIN von WEYMARN, PhD
MR Research Group, Cantonal Hospital,
Winterthur, Switzerland

MAURICIO ZAPPAROLI, MD
Department of Radiology, University of North
Carolina at Chapel Hill, Chapel Hill, North
Carolina

BODY MR IMAGING: 1.5T VERSUS 3T

Volume 15 • Number 3 • August 2007

Contents

A Review of MR Physics: 3T versus 1.5T   277

Brian J. Soher, Brian M. Dale, and Elmar M. Merkle

This article illustrates changes in the underlying physics concepts related to increasing the main magnetic field from 1.5T to 3T. The effects of these changes on tissue constants and practical hardware limitations is discussed as they affect scan time, quality, and contrast. Changes in susceptibility artifacts, chemical shift artifacts, and dielectric effects as a result of the increased field strength are also illustrated. Based on these fundamental considerations, an overall understanding of the benefits and constraints of signal-to-noise ratio and contrast-to-noise ratio changes between 1.5T and 3T MR systems is developed.

Cardiac MR Imaging: New Advances and Role of 3T   291

Kambiz Nael, Michael Fenchel, Roya Saleh, and J. Paul Finn

Over the last decade, cardiac magnetic resonance imaging has increasingly evolved into a useful diagnostic tool among the radiology and cardiology communities. Ongoing improvements in MR imaging hardware, processing speed, and pulse sequence development have laid the foundation for rapid progress in cardiac MR imaging. This article summarizes developing techniques and technique-related aspects, and the advantages and possible pitfalls of 3T in particular.

Abdominal and Pelvic MR Angiography   301

Henrik J. Michaely, Ulrike I. Attenberger, Harald Kramer, Kambiz Nael, Maximilian F. Reiser, and Stefan O. Schoenberg

Currently, 3T MR scanners hold 10% of the market with rising market share. Angiographic exams in particular benefit directly from the higher field strength. The theoretically doubled signal-to-noise ratio at 3T allows for abdominal magnetic-resonance angiography (MRA) exams with submillimeter spatial resolution with acquisition times of less than 20 seconds. Because of altered longitudinal relaxation times, MRA exams can be performed with a significantly reduced amount of contrast agents. This review describes the current technical concepts and outlines typical sequence parameters for abdominal and pelvic MRA. The choice of contrast agents for abdominal MRA is discussed in detail. This article also provides an outlook to new technical concepts that are already at the horizon of MRA.

For breast MR imaging, a high spatial resolution is important to resolve morphologic and architectural details of even small tumors. At the same time, fast imaging is required to account for the transient enhancement of breast cancers. This is the "temporal versus spatial dilemma" that current breast MR imaging protocols face. This article provides a short introduction to the clinical use of breast MR imaging, presents the different concepts that exist for breast MR imaging in general, and explains the advantages and disadvantages of the respective approaches. The specific high-field–induced physical changes and their effects on breast imaging are explained. A short overview is given on the current level of evidence regarding breast MR imaging at higher magnetic fields.

This article focuses on technical challenges in transferring 1.5T liver protocols to 3T systems and the overall comparison of MR sequences, highlighting the advantages and disadvantages of imaging at the higher field strength. An important benefit is the capacity of acquiring high-quality, thin-section postgadolinium T1-weighted three-dimensional gradientecho sequences, most clinically relevant for the detection and characterization of small hypervascular malignant diseases. Further research and development is necessary to overcome disadvantages, such as with in- and out-of phase T1-weighted gradient-echo sequences, and to minimize artifacts that appear at 3T.

Pancreatic cancer has an almost uniformly grim prognosis. Early detection has the potential to improve survival, however. One promising approach to increase detection rates is the use of MR imaging at 3T. Imaging at 3T improves temporal or spatial resolution for pancreatic evaluation. Known challenges of imaging at 3T, such as increased power deposition and B1 field inhomogeneity, are not significant limitations for pancreatic imaging. Preliminary results suggest that the signal-to-noise ratio can be as much as twice as high as at 1.5T, particularly after contrast administration. Evaluation of the hepatobiliary ducts is comparable or superior to that at 1.5T. Additional studies are needed to determine if the improved image quality translates into improved sensitivity for disease.

Soon after its introduction in 1991, MR cholangiopancreatography has become an established diagnostic tool for the evaluation of the pancreaticobiliary ductal system at a field strength of 1.5T. It remains unclear whether MR cholangiopancreatography performed at 3T will benefit from the higher magnetic field strength or whether a field strength of 1.5T should continue to be considered the gold standard for MR cholangiopancreatography. This article reviews the current literature on the benefits and drawbacks of MR cholangiopancreatography at 3T compared with a standard field strength of 1.5T. Field strength-related artifacts that affect MR cholangiopancreatography at 3T also are discussed.

from malignant disease with very high specificity, it can aid the selection of patients requiring further treatment and determine the level of urgency. Staging accuracy, which equals that obtained at laparotomy, allows appropriate clinical expertise to be organized before surgery or the deferment of surgery until later in the treatment pathway and is a cost-effective use of resources. This article compares and contrasts MR imaging of gynecologic conditions at 1.5 and 3T and defines a role for high field imaging for these clinical conditions.

Over the past several years, evidence supporting the use of MR imaging in the evaluation of prostate cancer has grown. Almost all this work has been performed at 1.5T. The gradual introduction of 3T scanners into clinical practice provides a potential opportunity to improve the quality and usefulness of prostate imaging. Increased signal to noise allows for imaging at higher resolution, higher temporal resolution, or higher bandwidth. Although this may improve the quality of conventional T2-weighted prostate imaging, which has been the standard sequence for detecting and localizing prostate cancer for years, the real potential for improvement at 3T involves more advanced techniques, such as spectroscopy, diffusion-weighted imaging, dynamic contrast imaging, and susceptibility imaging. This review presents the current data on 3T MR imaging of the prostate as well as the authors' impressions based on their experience at Yale–New Haven Hospital.

As investigators consider approaching the challenge of MR imaging at field strengths above 3T, do they follow the same paradigm, and continue to work around the same problems they have encountered thus far at 3T, or do they explore other ways of answering the clinical questions more effectively and more comprehensively? The most immediate problems of imaging at ultrahigh field strength are not unfamiliar, as many of them are still pressing issues at 3T: radiofrequency coils, B_1 homogeneity, specific absorption rate, safety, B_0 field homogeneity, alterations in tissue contrast, and chemical shift. In this article, these issues are briefly reviewed in terms of how they may affect image quality at field strengths beyond 3T. The authors propose various approaches to overcoming the challenges, and discuss potential applications of ultrahigh field MR imaging as it applies to specific abdominal, pelvic, peripheral vascular, and breast imaging protocols.

THE CLINICS ARE NOW AVAILABLE ONLINE!

Access your subscription at:
www.theclinics.com

GOAL STATEMENT

The goal of *Magnetic Resonance Imaging Clinics of North America* is to keep practicing physicians up to date with current clinical practice by providing timely articles reviewing the state of the art in patient care.

ACCREDITATION

The *Magnetic Resonance Imaging Clinics of North America* is planned and implemented in accordance with the Essential Areas and Policies of the Accreditation Council for Continuing Medical Education (ACCME) through the joint sponsorship of the University of Virginia School of Medicine and Elsevier. The University of Virginia School of Medicine is accredited by the ACCME to provide continuing medical education for physicians.

The University of Virginia School of Medicine designates this educational activity for a maximum of 15 *AMA PRA Category 1 Credits™*. Physicians should only claim credit commensurate with the extent of their participation in the activity.

The American Medical Association has determined that physicians not licensed in the US who participate in this CME activity are eligible for 15 *AMA PRA Category 1 Credits™*.

Credit can be earned by reading the text material, taking the CME examination online at http://www.theclinics.com/home/cme, and completing the evaluation. After taking the test, you will be required to review any and all incorrect answers. Following completion of the test and evaluation, your credit will be awarded and you may print your certificate.

FACULTY DISCLOSURE/CONFLICT OF INTEREST

The University of Virginia School of Medicine, as an ACCME accredited provider, endorses and strives to comply with the Accreditation Council for Continuing Medical Education (ACCME) Standards of Commercial Support, Commonwealth of Virginia statutes, University of Virginia policies and procedures, and associated federal and private regulations and guidelines on the need for disclosure and monitoring of proprietary and financial interests that may affect the scientific integrity and balance of content delivered in continuing medical education activities under our auspices.

The University of Virginia School of Medicine requires that all CME activities accredited through this institution be developed independently and be scientifically rigorous, balanced and objective in the presentation/discussion of its content, theories and practices.

All authors/editors participating in an accredited CME activity are expected to disclose to the readers relevant financial relationships with commercial entities occurring within the past 12 months (such as grants or research support, employee, consultant, stock holder, member of speakers bureau, etc.). The University of Virginia School of Medicine will employ appropriate mechanisms to resolve potential conflicts of interest to maintain the standards of fair and balanced education to the reader. Questions about specific strategies can be directed to the Office of Continuing Medical Education, University of Virginia School of Medicine, Charlottesville, Virginia.

The authors/editors listed below have identified no professional or financial affiliations for themselves or their spouse/partner:

Ersan Altun, MD; Ulrike I. Attenberger, MD; Susanne Booth, MRCOG; David D. Childs, MD; Daniel Cornfeld, MD; Michael Fenchel, MD; Elizabeth Hecht, MD; Vasco Herédia, MD; Harald Kramer, MD; Christiane Kuhl, MD; Thomas Lauenstein, MD; Ray F. Lee, PhD; Henrik Michaely, MD; Kambiz Nael, MD; Michael Patak, MD; Miguel Ramalho, MD; Maximilian Reiser, MD; Lisa Richman (Acquisitions Editor); Bettina Saar, MD; Roya Saleh, MD; Sebastian T. Schindera, MD; Stefan O. Schoenberg, MD; Daniel K. Sodickson, MD, PhD; Brian J. Soher, PhD; Bachir Taouli, MD; Lindsay Turnbull, FRCR, MD; Constantin von Weymarn, PhD; and, Mauricio Zapparoli, MD.

The authors/editors listed below identified the following professional or financial affiliations for themselves or their spouse/partner:

Brian M. Dale, PhD is employed by Siemens Medical Solutions.

Robert R. Edelman, MD receives research support from Siemens Medical Solutions

J. Paul Finn, MD is a consultant for Siemens Medical Solutions and serves on the speaker's bureau for Berlex Laboratories.

Johannes M. Froelich, PhD is a consultant for Guerbert AG

John R. Leyendecker, MD serves on the speaker's bureau for Bracco Diagnostics and GE Healthcare.

Diego R. Martin, MD, PhD performs investigator initiated research for Siemens Medical Systems, General Electric, Bracco Diagnostics, and Berlex.

Elmar M. Merkle, MD (Guest Editor) is a consultant, on the speaker's bureau, on the advisory committee, and owns stock in GE and Siemens Medical Solutions; is on the speaker's bureau and advisory committee for Bracco; and is on the speaker's bureau, advisory committee, and owns stock in Berlex.

Richard Semelka, MD is on the speaker's bureau for Bracco.

Jeffrey Weinreb, MD is a consultant for GE Health Care, Bayer and Covidien. He serves on the speaker's bureau for GE Health Care and Bayer.

Disclosure of Discussion of non-FDA approved uses for pharmaceutical products and/or medical devices:

The University of Virginia School of Medicine, as an ACCME provider, requires that all faculty presenters identify and disclose any "off label" uses for pharmaceutical and medical device products. The University of Virginia School of Medicine recommends that each physician fully review all the available data on new products or procedures prior to instituting them with patients.

TO ENROLL

To enroll in the Magnetic Resonance Imaging Clinics of North America Continuing Medical Education program, call customer service at 1-800-654-2452 or visit us online at www.theclinics.com/home/cme. The CME program is available to subscribers for an additional fee of $99.95.

MAGNETIC
RESONANCE
IMAGING CLINICS

Magn Reson Imaging Clin N Am 15 (2007) xi–xii

Preface

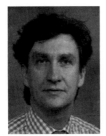

Elmar M. Merkle, MD
Center for Advanced MR Development
Department of Radiology
Duke University Medical Center
Erwin Road, Duke North, Room 1417
Durham, NC 27710, USA

E-mail address:
elmar.merkle@duke.edu

Elmar M. Merkle, MD
Guest Editor

The intent of this issue of the *Magnetic Resonance Imaging Clinics of North America* is to provide a closer look at various magnetic resonance applications within the chest, abdomen, and pelvis with specific emphasis on the effects of a higher 3 Tesla (T) magnetic field strength.

Since the inception of MR imaging in the 1970s, radiologists have searched intensively for the optimal magnetic field strength, and this quest continues. In the early 1980s, a magnetic field strength of 0.3T was considered optimal. During the 1990s, the radiologic community saw a shift toward 1T and 1.5T; during the last five years, a substantial trend toward 3T MR imaging could be observed. The search for higher field strength has been driven by the desire for an increase in signal-to-noise ratio, which can be kept to improve image quality, or traded for increased spatial resolution, improved temporal resolution, or both. Besides a gain in signal-to-noise ratio, other factors such as safety issues, image artifacts, and efficiency of contrast agents (to name a few) also have to be considered.

For this issue, I am fortunate to have the contributions of many colleagues, all of who were chosen as clinicians and scientists involved in the early adoption of 3T scanners in their practice. In the first article, Dr. Soher and colleagues cover the basic concepts of magnetic resonance physics relevant to the switch from 1.5T to 3T. Following this article, two cardiovascular research groups based in Los Angeles and Munich discuss cardiac and thoracoabdominal vascular MR imaging. Dr. Kuhl contributed the article on breast MR imaging, where early results at 3T have been both, promising and challenging. The article by Dr. Kuhl is followed by organ-specific contributions that examine in greater detail MR imaging of the liver, biliary system, pancreas, adrenals, kidneys, small bowel, and large bowel. Drs. Turnbull and Cornfeld provide their insights of the advantages of 3T MR imaging of the female and male pelvis, respectively, which is followed by Dr. Hecht's article, which looks beyond 3T to explore the even greater challenges of body MR imaging at 7T.

As you read this issue, it is my hope that you realize how little is proven scientifically about the advantages of 3T over 1.5T MR imaging. None of the contributors had a wealth of scientific literature to rely on, and there are topics such as renal MR

1064-9689/07/$ – see front matter © 2007 Elsevier Inc. All rights reserved.
mri.theclinics.com

doi:10.1016/j.mric.2007.08.004

imaging, where not a single comparison study is available currently. This is surprising, since the Federal Drug Administration approved 3T magnetic resonance systems for clinical use in 2002. Thus, despite the mostly marketing-driven hype about 3T, it currently remains unclear whether body MR imaging at 3T is superior to standard 1.5T MR imaging. Notwithstanding radiologists' continued faith in the advantages of 3T, perhaps this issue will provide the necessary guidance to make an informed choice between 3T and 1.5T body MR imaging, rather than simply following Theodore Roosevelt, who once advised "Do what you can, with what you have, where you are."

MAGNETIC
RESONANCE
IMAGING CLINICS

Magn Reson Imaging Clin N Am 15 (2007) 277–290

A Review of MR Physics: 3T versus 1.5T

Brian J. Soher, PhD[a],*, Brian M. Dale, PhD[b], Elmar M. Merkle, MD[a]

- Tissue relaxation rates
- Pulse sequence changes: timings, radiofrequency, and specific absorption rate
  Pulse sequence optimization
  Radiofrequency pulse limitations and specific absorption rate
- So what about signal to noise?
- Susceptibility
- Contrast agents

- Specific artifacts
  Chemical shift artifacts of the first and second kinds
  B_1 inhomogeneity and standing wave artifacts
  Steady-state pulse sequence banding artifacts
- Summary
- References

Since their development in the early 1990s, high-field whole-body 3T MR systems have been installed in numerous institutions, and are being increasingly used clinically. As of summer 2006, approximately 10% of installed MR systems in the United States were 3T systems. Besides market considerations, such as strategic marketing and/or to stay competitive, the main argument for purchasing a high-field MR system is the expected increase in MR signal-to-noise ratio (SNR) of up to twofold [1] as compared with a standard 1.5T MR scanner. This gain in SNR can be kept or traded for either speed or spatial resolution, or both.

The actual gain in SNR attained by 3T MR systems is dependent on many inherent and external factors. Changes in tissue relaxation times, specifically significant increases in tissue T_1 times [2–4], effectively reduce SNR for equivalent scanning times. Radiofrequency (RF) power deposition increases at higher field strength, reaching or exceeding specific absorption rate (SAR) limits more quickly for typical pulse sequence parameter ranges. Pulse sequence parameters at 3T need to be reoptimized from 1.5T values to maintain desired image contrast. Image artifacts because of changes in tissue susceptibility, chemical shift, RF effects, and/or pulse sequence physics are more noticeable and sometimes harder to suppress at high field. Field strength–related changes of the relaxivity values of MR contrast agents (a measure of their effectiveness) need to be considered and recharacterized as these values decrease with magnetic field strength [5–10]. And finally, until recently the number of accessory receiving coils had been limited; however, the spectrum of dedicated receiver coils offered by vendors has increased substantially, which allows almost all of the standard MR examinations to be performed on a 3T whole-body MR system.

Despite various difficulties and challenges, much work has already been done to demonstrate the performance of 3T high-field MR systems for various indications in the brain, musculoskeletal system, chest, abdomen, and pelvis as compared with

a Center for Advanced MR Development, Duke University Medical Center, Box 3808, Durham, NC 27710, USA
b Siemens Medical Solutions, 402 Park York Lane, Cary, NC 27519, USA
* Corresponding author.
E-mail address: brian.soher@duke.edu (B.J. Soher).

1064-9689/07/$ – see front matter © 2007 Elsevier Inc. All rights reserved.
mri.theclinics.com

doi:10.1016/j.mric.2007.06.002

standard high-field 1.5T MR systems [3,8,9,11–36]. Unfortunately, insights gained in one organ system or application, such as musculoskeletal or neuroimaging, cannot simply be transferred to another, such as body MR imaging, since MR sequence protocols as well as object size differ substantially. Additionally, some high-field artifacts are unique to specific anatomical locations for 3T MR imaging, and are not seen in other regions of the body. Investigations are currently ongoing about which patient groups will benefit from MR studies at high field versus scans acquired on a 1.5T MR scanner.

This article will illustrate changes in the underlying physics concepts related to increasing the main magnetic field from 1.5T to 3T. The effects of these changes on tissue constants and practical hardware limitations will be discussed as they affect scan time, quality, and contrast. Changes in susceptibility artifacts, chemical shift artifacts, and dielectric effects as a result of the increased field strength will also be illustrated. Based on these fundamental considerations, an overall understanding of the benefits and constraints of SNR and contrast-to-noise ratio (CNR) changes between 1.5T and 3T MR systems will be developed.

Tissue relaxation rates

It is well known that the longitudinal relaxation time, T_1, is longer at higher magnetic field than at lower magnetic field [2–4,12,19,37–43]. T_1 relaxation is defined as the transfer of energy from excited protons to the surrounding structure (or lattice). This energy transfer occurs most easily when there is good "contact" between the spins and the lattice. As the main B_0 field strength increases, the resonance frequency of the excited spins also increases (from approximately 64 MHz at 1.5T to 128 MHz at 3T). The higher frequency of the spins reduces the efficiency of energy transfer, resulting in longer T_1 relaxation times at 3T. Examples of reported T_1 tissue changes include up to 40% increase in skeletal muscle, up to 62% increase for gray matter and 42% for white matter in brain, 41% increase in liver, and up to 73% increase for kidney [4]. In general, an increase in tissue T_1 will cause a decrease in image SNR (as discussed in the SNR section). The T_1 of lipids at 3T has been shown to increase by only approximately 20% [3,43], which is somewhat less than increases reported for other tissues, thus lipid signal in images remains strong at 3T resulting in increased artifacts (eg, chemical shift artifacts of the first kind, more distinct ghosting artifacts in relation to Gibbs ringing).

The transverse relaxation time T_2, on the other hand, has been reported to be mostly independent of the main magnetic field strength [2]. However, more recently published studies by de Bazelaire and colleagues [3], Gold and colleagues [19], and Stanisz and colleagues [4] suggest a small, statistically insignificant, decrease of the transverse relaxation time T_2 in certain tissues by up to 10% or more at higher magnetic field strengths, which would further reduce the gain in SNR at high-field MR imaging for long echo time (TE) protocols. Of greater concern is the increased effect of T_2^* (transverse signal decay due to spin-spin interactions, field inhomogeneities, and susceptibility effects) at 3T. As discussed further below, field inhomogeneity and shimming difficulty both increase because of tissue susceptibility effects at high field. This causes T_2^* to shorten significantly, changing image contrast owing to decay of transverse magnetization. The effect of this relaxation constant change is seen mainly in gradient-recalled sequences, but can also be seen in fast imaging sequences that yield a mixture of T_1/T_2 image contrast such as true-FISP (fast imaging with steady state precession).

In addition to the absolute change in the T_1 relaxation time as a function of magnetic field strength, there are also relative changes where the T_1 relaxation time for one tissue increases at a different rate than the T_1 relaxation time of another tissue. For example, according to Bottomley and colleagues [2], at 1.5T the T_1 relaxation time of the kidney is 32% greater than the T_1 relaxation time of liver (652 ms kidney, 493 ms liver) but at 3T that difference shrinks to 21% (774 ms kidney, 641 ms liver). For other tissue pairs the relative T_1 dispersion may actually increase at high field, rather than decreasing as shown here for kidney and liver (Fig. 1). In any case, this example should illustrate why the contrast between various tissues on T_1-weighted images at 3T MR imaging cannot be identical to the contrast seen on standard 1.5T

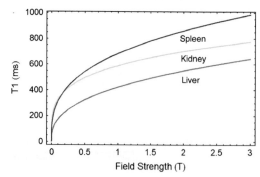

Fig. 1. Estimated T_1 relaxation times for liver, kidney, and spleen with increasing main magnetic field strength, based on theoretical models by Bottomley and colleagues [2]. Relative tissue contrasts at 1.5T versus 3T must be different due to variations in T_1 changes between tissues.

T_1-weighted MR imaging. However, many of contrast changes caused by the switch to 3T imaging may either not be significantly visible [25] or can be ameliorated by changes to pulse sequence parameters.

Pulse sequence changes: timings, radiofrequency, and specific absorption rate

Pulse sequence optimization

Possibly the most important practical effect of the changes to the relaxation times is in the need to re-optimize pulse sequence parameter settings at 3T to maintain or improve on image CNR and SNR seen at 1.5T. One simple example is for T_1-weighted images and the effects of increased T_1 relaxation times at 3T. If sequence timings are not changed from 1.5T to 3T, then it has been shown [14] that T_1-weighted contrast at 3T can actually be worse than for images taken at 1.5T. In this case, an extension in repetition time (TR) to match the T_1 increase is one way to overcome signal and contrast changes; however, it may also prove effective to use inversion recovery methods to maintain T_1 image weighting while maintaining overall scan time. In a similar fashion, because of changes in transverse relaxation time (T_2) and T_2* at 3T, TE values in various sequences may also need to be reoptimized.

Changes necessitated in pulse sequences because of a desire to improve SNR or CNR at 3T versus 1.5T can have substantial effects on overall MR image scan effectiveness. Increased TR alone can lead to longer scan times, increased motion artifacts, decreased patient compliance, fewer scan options for complex patient pathologies, and possibly decreased overall patient throughput. Under certain conditions, other sequence parameters, such as the number of signal averages, phase encodes, or echo train length for fast-imaging sequences, can be altered to decrease the overall scan time. Tradeoffs like these result in decreased gain of SNR, such as reducing the signal averages and acquisition time by a factor of two for a signal loss of approximately 30% relative to the theoretical twofold gain, or a gain of only approximately 70% relative to the SNR at 1.5T.

Two promising technologies for maintaining reasonable scan times while maximizing SNR are fast three-dimensional (3D) pulse sequences and parallel imaging techniques [36]. The first category, fast 3D data acquisition schemes, has benefited greatly from higher gradient amplitudes and switching speeds that are available for most new high-field scanners. By exciting a slab of spins and encoding along the slice dimension, rather than acquiring images slice by slice, these sequences take advantage of the increase in SNR due to averaging obtained

from increasing the total scan time for each slice. Increased gradient performance permits longer echo pulse trains or faster repetition times, allowing 3D volumes to be acquired with acquisition times similar to those for multislice 2D data. Parallel imaging techniques take advantage of the higher SNR achieved at 3T and increased availability of phased array coils to acquire fewer phase encodes, thus shortening total acquisition times, while maintaining equivalent image resolution to standard scan techniques. This effectively allows the increased SNR at 3T to be traded for spatial or temporal resolution for applications that are not SNR limited.

Radiofrequency pulse limitations and specific absorption rate

Another effect with major impact on the gain in SNR at 3T is in regard to SAR. SAR is a measure for energy deposition within the human body and is defined in equation 1 as:

$$\text{SAR} = \frac{\sigma |E|^2}{2\rho}\left(\frac{\tau}{\text{TR}}\right)N_p N_s \tag{1}$$

Where σ is the conductivity, E the electric field, ρ the tissue density, τ is pulse duration and N_p and N_s are pulse number and number of slices [34]. Since E is proportional to the magnetic field, by doubling the main magnetic field strength, the SAR required at 3T increases by a factor of four. While the energy deposited at 3T is still nonionizing, a small part of the total energy used is absorbed by the subject and can cause increased tissue temperature. Although SAR is not a direct measure of tissue heating, the goal of the federally mandated SAR limits is to avoid temperature increases in the body of more than 1°C. The calculation of SAR depends on many things, including the field strength, the pulse sequence, the RF transmit coil used, and the patient position inside the coil. In addition to the increased power requirements at 3T, the RF wavelength used at 3T is shorter than that used for 1.5T, which can result in inhomogeneous power deposition and the formation of localized "hot spots," particularly in the locale of medical implants. Thus, the increased SAR requires an increased concern for patient safety and may additionally limit the optimization of pulse sequences.

Imaging protocols most affected by SAR limitations at 3T are those using spin-echo and turbo spin-echo (TSE) sequences. These sequences typically make use of closely spaced refocusing pulses or pulse trains that can quickly exceed SAR thresholds. Initial workarounds modified TR or pulse train lengths to decrease SAR. More recent technical solutions include the use of "variable flip angle" or "hyper-echo" RF pulse train techniques that can lower RF energy absorption by factors of 2.5 to 6.0 [44–46] while maintaining acceptable SNR and CNR levels or VERSE (Variable Rate Selective Excitation) pulses, which can reduce energy deposition without decreasing the flip angle or increasing the excitation time [47]. Parallel imaging techniques can also be useful for alleviating SAR levels, either on their own or in conjunction with new RF technologies [36,48,49]. By reducing the number of repetitions, and thus shortening the total data acquisition time, the total amount of energy absorbed for a given data acquisition is reduced.

Other areas where SAR limitations have had effects are for magnetization preparation pulses. Inversion recovery pulses, magnetization transfer pulses, and fat and other saturation pulses all contribute to overall energy deposition. At 3T, these preparation pulses are being used more frequently and for a variety of new purposes such as using inversion recovery (IR) pulses in an MP-RAGE (magnetization preparation rapid gradient echo) sequence to improve T_1-weighted contrast [50], or fat saturation pulses to minimize chemical shift artifact.

MR body imaging is particularly impacted by changes in SAR at 3T [25]. Because body MR imaging at 3T almost always runs at the upper limits of the allowed SAR deposition, patients are more likely to experience an uncomfortable sensation of warmth or heating. To minimize SAR effects, protocol adjustments are frequently necessary such as an increase of the TR, decrease in the number of slices, or decrease of the flip angle. These adjustments are all undesirable as they increase scan time, reduce anatomical coverage, alter contrast, and/or further reduce the gain in SNR at 3T when compared with a standard 1.5T MR system.

So what about signal to noise?

The idea that twice the magnetic field will give twice the SNR is very appealing, and at first it seems correct since the intrinsic SNR in MR imaging is approximately proportional to the main magnetic field strength B_0 (equations 2 and 3) [1,25].

$$SNR_{SE} \propto B_0 V \sqrt{\frac{N_{PE} N_{PA} N_{AV}}{BW}} \left(1 - e^{-TR/T1}\right) e^{-TE/T2} \quad (2)$$

(Equation 2 for spin-echo-based MR sequences)

$$SNR_{GRE} \propto$$

$$B_0 V \sqrt{\frac{N_{PE} N_{PA} N_{AV}}{BW}} \frac{\sin(\theta)\left(1 - e^{-TR/T1}\right)}{\left(1 - e^{-TR/T1}\cos(\theta)\right)} e^{-TE/T2^*} \quad (3)$$

(Equation 3 for gradient-echo-based MR sequences), where, SNR_{SE} = signal-to-noise ratio for a spin echo pulse sequence; SNR_{GRE} = signal-to-noise ratio for a spoiled gradient echo sequence; B_0 = main

magnetic field strength; V = voxel volume; N_{PE} = number of acquired phase encode lines; N_{PA} = number of acquired partitions; N_{AV} = number of signals averaged; BW = receiver band width per pixel; TR = repetition time; T_1 = longitudinal relaxation time; TE = echo time; T_2 = transverse relaxation time; and θ = flip angle.

Note that, in both equations 2 and 3, the term under the square root is simply the total time spent acquiring data. Therefore, SNR is proportional to the main magnetic field strength, the voxel volume, the square root of the total sampling time, and some sequence-specific contrast-related terms. Some of these factors, such as the longitudinal relaxation time T_1 and receiver bandwidth, as well as specific absorption rate limitations can affect the SNR in a somewhat complicated manner by impacting other sequence-specific parameters (eg, changes to TR or flip angle to reach an allowable SAR).

As mentioned previously, if we accept the admittedly optimistic assumption that the transverse relaxation time T_2 is independent of the main magnetic field strength and assuming only an increase of the longitudinal relaxation time T_1, equations 2 and 3 can be used to determine the theoretical maximum relative gain in SNR during liver MR. For TSE-based T_2-weighted sequences with sequential acquisition such as HASTE (half Fourier single-shot turbo spin-echo) a factor of approximately 1.8 increase in SNR can be obtained. For gradient-echo-based T_1-weighted sequences such as in- and opposed-phase 2D dual echo and 3D VIBE (volume interpolated breath hold examination) a factor of about 1.6 to 1.7 increase in SNR can be obtained. Thus, the theoretical twofold increase in SNR at 3T compared with 1.5T MR imaging will not generally be obtained without additional sequence modifications [30].

Other factors, however, also lead to a degradation of SNR at 3T from theoretical maximums. These include practical limitations on sequence optimization due to SAR limits, conservation of contrast, various competing sequence parameter interactions, and/or a lack of certain specialized RF coils at 3T [32]. All these reasons contribute to a gain in SNR that is less than the factor of 2.0 originally expected. This may help explain why reports of 1.5T and 3T imaging comparisons of various anatomic locations [13,27,51–54] have found that, at least visually, when applying a protocol with similar spatial and temporal resolution the resultant images appear equal in SNR. Alternatively, it could be because many applications are not SNR-limited even at 1.5T, so it becomes difficult to visually detect further improvements in SNR regardless of the quantitative improvement in SNR.

Susceptibility

Magnetic susceptibility is the extent to which a material becomes magnetized when placed within a magnetic field. Susceptibility artifacts occur as the result of microscopic gradients or variations in the magnetic field strength that occur near the interfaces of materials of different magnetic susceptibility, such as bone-soft tissue or air-tissue interfaces. These artifacts can especially be caused by metallic objects from previous surgical/interventional procedures or iron deposition in tissues, since the susceptibility of metal is much higher than that of soft tissue. The variations in the main field caused by susceptibility can result in image nonuniformities, including in-plane image distortion, nonplanar 2D image slices, localized regions of high or low signal intensity, and localized signal drop-outs caused by $T_2{}^*$ shortening.

Susceptibility artifacts also occur next to gas-filled structures, such as the gas-filled bowel or sinuses in the head, since the susceptibility of gas is much smaller than that of soft tissue (Fig. 2). In some cases, this can make imaging studies at 3T more difficult, such as for bowel wall imaging in patients with inflammatory bowel disease, patients referred for MR colonography or studies in the brain that need to observe the frontal lobes in proximity to the sinuses. However, enlarged susceptibility artifacts because of a gas/soft tissue interface may also be helpful, eg, for detecting gas as in intrahepatic pneumobilia or free intraperitoneal gas (Fig. 3).

Susceptibility artifacts increase with the main magnetic field strength, and are slightly larger at 3T compared with standard 1.5T MR imaging [55]. This may be advantageous in selected cases such as improved visualization in $T_2{}^*$-weighted perfusion studies or using metal-related susceptibility artifacts from surgical clips or surgical debris (eg, prior cholecystectomy or prior hepatic resection) to improve body imaging studies. However, it is possible that enlarged susceptibility artifacts may obscure important findings at 3T MR imaging that may have been visualized at standard 1.5T MR imaging (Fig. 4) [11,56,57]. It must be clearly stated here that metal-containing devices that are considered MR safe at a field strength of 1.5T are not necessarily safe at 3T [58–63]. All these devices need to be rigorously tested at 3T as well before affected patients can undergo an MR examination at this field strength. An excellent source of information is available free of charge online through www.mrisafety.com.

One final aspect of localized susceptibility fields are their effect on magnetization preparation such as inversion recovery pulses. Regions of sufficiently high field variability due to susceptibility can cause incomplete inversion of the spin magnetization since the local spins may lie outside the pulse bandwidth. Many protocols at both 3T and 1.5T make use of IR pulses (eg, fluid attenuation inversion recovery [FLAIR] and magnetization preparation rapid gradient echo [MPRAGE]) to achieve desired contrasts or the suppression of fat signal [64].

A variety of techniques can be used to minimize the influence of susceptibility artifacts. The readout direction can be changed to alter the location of the artifact, voxel size can be reduced, or the shimming of the main magnetic field can be optimized to even out field variations. Gradient echo, and particularly echo-planar sequences, are most affected by susceptibility since they do not have 180° refocusing pulses and do have long echo trains, respectively. Using short echo times with increased receiver bandwidth can help to minimize these artifacts for GRE sequences. Implementing a parallel imaging technique with an echo-planar imaging sequence can reduce these artifacts since shorter echo trains can be used.

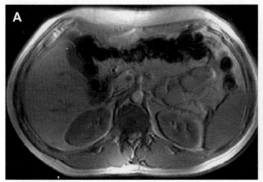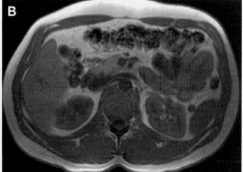

Fig. 2. Susceptibility artifacts in the transverse colon in the same patient at 3T (*A*) and 1.5T (*B*). Gas-filled bowel causes susceptibility artifacts at the tissue-gas interface that at 3T are more pronounced in gradient echo acquisitions than at 1.5T.

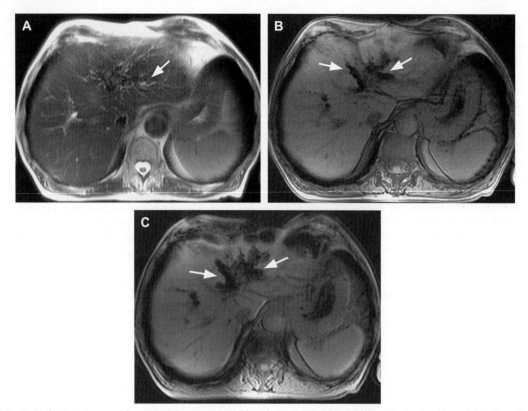

Fig. 3. Patient status post-hepaticojejunostomy with subsequent pneumobilia. Bile in the T$_2$-weighted, turbo spin-echo image (*A*) displays as bright signal (*arrow*). Corresponding dual-echo GRE images, acquired at echo times of 1.5 ms (*B*) and 4.9 ms (*C*), demonstrate gas within the biliary system causing a marked susceptibility artifact (*arrows*). Note also that these susceptibility artifacts increase on the images with the longer echo time.

Contrast agents

The behavior and effectiveness of contrast agents at 3T versus 1.5T depend on the relaxivity of the paramagnetic ion complex and tissue relaxation times, both of which vary with field strength. The relaxivity of chelated gadolinium contrast agents decrease only on the order of 5% to 10% [12,65,66] from 1.5 T to 3T. T$_1$ values for tissues, as described previously, can lengthen by 40% or more at 3T. The

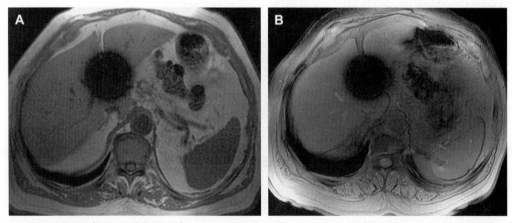

Fig. 4. Comparison of susceptibility artifacts at 1.5T and 3T due to metal clip from a prior cholecystectomy. (*A*) Gradient echo image at 1.5T with TE = 5.2 ms showing a large circular susceptibility artifact. (*B*) Gradient echo image at 3T shows a similar-sized artifact despite a shorter TE = 4.4 ms.

relationship between contrast and its effect on tissue T_1 can be given by:

$$\frac{1}{T_1(C)} = \frac{1}{T_1(0)} + RC \qquad (4)$$

where C is the in vivo contrast agent concentration, R is the relaxivity of the contrast agent, $T_1(0)$ is baseline tissue T_1 relaxation time without contrast, and $T_1(C)$ is the T_1 relaxation of the tissue after contrast administration [7]. Because T_1 times at 1.5T are shorter than at 3T, an equivalent dose of contrast at 3T appears to cause more of a contrast difference. This apparent increase in effectiveness of contrast agents at higher field can be used clinically to either reduce the amount of contrast given in routine studies or to improve CNR. Also of value is the increased effectiveness of contrast-enhanced MR angiography (MRA) techniques at 3T because of the further increases in T_1 times for blood and better suppression of the background signal from fat [67].

Specific artifacts

It is important to note here that in general every artifact that is present at 1.5T is also present at 3T. In some cases, as will be presented below, the increase in field strength actually causes artifacts to be more of a problem, either in absolute terms or because effective workarounds have not yet been developed or extensively implemented. In other cases, it is only the increased SNR, CNR, or resolution that is afforded by 3T systems that make some artifacts visible at all by comparison to 1.5T systems. Examples of these latter artifacts might include Gibbs ringing ghosting [68], fine-line artifacts [12], or the one half FOV ghosting artifacts inherent to parallel imaging methodologies [69]. At any rate, while a full review of MR imaging artifacts is beyond the scope of this report, a fuller discussion of these topics can be found particularly in Bernstein and colleagues [12] and in references [64,70–77]. The following sections concentrate on a few artifacts that are particularly problematic at 3T or specifically related to the change in field strength.

Chemical shift artifacts of the first and second kinds

The chemical shift artifact of the first kind is a result of a difference in the resonant frequency between water and fat and is seen only along the frequency encoding axis and the slice selection dimension [78]. This difference in resonant frequency is directly proportional to the main magnetic field strength, and has been measured to be approximately 3.5 ppm, resulting in a difference of about 225 Hz at 1.5T, or a difference of about 450 Hz at 3T. This difference causes a chemical shift misregistration, which is most easily seen around the kidneys (Fig. 5). The chemical shift artifact of the first kind appears as a hypointense band, one to several pixels in width, toward the lower part of the readout gradient field, and as a hyperintense band toward the higher part of the readout gradient field. At a constant field of view, base resolution, and receiver bandwidth, the chemical shift artifact of the first kind will be twice as wide at 3T compared with standard 1.5T imaging. Usually this enlarged artifact does not cause substantial problems in clinical MR imaging at 3T; however, it may be problematic in selected cases such as in body MR for a search for a small subcapsular renal hematoma or an intramural aortic hematoma. In these cases, the receiver bandwidth can be increased to minimize the chemical shift artifact of the first kind. Unfortunately, this comes at the expense of SNR—doubling the receiver bandwidth will decrease the SNR by approximately 30%, (see Equations 2 and 3) (see Fig. 5). Another option is to repeat the MR pulse sequence with either a chemical shift fat saturation, inversion nulling, or water excitation, which will eliminate chemical shift artifacts effectively, allow imaging at the lower bandwidth, and return the 30% loss in SNR.

The chemical shift artifact of the second kind is not limited to the frequency encoding axis, but may be seen in all pixels along a fat/water interface as it is based on an intravoxel phase-cancellation effect where fat and water exist in the same voxel [78]. The size of this artifact does not increase with the main magnetic field strength and is defined by the spatial resolution of the MR sequence (Fig. 6). However, the echo time needs to be adjusted as the frequency difference is twice as large compared with standard 1.5T MR systems [79] as described in the section on chemical shift artifact of the first kind. Using a 3T MR system, both fat and water protons are in-phase at 2.2 ms, 4.4 ms, 6.6 ms, and so on, and out-of-phase (also referred to as opposed-phase) at 1.1 ms, 3.3 ms, 5.5 ms, and so on. Note that at 1.5T, the fat and water are phase opposed at 2.2 ms and in phase at 4.4 seconds (nominal values). In short, by doubling the field strength we have halved the echo times needed for in-phase and opposed phase imaging.

Fortunately, the increased difference in resonant frequency between water and fat at 3T may also be advantageous as it allows for a better separation of the fat and water peak during MR spectroscopy, and for a better or faster fat suppression using other chemical shift techniques as well, eg, fat saturation and water excitation.

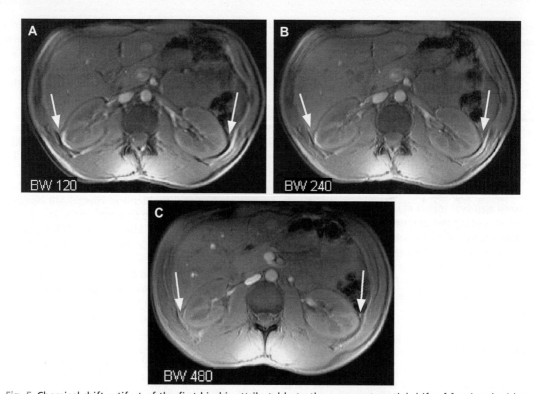

Fig. 5. Chemical shift artifact of the first kind is attributable to the apparent spatial shift of fat signal with respect to water because of the fat signal being off-resonance. The resultant artifact displays as light and dark bands in the image, as indicated by the arrows in (*A–C*). These bands occur in the direction of the readout gradient, which increases right to left in these images. This artifact is dependent on the receiver bandwidth and the readout gradient applied. Increasing the receiver bandwidth, eg, 120 Hz/pixel (*A*), 240 Hz/pixel (*B*), and 480 Hz/pixel (*C*), will decrease the artifact, but at the expense of additional noise in the image.

B_1 inhomogeneity and standing wave artifacts

In addition to the exacerbation of artifacts that are seen at 1.5T, there are also some "new" artifacts that begin to appear at 3T. In all fairness, however, these artifacts are not "new" at all, but have just not caught any attention at 1.5T (Fig. 7). These artifacts are much more pronounced at 3T as they are related to the higher frequency B_1 transmit fields that are used at 3T. RF transmit and transmit/receive coils

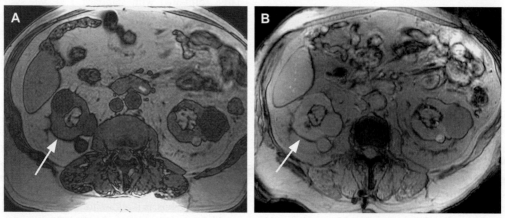

Fig. 6. Chemical shift artifact of the second kind, or India ink artifact, is caused by signals from fat and water from the same voxel interacting destructively to result in dark bands of signal cancellation. This artifact appears similar at both 1.5T (*A*) and 3T (*B*), as it is independent of the main magnetic field strength. Note also the difference in image contrast for these two opposed-phase images.

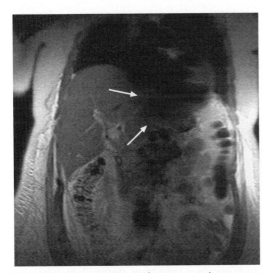

Fig. 7. B₁ inhomogeneity artifacts are much more pronounced at 3T as they are related to the higher frequency B₁ transmit fields that are used at 3T. However, they are occasionally distinct enough at 1.5T to be seen. Compare the signal drop out for a patient with anasarca and ascites in this figure, indicated by the white arrows, to the signal drop out due to similar B₁ inhomogeneity artifacts at 3T shown in Fig. 8.

used at 3T have been redesigned for use at 128 MHz rather than the 64 MHz of 1.5T systems. This redesign was not trivial due to nonlinear power deposition, dielectric effects, and other engineering considerations. Only recently have a similar range of RF coils at 3T have become as available as those for use at 1.5T.

A particular difficulty for designing RF coils at the higher frequency is achieving a homogeneous B₁ RF field. While T₁-weighted gradient-echo imaging is usually not compromised by B₁-inhomogeneity artifacts, this kind of artifact is oftentimes problematic in T₂-weighted TSE imaging [29,80]. The wavelength of the RF field at 128 MHz is 234 cm in free space, which is much larger than the field-of-view (FOV) for clinical body imaging. However, water (and most body tissue) has a rather high dielectric constant, which reduces both the speed and wavelength of electromagnetic radiation [81,82]. This effect reduces the RF field wavelength from 234 cm in free space to about 30 cm in most human tissues, ie, water containing [81]. This is approximately the size of the FOV for many body applications and can result in a so-called "standing wave" effect (often incorrectly called a "dielectric resonance" effect Refs. [81,83]). As a result, strong signal variations across an image can be seen, especially brightening or dark "holes" in regions away from the receive coil caused by constructive or destructive interference from the standing waves (Fig. 8). These artifacts become more pronounced the larger the region of interest is relative to the wavelength, ie, they are seen more in obese patients with a distended abdomen than in thin patients.

Several approaches have been proposed to overcome the B₁ inhomogeneity challenge, eg, special RF pulse designs or coil designs such as multichannel RF transmission techniques where the phase and amplitude of the various elements can be adjusted to obtain a uniform B₁ field [80,84]. Another option is the passive coupling of coils to improve B₁-homogeneity [85]. While most of these methods are technically demanding, the use of dielectric pads or RF cushions is both noninvasive and not technically demanding and has thus emerged as a viable method to improve the homogeneity of

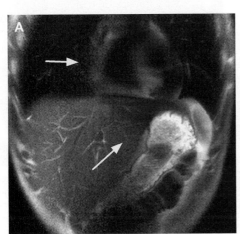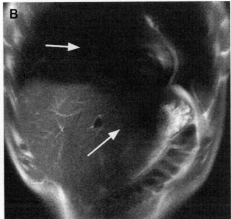

Fig. 8. B₁ inhomogeneity artifacts that cause shading across the torso can be minimized or even eliminated by the use of an RF cushion as shown in these 3T coronal HASTE images of the torso both (*A*) with and (*B*) without the RF cushion present. See Fig. 9 for the composition and usage of the RF cushion.

the B_1-field during abdominal MR imaging at 3T [25,86]. RF cushions may be used in conjunction with the body coil, as well as a dedicated receive-only torso array coil, and consist of a gel encapsulated in synthetic material (Fig. 9). The gel is usually ultrasound gel, which has a high dielectric constant, and is mixed with a highly concentrated gadolinium- or manganese-based MR contrast agent to eliminate the MR signal from the gel itself [25]. The B_1-inhomogenity artifact is strongly affected by the presence of dielectric materials. The RF cushion has a higher dielectric constant with subsequent shorter wavelength than body tissues, and therefore it alters these interference patterns and potentially reduces or eliminates the destructive interference that would otherwise occur in the body [87].

Shielding effects are another cause of B_1 inhomogeneity. A rapidly changing magnetic field, like the RF transmit field, will induce a circulating electric field (Fig. 10). When this happens in a conductive medium, a circulating electric current is established. This current in turn acts like an electromagnet that opposes the changing magnetic field, reducing the amplitude and dissipating the energy of the RF field. The more conductive the medium, eg, ascites, the stronger the opposing electromagnet and therefore the greater the attenuation of the RF field. Large

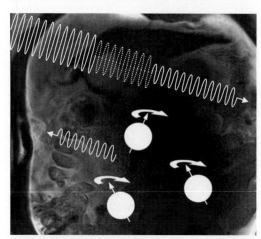

Fig. 10. RF shielding effects occur because an RF transmit field creates a rapidly changing magnetic field, which induces a circulating electric field. When this happens in a conductive medium, eg, ascites, a circulating electric current is established that in turn acts like an electromagnet that opposes the changing magnetic field, reducing the amplitude and dissipating the energy of the RF field. This shielding effect results in hypointense areas in the image where the RF field is partially attenuated.

amounts of relatively highly conductive tissues can cause this shielding effect resulting in hypointense areas in the image where the RF field is partially attenuated [81].

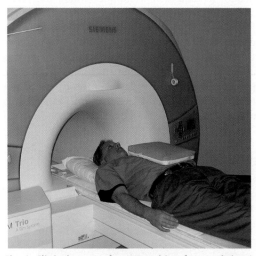

Fig. 9. Clinical setup of an RF cushion for an abdominal MR scan. RF cushions may be used in conjunction with the body coil, as well as a dedicated receive-only torso array coil. RF cushions consist of a gel encapsulated in synthetic material that has a higher dielectric constant with subsequent shorter wavelength than body tissues. It alters interference patterns and potentially reduces or eliminates the destructive interference that would otherwise occur in the body at 3T. The gel is mixed with a highly concentrated MR contrast agent to eliminate the MR signal from the gel itself.

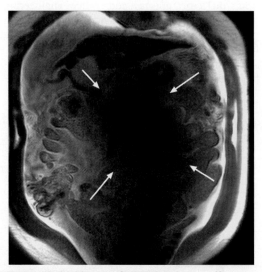

Fig. 11. RF shielding artifact and dielectric effects can combine to cause particularly strong inhomogeneity artifacts for 3T body MR imaging as shown here for a patient with ascites. The standing wave effects are more pronounced because of the large body size, and there is greater RF field attenuation because of the increased amounts of highly conductive ascitic fluid (*arrows*).

These two effects combine to cause particularly strong artifacts for 3T body MR imaging in pregnant patients and in patients with ascites (Fig. 11). In both cases, not only are the standing wave effects more pronounced because of the enlarged abdomen, but there is also greater RF field attenuation because of the increased amounts of highly conductive amniotic or ascitic fluid.

Steady-state pulse sequence banding artifacts

Pulse sequences based on the principles of steady-state free precession (SSFP) have gained in popularity recently because they provide both higher CNR and SNR and motion compensation as compared with other fast-imaging methods. Cardiac imaging has taken particular advantage of these methods, but they are being used increasingly in MR imaging to achieve preferred image contrast in other areas of the body with 3D acquisitions that take roughly equivalent scan times as previous 2D multislicemethods [88–96]. Clinical names for these sequences include SSFP, or balanced-SSFP (bSSFP), fast-imaging employing steady-state acquisition (FIESTA), and fast imaging with steady precession (true FISP).

SSFP sequences are vulnerable to banding artifacts because of off-resonance effects, which cause variations in signal intensities across images. Whenever the local off-resonance frequency is equal to a multiple of $1/TR$, dark stripes appear in images (Fig. 12). These artifacts occur since SSFP sequences are both spatially and spectrally selective. These artifacts have been minimized at 1.5T by keeping TR

as short as possible [88] to shift these stripes outside of the FOV or by summing frequency modulated acquisitions to average images over multiple spectral offsets [88,96,97].

At higher field, difficulties with shimming and increased susceptibility effects increase B_0 inhomogeneity and exacerbate the conditions that cause banding artifacts. Increases in tissue T_1 values make it less desirable to shorten TR to remove the bands from the FOV, and the larger spectral offsets caused by the higher field make it difficult to achieve a sufficiently short TR; although this requirement can be lessened with improved shimming optimization. Despite these requirements, under certain conditions the short TR method can be used to reduce artifacts. The trade-offs are increased gradient switching speed for patients. The advantage to using frequency-averaging methods at 3T to reduce banding artifacts is that it is not limited by a need for short TR spacing [97].

Summary

Body MR imaging at 3T has improved substantially over the past 5 years. The image quality of T_1-weighted 3D gradient echo imaging with chemical shift fat saturation at 3T now is equal to the one at 1.5T before the administration of contrast, and is even superior post–contrast administration because of the increase in CNR. Also, in- and opposed phase gradient echo imaging has been improved recently, and new prototype 3D dual-echo sequences are currently being developed [79,98]. T_2-weighted fast spin-echo imaging including magnetic resonance cholangiopancreatography on the other hand still suffers from dielectric artifacts, and no robust solution is currently available; however, we are hopeful that the approach of multiple transmit coils will solve this problem. Steady-state imaging with free precession at 3T also is still problematic, and no sufficient solution is on the horizon. Finally, diffusion-weighted imaging, which has become rather popular at 1.5T lately, currently suffers from increased susceptibility artifacts at 3T. Here, the implementation of parallel imaging algorithms seems to be a promising approach to improve the image quality substantially over the next few years.

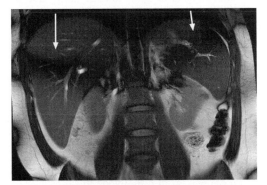

Fig. 12. Steady-state free precession sequences are vulnerable to banding artifacts because of off-resonance effects that cause variations in signal intensities across images. Whenever the local off-resonance frequency is equal to a multiple of $1/TR$, dark stripes appear in images, as indicated by the arrows in this coronal torso image. At 3T, difficulties with shimming and increased susceptibility effects increase B_0 inhomogeneity and exacerbate the conditions that cause banding artifacts.

References

[1] Edelstein W, Glover G, Hardy C, et al. The intrinsic signal-to-noise ratio in NMR imaging. Magn Reson Med 1986;3:604–18.

[2] Bottomley P, Foster T, Argersinger R, et al. A review of normal tissue hydrogen NMR relaxation times and relaxation mechanisms from 1-100 MHz: dependence on tissue type, NMR

frequency, temperature, species, excision, and age. Med Phys 1984;11:425–48.

[3] de Bazelaire C, Duhamel G, Rofsky N, et al. MR imaging relaxation times of abdominal and pelvic tissues measured in vivo at 3.0 T: preliminary results. Radiology 2004;230:652–9.

[4] Stanisz G, Odrobina E, Pun J, et al. T1, T2 relaxation and magnetization transfer in tissue at 3T. Magn Reson Med 2005;54:507–12.

[5] Lee T, Stainsby J, Hong J, et al. Blood relaxation properties at 3T—effects of blood oxygen saturation. Presented at the 11th Annual Meeting of ISMRM. July 10–16, 2003, Toronto, Canada.

[6] Rinck P, Muller R. Field strength and dose dependence of contrast enhancement by gadolinium-based MR contrast agents. Eur Radiol 1999;9:998–1004.

[7] Rohrer M, Bauer H, Mintorovitch J, et al. Comparison of magnetic properties of MRI contrast media solutions at different magnetic field strengths. Invest Radiol 2005;40:715–24.

[8] Trattnig S, Ba-Ssalamah A, Noebauer-Humann I, et al. MR contrast agent at high-field MRI (3 tesla). Top Magn Reson Imaging 2003;14:365–75.

[9] Trattnig S, Pinker K, Ba-Ssalamah A, et al. The optimal use of contrast agents at high field MRI. Eur Radiol 2006;16:1280–7.

[10] Weinmann H, Bauer H, Ebert W, et al. Comparative studies on the efficacy of MRI contrast agents in MRA. Acad Radiol 2002;9:135–6.

[11] Allkemper T, Schwindt W, Maintz D, et al. Sensitivity of T2-weighted FSE sequences towards physiological iron depositions in normal brains at 1.5 and 3.0 T. Eur Radiol 2004;14:1000–4.

[12] Bernstein M, Huston J III, Ward H. Imaging artifacts at 3.0 T. J Magn Reson Imaging 2006;24:735–46.

[13] Beyersdorff D, Taymoorian K, Knosel T, et al. MRI of prostate cancer at 1.5 and 3.0 T: comparison of image quality in tumor detection and staging. Am J Roentgenol 2005;185:1214–20.

[14] Bolog N, Nanz D, Weishaupt D. Muskuloskeletal MR imaging at 3.0 T: current status and future perspectives. Eur Radiol 2006;16:1298–307.

[15] Briellmann R, Pell G, Wellard R, et al. MR imaging of epilepsy: state of the art at 1.5 T and potential of 3 T. Epileptic Disord 2003;5:3–20.

[16] Campeau N, Huston J 3rd, Bernstein M, et al. Magnetic resonance angiography at 3.0 tesla: initial clinical experience. Top Magn Reson Imaging 2001;12:183–204.

[17] Edelman R, Salanitri G, Brand R, et al. Magnetic resonance imaging of the pancreas at 3.0 tesla. Invest Radiol 2006;41:175–80.

[18] Gibbs G, Huston J 3rd, Bernstein M, et al. Improved image quality of intracranial aneurysms: 3.0-T versus 1.5 T time-of-flight MR angiography. AJNR Am J Neuroradiol 2004;25:84–7.

[19] Gold G, Han E, Stainsby J, et al. Musculoskeletal MRI at 3.0 T: relaxation times and image contrast. Am J Roentgenol 2004;183:343–51.

[20] Gold G, Suh B, Sawyer-Glover A, et al. Musculoskeletal MRI at 3.0 T: initial clinical experience. Am J Roentgenol 2004;183:1479–86.

[21] Greenman R, Shirosky J, Mulkern R, et al. Double inversion black-blood fast spin-echo imaging of the human heart: a comparison between 1.5T and 3.0T. J Magn Reson Imaging 2003;17:648–55.

[22] Hugg J, Rofsky N, Stokar S, et al. Clinical whole body MRI at 3.0 T—initial experience. Presented at the 10th Annual Meeting of ISMRM. May 18–24, 2002, Honolulu, Hawaii.

[23] Katz-Brull R, Rofsky N, Lenkinski R. Breathhold abdominal and thoracic proton MR spectroscopy at 3 T. Magn Reson Med 2003;50:461–7.

[24] Martin D, Friel H, Danrad R, et al. Approach to abdominal imaging at 1.5 tesla and optimization at 3 tesla. Magn Reson Imaging Clin N Am 2005;13:241–54.

[25] Merkle E, Dale B. Abdominal MR imaging at 3.0 tesla—the basics revisited. Am J Roentgenol 2006;186:1524–32.

[26] Merkle E, Haugan P, Thomas J, et al. MR cholangiography: 3.0 tesla versus 1.5 tesla—a pilot study. Am J Roentgenol 2006;186:516–21.

[27] Morakkabati-Spitz N, Gieseke J, Kuhl C, et al. 3.0-T high-field magnetic resonance imaging of the female pelvis: preliminary experiences. Eur Radiol 2005;15:639–44.

[28] O'Regan D, Fitzgerald J, Allsop J, et al. A comparison of MR cholangiopancreatography at 1.5 and 3.0 tesla. Br J Radiol 2005;78:894–8.

[29] Schick F. Whole-body MRI at high field: technical limits and clinical potential. Eur Radiol 2005;15:946–59.

[30] Schindera S, Merkle E, Dale B, et al. Abdominal magnetic resonance imaging at 3.0 T: what is the ultimate gain in signal-to-noise ratio? Acad Radiol 2006;13:1236–43.

[31] Schmitz B, Aschoff A, Hoffmann M, et al. Advantages and pitfalls in 3 T MR brain imaging: a pictorial review. AJNR Am J Neuroradiol 2005;26:2229–37.

[32] Sosna J, Pedrosa I, Dewolf W, et al. MR imaging of the prostate at 3 tesla: comparison of an external phased-array coil to imaging with an endorectal coil at 1.5 tesla. Acad Radiol 2004;11:857–62.

[33] Sosna J, Rofsky N, Gaston S, et al. Determinations of prostate volume at 3-tesla using an external phased array coil: comparison to pathologic specimens. Acad Radiol 2003;10:846–53.

[34] Takahashi M, Uematsu H, Hatabu H. MR imaging at high magnetic fields. Eur J Radiol 2003;46:45–52.

[35] Uematsu H, Takahashi M, Dougherty L, et al. High field body MR imaging: preliminary experiences. Clin Imaging 2004;28:159–62.

[36] van den Brink J, Watanabe Y, Kuhl C, et al. Implications of SENSE MR in routine clinical practice. Eur Radiol 2003;46:3–27.

[37] Duewell S, Ceckler T, Ong K, et al. Musculoskeletal MR imaging at 4 T and at 1.5 T: comparison of relaxation times and image contrast. Radiology 1995;196:551–5.

[38] Fischer H, Rinck P, Van Haverbeke Y, et al. Nuclear relaxation of human brain gray and white matter: analysis of field dependence and implications for MRI. Magn Reson Med 1990;16: 317–34.

[39] Jezzard P, Duewell S, Balaban R. MR relaxation times in human brain: measurement at 4 T. Radiology 1996;199:773–9.

[40] Kangarlu A, Abduljalil A, Robitaille P. T1- and T2-weighted imaging at 8 tesla. J Comput Assist Tomogr 1999;23:875–8.

[41] Kim S, Hu X, Ugurbil K. Accurate T1 determination from inversion recovery images: application to human brain at 4 tesla. Magn Reson Med 1994;31:445–9.

[42] Maubon A, Ferru J, Berger V, et al. Effect of field strength on MR images: comparison of the same subject at 0.5, 1.0, and 1.5 T. Radiographics 1999;19:1057–67.

[43] Rakow-Penner R, Daniel B, Yu H, et al. Relaxation times of breast tissue at 1.5T and 3T measured using IDEAL. J Magn Reson Imaging 2006;23:87–91.

[44] Busse R. Reduced RF power without blurring: correcting for modulation of refocusing flip angle in FSE sequences. Magn Reson Med 2004; 51:1031–7.

[45] Hennig J. Multiecho imaging sequences with low refocusing flip angles. J Magn Reson 1988;78: 397–407.

[46] Hennig J, Scheffler K. Hyperechoes. Magn Reson Med 2001;46:6–12.

[47] Hargreaves B, Cunningham C, Nishimura D, et al. Variable-rate selective excitation for rapid MRI sequences. Magn Reson Med 2004;52:590–7.

[48] Pruessmann K. Parallel imaging at high field strength: synergies and joint potential. Top Magn Reson Imaging 2004;15:237–44.

[49] Pruessmann K, Weiger M, Scheidegger M, et al. SENSE: sensitivity encoding for fast MRI. Magn Reson Med 1999;42:952–62.

[50] Mugler J 3rd, Brookeman J. Rapid three-dimensional T1-weighted MR imaging with the MP-RAGE sequence. J Magn Reson Imaging 1991;1: 561–7.

[51] Barker P, Hearshen D, Boska M. Single-voxel proton MRS of the human brain at 1.5T and 3.0T. Magn Reson Med 2001;45:765–9.

[52] Kantarci K, Reynolds G, Petersen R, et al. Proton MR spectroscopy in mild cognitive impairment and Alzheimer disease: comparison of 1.5 and 3 T. AJNR Am J Neuroradiol 2003;24: 843–9.

[53] Michaely H, Nael K, Schoenberg S, et al. Analysis of cardiac function—comparison between 1.5 tesla and 3.0 tesla cardiac cine magnetic resonance imaging: preliminary experience. Invest Radiol 2006;41:133–40.

[54] Morakkabati-Spitz N, Gieseke J, Kuhl C, et al. MRI of the pelvis at 3 T: very high spatial resolution with sensitivity encoding and flip-angle sweep technique in clinically acceptable scan time. Eur Radiol 2005;16:634–41.

[55] Lewin J, Duerk J, Jain V, et al. Needle localization in MR-guided biopsy and aspiration: effects of field strength, sequence design, and magnetic field orientation. Am J Roentgenol 1996;166: 1337–45.

[56] Heindel W, Friedmann G, Bunke J, et al. Artifacts in MR imaging after surgical intervention. J Comput Assist Tomogr 1986;10:596–9.

[57] Tien R, Buxton R, Schwaighofer B, et al. Quantitation of structural distortion of the cervical neural foramina in gradient-echo MR imaging. J Magn Reson Imaging 1991;1:683–7.

[58] Baker K, Nyenhuis J, Hrdlicka G, et al. Neurostimulation systems: assessment of magnetic field interactions associated with 1.5- and 3-tesla MR systems. J Magn Reson Imaging 2005;21:72–7.

[59] Shellock F. Biomedical implants and devices: assessment of magnetic field interactions with a 3.0-tesla MR system. J Magn Reson Imaging 2002;16:721–32.

[60] Shellock F, Forder J. Drug eluting coronary stent: in vitro evaluation of magnet resonance safety at 3 tesla. J Cardiovasc Magn Reson 2005;7:415–9.

[61] Shellock F, Gounis M, Wakhloo A. Detachable coil for cerebral aneurysms: in vitro evaluation of magnetic field interactions, heating, and artifacts at 3T. AJNR Am J Neuroradiol 2005;26: 363–6.

[62] Shellock F, Tkach J, Ruggieri P, et al. Cardiac pacemakers, ICDs, and loop recorder: evaluation of translational attraction using conventional (long-bore) and short-bore 1.5- and 3.0-tesla MR systems. J Cardiovasc Magn Reson 2003;5: 387–97.

[63] Sommer T, Maintz D, Schmiedel A, et al. [High field MR imaging: magnetic field interactions of aneurysm clips, coronary artery stents and iliac artery stents with a 3.0 tesla MR system]. Rofo 2004;176:731–8 [in German].

[64] Peh W, Chan J. Artifacts in musculoskeletal magnetic resonance imaging: identification and correction. Skeletal Radiology 2001;30:179–91.

[65] Fernandez-Seara M, Wehrli F. Postprocessing technique to correct for background gradients in image-based R*2 measurements. Magn Reson Med 2000;44:358–66.

[66] Wood M, Hardy P. Proton relaxation enhancement. J Magn Reson Imaging 1993;3:149–56.

[67] Merkle E, Dale B, Barboriak D. Gain in signal-to-noise for first-pass contrast-enhanced abdominal MR angiography at 3 Tesla over standard 1.5 Tesla: prediction with a computer model. Acad Radiol 2007;14:795–803.

[68] Oppenheim A, Schafer R, Buck J. Discrete-time signal processing. Englewood Cliffs (NJ): Prentice Hall; 1999.

[69] Glockner J, Hu H, Stanley D, et al. Parallel MR imaging: a user's guide. Radiographics 2005;25: 1279–97.

[70] Arena L, Morehouse H, Safir J. MR imaging artifacts that simulate disease: how to recognize and eliminate them. Radiographics 1995;15: 1373–94.

[71] Hahn F, Chu W, Coleman P, et al. Artifacts and diagnostic pitfalls on magnetic resonance imaging: a clinical review. Radiol Clin North Am 1988;26:717–35.

[72] Henkelman R, Bronskill M. Artifacts in magnetic resonance imaging. Reviews of Magnetic Resonance in Medicine 1987;2:1–126.

[73] Herrick R, Hayman L, Taber K, et al. Artifacts and pitfalls in MR imaging of the orbit: a clinical review. Radiographics 1997;17:707–24.

[74] Hinks R, Quencer R. Motion artifacts in brain and spine MR. Radiol Clin North Am 1988;26: 737–53.

[75] Pusey E, Lufkin R, Brown R, et al. Magnetic resonance imaging artifacts: mechanism and clinical significance. Radiographics 1986;6.891–911.

[76] Taber K, Herrick R, Weathers S, et al. Pitfalls and artifacts encountered in clinical MR imaging of the spine. Radiographics 1998;18:1499–521.

[77] Wood M, Henkelman R. MR image artifacts from periodic motion. Med Phys 1985;12:143–51.

[78] Elster A, Burdette J. Questions and answers in magnetic resonance imaging. 2nd edition. St. Louis (MO): Mosby; 2001. p. 128.

[79] Dale B, Merkle E. A new 3D approach for clinical in- and opposed-phase MRI at 3 T. Presented at the 15th Annual Meeting of ISMRM. May 19–25, 2007, Berlin, Germany.

[80] Thesen S, Krueger G, Mueller E. Compensation of dielectric resonance effects by means of composite excitation pulses. Presented at the 11th Annual Meeting of ISMRM. July 10–16, 2003, Toronto, Canada.

[81] Haacke E, Brown R, Thompson M, et al. Magnetic resonance imaging: physical principles and sequence design. New York: Wiley-Liss, Inc.; 1999. p. 1–868.

[82] Serway R. Physics for scientists & engineers. 3rd edition. Philadelphia: Harcourt Brace College Publishers; 1992. p. 955–77.

[83] Collins C, Liu W, Schreiber W, et al. Central brightening due to constructive interference with, without, and despite dielectric resonance. J Magn Reson Imaging 2005;21:192–6.

[84] Alsop D, Connick T, Mizsei G. A spiral volume coil for improved RF field homogeneity at high static magnetic field. Magn Res Med 1998;40: 49–54.

[85] Schmitt M, Feiweier T, Voellmecke E, et al. B1-homogenization in abdominal imaging at 3T by means of coupling coils. Presented at the 13th Annual Meeting of ISMRM. May 7–13, 2005, Miami Beach, Florida.

[86] Schmitt M, Feiweier T, Horger W, et al. Improved uniformity of RF-distribution in clinical whole body imaging at 3T by means of dielectric pads. Presented at the 12th Annual Meeting of ISMRM. May 15–21, 2004, Kyoto, Japan.

[87] Franklin K, Dale B, Merkle E. Improvement in B1-inhomogeneity artifacts in the abdomen at 3 tesla MR imaging using a radiofrequency cushion. J Magn Reson Imaging, in press.

[88] Duerk J, Lewin J, Wendt M, et al. Remember true FISP? A high SNR, near 1-second imaging method for T2-like contrast in interventional MRI at 0.2T. J Magn Reson Imaging 1998;8:203–8.

[89] Hargreaves B, Vasnawala S, Pauly J, et al. Characterization and reduction of the transient response in steady state MR imaging. Magn Reson Med 2001;46:149–58.

[90] Mansfield P, Morris P. NMR imaging in biomedicine. In: Waugh JS, editor. Advances in magnetic resonance. New York: Academic Press; 1982. p. 41–77.

[91] Oppelt A, Graumann R, Barfuss H, et al. FISP: a new fast MRI sequence. Electromedica 1986; 54:15–8.

[92] Redpath T, Jones R. FADE: a new fast imaging sequence. Magn Reson Med 1988;6:224–34.

[93] Vasnawala S, Pauly J, Nishimura D. Fluctuating equilibrium MRI. Magn Reson Med 1999;42: 876–83.

[94] Vasnawala S, Pauly J, Nishimura D. Linear combination steady state free precession MRI. Magn Reson Med 2000;43:82–90.

[95] Zur Y, Stokar S, Bendel P. An analysis of fast imaging sequences with steady state transverse magnetization refocusing. Magn Reson Med 1988;6: 175–93.

[96] Zur Y, Wood M, Neuringer L. Motion-insensitive, steady-state free precession imaging. Magn Reson Med 1990;16:444–59.

[97] Foxall D. Frequency-modulated steady-state free precession imaging. Magn Reson Med 2002;48: 502–8.

[98] Ma J, Vu A, Son J, et al. Fat-suppressed three-dimensional dual echo dixon technique for contrast agent enhanced MRI. J Magn Reson Imaging 2006;23:36–41.

MAGNETIC
RESONANCE
IMAGING CLINICS

Magn Reson Imaging Clin N Am 15 (2007) 291–300

Cardiac MR Imaging: New Advances and Role of 3T

Kambiz Nael, MD*, Michael Fenchel, MD, Roya Saleh, MD, J. Paul Finn, MD

- Potential advantages of 3T
- Potential disadvantages of 3T
  Radiofrequency energy deposition
  Field inhomogeneity
  Dielectric resonance and radiofrequency inhomogeneity
- Clinical applications

Dark-blood anatomic imaging
Cine imaging
Myocardial tagging
Perfusion imaging
Delayed enhancement imaging
Coronary MR angiography
- Summary
- References

   This article underscores some of the more recent advances that are likely to impact cardiac MR imaging in the future. Developing techniques and technique-related aspects, and the advantages and possible pitfalls of 3T in particular, are highlighted. Finally, existing clinical experiences, including functional and anatomical imaging, myocardial viability and perfusion imaging, and coronary artery imaging are summarized.

   Cardiovascular magnetic resonance (MR) imaging has gained broad clinical acceptance over the past several years [1–4]. Cardiac MR imaging must deal with physiologic cardiac and respiratory motion, and must balance the competing demands of high spatial and temporal resolution, while maintaining sufficient contrast-to-noise ratio (CNR) and signal-to-noise ratio (SNR). The development of parallel acquisition technology [5–7] and advances in pulse sequences, such as steady-state free-precession (SSFP) [8,9], have resulted in substantial improvement in image quality and speed for cardiac MR applications [1,2,10,11].

   At 3T, more baseline SNR is available than at 1.5T, and the extra signal can be used to reduce acquisition time and improve spatial resolution. The added SNR is of particular advantage when parallel acquisition with high acceleration factors is employed [12–14]. Cardiac MR imaging at 3T holds promise to overcome some of the SNR limitations for techniques with borderline SNR at 1.5T, such as myocardial perfusion, delayed enhancement imaging, or imaging of coronary arteries. On the other hand, specific absorption rate (SAR) limitations and susceptibility effects remain challenging and may occasionally impede the progress of cardiac MRI imaging at 3T.

   In this article, some of the fundamental changes of cardiac MR imaging at 3T, in comparison to 1.5T, and some of the advantages and limitations of MR imaging at 3T are outlined. The authors emphasize those techniques for which there are established clinical applications or that might have a clinical role in the near term. It seems likely that the SNR advantages at 3T will fuel further

Department of Radiological Sciences, David Geffen School of Medicine, University of California Los Angeles, 10945 Le Conte Avenue, Suite # 3371, Los Angeles, CA 90095–7206, USA
* Corresponding author.
E-mail address: nkambiz@mednet.ucla.edu (K. Nael).

1064-9689/07/$ – see front matter © 2007 Elsevier Inc. All rights reserved.
mri.theclinics.com

doi:10.1016/j.mric.2007.08.002

developments in high magnetic field cardiac MR imaging and pave the way for further novel and promising imaging techniques.

Potential advantages of 3T

The main advantage of MR imaging at higher magnetic field is the potential SNR gain. Theoretically, imaging at 3T leads to a two-fold increase in SNR, as compared with 1.5T, as the signal increases with B_0^2, whereas noise contributions increase with B_0 [15]. These theoretical SNR advantages at 3T are of the most relevance for applications with borderline SNR at 1.5T, such as contrast-enhanced MR angiography, coronary MR angiography, and assessment of myocardial perfusion and viability.

In practice, SNR represents a fundamental challenge for parallel imaging and is increasingly limiting as acceleration factors increase and in this situation, 3T is helpful. In fact, there is a reciprocal synergy between high magnetic field strengths and parallel imaging:

On one hand, higher SNR base at 3T has the promise of sufficient support for faster parallel acquisition [13,16,17] and reduction in the noise amplification associated with parallel imaging techniques [18,19]. Higher acceleration factors shorten acquisition windows and support more robust segmented acquisition schemes, which are suitable for very high heart rates, for example in pediatric patients or in examinations with injection of pharmacologic stress agents (eg, stress perfusion studies).

On the other hand, the increased speed and efficiency associated with parallel imaging may be converted into extra diagnostic value for high field cardiovascular MR imaging in two ways. First, by reducing echo train length for any given acquisition time, parallel imaging helps to limit T2* artifact (relaxation-related blurring) associated with high magnetic field, improving the over all image quality. Second, by omitting some of the phase-encoding steps and corresponding radiofrequency (RF) refocusing pulses, parallel imaging helps to reduce the total power deposition, overcoming some of the physiologic limitations (RF power deposition, peripheral nerve stimulation, acoustic noise) and physical constraints (eg, gradient switching rate dB/dt) [20].

The integration of parallel imaging with 3T and the aforementioned mutual relationship may be the most essential contributing factor of high magnetic field to enhance the cardiovascular MR applications, and may pave the way for further development of promising cardiac MR imaging techniques.

Potential disadvantages of 3T

Radiofrequency energy deposition

SAR increases almost quadratically with field strength ($SAR \propto B_0^2$). This limits the maximum allowable flip angles and the minimum achievable repetition time (TR), which in turn can restrict RF intensive techniques at 3T, such as SSFP cine and spin-echo train imaging.

Field inhomogeneity

Increased B_0 inhomogeneity and $T_2^*\backslash$ susceptibility effects are well known anticipated problems at higher magnetic field [21–23]. These factors may result in regional shading and focal T2*-induced signal loss (dark banding) or ghosting of flow in the image (Fig. 1). Magnetic field inhomogeneities increase linearly with field strength, leading to faster dephasing of the contributing frequency components, and therefore to areas with pronounced signal loss. This increasingly rapid dephasing for higher field strength is especially important for tissue types with marked inherent structural inhomogeneities, such as lung with lung-air interfaces or at tissue boundaries, such as the heart-lung interface. Several strategies have been described to modulate these artifacts, including adjusting synthesizer frequency [24], summing frequency-modulated acquisitions [25], and applying localized linear or second order shimming corrections [26].

Dielectric resonance and radiofrequency inhomogeneity

The wavelength of RF pulse decreases with frequency, and at 3T the effective wavelength of RF

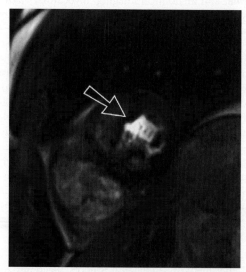

Fig. 1. Steady-state free-precession cine sequence in short-axis plane acquired at 3T. Reduced B_0 homogeneity at 3T can cause dark banding artifacts (*arrow*), degrading the diagnostic image quality.

pulses becomes comparable to the size of human organs. As it is difficult to achieve good RF field homogeneity in large field of view at higher fields because of RF penetration effects, this might cause an inhomogeneous RF transmit field and, as a result, lead to location dependent flip angles, receiver-coil sensitivity, and ultimately to suboptimal parameters throughout the imaging volume. Further RF effects might arise from induced eddy currents and compromise the performance of selective profile of RF pulses or accumulate additional phase error in SSFP sequences.

Dielectric resonance artifacts typically manifest as bright regions near the center of the imaged object, and the resulting signal and contrast behavior may negatively affect the diagnostic information in the cardiac MR images, for example in myocardial perfusion series. To modulate these artifacts, several measures, such as signal intensity normalization, use of B_1 insensitive RF pulses (eg, adiabatic pulses) [27,28], or application of dielectric pads may be beneficial to increase the signal homogeneity of the acquired images.

Considering the above mentioned difficulties, cardiac MR imaging at 3T, although feasible [12,14,29,30], remains to be challenging, particularly in relation to SSFP cine methods. The restricting effect of SAR on maximum allowable flip angle and minimum achievable TR, and increased magnetic susceptibility effects (heighten sensitivity to off-resonance artifacts), make SSFP cine imaging more challenging at higher field strengths. Introduction of intravascular contrast agents may provide an alternative approach for cardiac cine imaging independent of SSFP techniques [31]. If the T1 of the blood is short, then spoiled gradient recalled echo (GRE) cine imaging with a very short TR becomes practical, with performance characteristics similar to those of SSFP.

Clinical applications

Dark-blood anatomic imaging

After integration of ECG-gating with spin-echo imaging, the resulted dark blood images of the myocardium and cardiac chambers has gained broad acceptance in cardiac MR clinical applications [32–35]. Black-blood preparation schemes for spin-echo imaging of the heart and blood vessels routinely involve a double inversion pulse pair [36,37].

Dark blood imaging may benefit at 3T for two reasons:

1. The higher readout bandwidth allows for shorter minimal echo times in spin-echo sequences, and for narrower echo spacing in turbo-spin-echo sequences. As a result, an SNR boost ranging from 30% in dark-blood prepared techniques to 75% for dark-blood prepared fat-saturated imaging can be achieved [30].

2. Implementation of faster parallel acquisition at 3T helps to limit relaxation-related blurring by allowing a reduced echo train length for any given acquisition time. This will also reduce the total power deposition by omitting phase encoding steps and corresponding RF refocusing pulses.

Although today spin-echo imaging plays a more secondary role, for many protocols—including anatomic surveys involving structural abnormalities of the ventricles and the pericardium—single-shot spin-echo imaging can be a valuable supplement [38,39]. Newer approaches, such as application of variable flip angles and hyperechoes [27], in addition to integration of highly accelerated parallel acquisition at high magnetic field, have the promise to increase the performance and potential applications of dark-blood cardiac imaging, eliminating the risk of slice misregistration and long examination time [40–42].

Cine imaging

Cardiac cine imaging remains the cornerstone of functional cardiac MR imaging. In this regard, the early work involved the use of spoiled GRE pulse sequences to generate gated cine imaging [43,44]. Breath-hold cine MR imaging with a spoiled GRE sequence remained the standard for functional imaging of the heart until the introduction of steady-state techniques at the turn of the century.

The main limitation of spoiled GRE cine MR as a T1-weighted sequence is its dependence on through-plane flow enhancement to generate contrast between the blood and the myocardium. Therefore, if the TR is too short or the flow is too slow, the blood becomes saturated. This is particularly the case for long-axis imaging, where blood may linger in the section, and even for short-axis imaging if myocardial function is poor. Introduction of SSFP cine imaging [8,45] has substantially enhanced the image quality and performance of cardiac cine imaging, and has largely replaced spoiled GRE cine MR imaging for all routine applications.

Recently, cardiac cine imaging has been applied at 3T and initial reports suggest they may have a role in clinical cardiac imaging [12,29,30]. The integration of highly accelerated parallel acquisition technique with higher field strengths and multichannel MR imaging at 3T exceeds the performance of 1.5T applications [12,14]. The SNR benefit at 3T, in conjunction with accelerated acquisition strategies, may be used to increase the number of cardiac phases, resulting in an improved temporal resolution without exceeding breath-hold constraints (Fig. 2). Higher temporal resolution improves accurate wall motion tracking, enhancing the accuracy of cardiac function analysis [46]. Furthermore, by better tracking of small, rapidly moving structures, such as valve cusps throughout the cardiac cycle, this may be beneficial for more accurate assessment of patients with valvular disease.

There are however, several technical challenges for cardiac SSFP cine imaging at 3T caused by high B_0 inhomogeneities and shorter T_2^* values [47]. These can cause dark banding artifacts overlying cardiac structures (see Fig. 1), severely degrading image quality and hampering diagnosis of cardiac pathology. SSFP cine works best with the constant high flip angle excitations, short repetition times, and very homogenous magnetic fields. All premises seem not to be ideally fulfilled at 3T because of SAR limitations, higher patient induced susceptibility effects as compared with 1.5T, and dielectric resonance effects. Furthermore, in contrast to spin-echo approaches, gradient-echo techniques are very sensitive to intravoxel spin dephasing. With SSFP, the blood signal is dependent on its relaxation time (specifically, the T2*/T1 ratio). At higher magnetic field, the T_2^* values of the tissues are clearly shortened, therefore shorter echo times are necessary to obtain similar tissue depiction as at 1.5T.

By using localized linear or second-order shimming, a local optimization of the resonance frequency can be achieved [26]. Similarly, by using a scout sequence which acquires several images, each with a different center frequency, the optimal center frequency for the region of interest can be determined to minimize banding artifacts overlying cardiac structures [48]. Therefore, although SSFP cine imaging at 3T is feasible, occasionally—and especially in long axis views—it may be impossible to shift banding artifacts completely from cardiac structures. Furthermore, residual off-resonance artifacts after determination of the optimal center frequency were often observed, especially in the lateral and inferior wall of the left ventricle at the heart-lung interface [49].

Myocardial tagging

Myocardial tagging refers to methods that track the deformation of a presaturation grid as a function of displacement and monitor the deformations of these lines subsequent to myocardial contraction [50]. When combined with cine imaging, myocardial tagging could be extremely powerful as a tool to study cardiac mechanics, providing complementary or supplementary information about cardiac wall motion.

A limitation of tagging is that the tag lines fade and the edges blur because of longitudinal relaxation. Consequently, the CNR between the saturation tags and surrounding myocardium is diminished during end-diastole. Recent results suggest that myocardial tagging techniques may benefit at 3T [30,51]. This can be attributed to the elevated baseline SNR, but primarily to the T_1 prolongation of myocardial tissue at 3T, which in return translates into a significant CNR increase at end-diastole at 3T versus 1.5T. The improved CNR and reduced fading of the tags at 3T, in combination with faster parallel acquisition, may enhance the performance of myocardial tagging, tracking the myocardial wall motion throughout the entire R-R interval (Fig. 3).

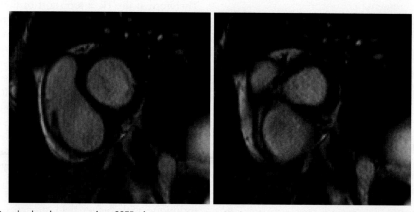

Fig. 2. Short axis cine images using SSFP cine sequence at 3T, integrated with parallel acquisition with acceleration factor of 4. Note the high diagnostic image quality with good contrast between the blood pool and myocardial wall. These images are acquired with spatial resolution of 1.5 × 1.2 × 5 mm³ during 6 seconds breath-hold.

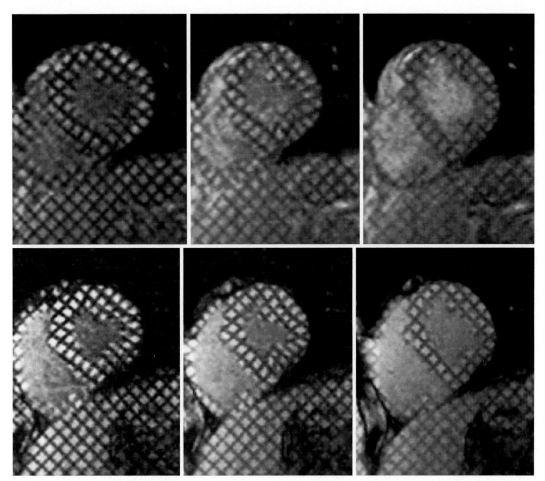

Fig. 3. Myocardial tagging experiment at 1.5T (*upper row*) and 3T (*lower row*). Note the improved image quality and reduced fading of the myocardial tags at 3T.

Perfusion imaging

The initial reports of myocardial perfusion MR imaging in human beings, performed with first-pass contrast enhancement, were published in the early 1990s [52,53]. Rapid contrast-enhanced MR imaging has become a valuable tool for the assessment of myocardial perfusion. By using a T1-weighted inversion-recovery fast GRE technique to capture first passage of the contrast agent with temporal resolution equal to one heart beat, cardiac MR perfusion has become a valuable and broadly accepted diagnostic tool [52,54–56].

Nonetheless, the task of capturing the first-pass perfusion MR imaging with sufficient spatial and temporal resolution and absence of artifact (Gibbs ringing artifact) is challenging [57]. In addition, the required high temporal resolution imposes a significant limitation on anatomic coverage and SNR. Moreover, variability in the shape of the bolus resulting from the patient's hemodynamic may be troublesome for standardization [58,59].

Myocardial perfusion imaging is one of the applications that may benefit the most from higher magnetic field strengths. Substantial SNR, CNR, and overall image quality improvements were reported for first-pass cardiac MR perfusion imaging at 3T [30,60,61]. The performance of myocardial MR perfusion protocols in terms of temporal resolution, spatial resolution, and coverage can be further enhanced by integration of faster parallel acquisition at 3T, as illustrated in Figs. 4 and 5.

Delayed enhancement imaging

Over the last several years, myocardial delayed contrast enhanced imaging has gained broad acceptance for the detection and characterization of acute and chronic myocardial infarction [62]. Because of improved spatial resolution of MR imaging, some investigators have suggested that MR imaging may be even more advantageous than nuclear tomography, in particular for nontransmural infarction [63,64].

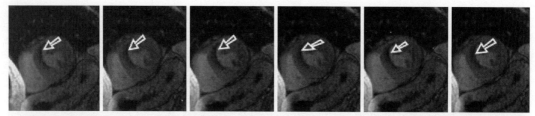

Fig. 4. 3T MR stress perfusion examination is performed as presurgical workup (cardiac risk stratification) on a 63-year-old male patient with bronchial carcinoma. Six selected images taken from the stress perfusion series are presented (saturation-recovery GRE sequence in short-axis orientation) after contrast injection, showing stress induced perfusion deficit in antero-septal part of the left ventricle (*arrows*). (*Courtesy of* M. Fenchel, MD, Tubingen, Germany.)

Gadolinium-based agents tend to accumulate in nonviable myocardium within several minutes and to wash slower than normal myocardium. The interval between injection and imaging should be long enough for the contrast agent to localize in scar and for the blood level to drop, but not so long that the imaging acquisition is unreasonably prolonged. Imaging windows of 10 to 30 minutes after injection are probably acceptable. This localization can be made conspicuous with an appropriate T1-weighted imaging technique. In this contest the most established and well-documented technique is segmented k-space inversion-recovery (IR) GRE sequence [65], which can provide high contrast between nonviable and healthy myocardium.

However, the relatively lower SNR associated with this technique, caused by suppression of background and healthy myocardial signal, maybe limiting for using this technique with higher required speed and coverage; in addition, higher SNR at 3T may directly benefit cardiac viability imaging (Fig. 6). Reported unaccelerated delayed enhancement approaches may be limited, with spatial coverage of only one to two slices per breath-hold, resulting in prolonged examination times of 10 to 15 minutes, corresponding with patient discomfort and decay of contrast agent concentration over the course of the exam.

Parallel imaging at 3T can overcome these difficulties by supporting accelerated delayed enhancement imaging, allowing whole-heart coverage in a single breath-hold, leading to uniform suppression of healthy myocardium for all imaged sections and increased patient comfort. Higher B_1-field inhomogeneities at 3T may result in an inhomogeneous signal suppression of healthy myocardium, using standard inversion pulses. Applying more homogenous inversion flip angles using an adiabatic inversion preparation pulse may be beneficial in this regard [30].

More recently, variants of SSFP, such as inversion-recovery SSFP, have been successfully used to address myocardial viability with some promising results [66,67]. Considering the known limitations

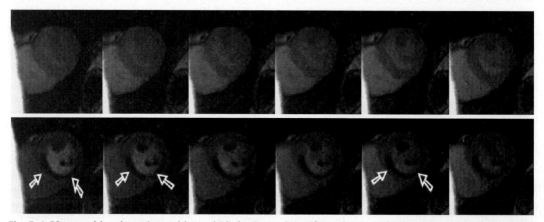

Fig. 5. A 33-year-old male patient with morbid obesity and significant history of atherosclerosis presented with angina. Coronary catheter angiography revealed three vessel disease with high grade stenosis in right coronary and circumflex arteries. Six selected myocardial perfusion images (midventricular short-axis slice) obtained at rest (*upper row*) and stress (adenosine) perfusion series (*lower row*) are presented (saturation-recovery GRE sequence in short-axis orientation) after injection of 0.1-mmol Gd-DTPA/kg body weight. Note the stress induced perfusion defects in infero-septal, posterior, and lateral walls (*arrows*).

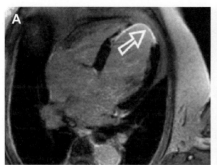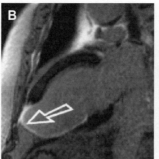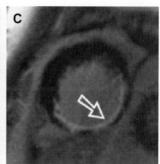

Fig. 6. Delayed 3T enhancement images in a 59-year-old male patient with coronary artery disease and myocardial infarction. IR-GRE sequence at 3T, using integrated parallel acquisition techniques in 4-chamber (*A*), long axis (*B*), and short axis (*C*) plane after administration of 0.1-mmol Gd-DTPA/kg body weight. There is delayed enhancement (*arrows*) in the septum, posterior, and lateral myocardial wall representing of myocardial infarction as well as an apical aneurysm. (*Courtesy of* M. Fenchel, MD, Tubingen, Germany.)

of SSFP at high magnetic field, it seems unlikely that this technique will develop into substantial clinical use at 3T. A phase sensitive reconstruction of inversion recovery (PSIR) has been shown to enhance the contrast between healthy and infarcted myocardial tissue and to avoid the individual adaptation of the inversion time [68]. At 1.5T, however, PSIR image quality may be hampered by higher image noise and artifacts because of the ambiguousness of the phase information at relatively lower SNR. The image quality and performance of PSIR single-shot fast imaging with steady-state precession (TrueFISP) can be significantly improved at 3T [69].

Coronary MR angiography

MR imaging of coronary arteries is challenging for a variety of reasons, including cardiac and respiratory motion, the size and tortuosity of the coronary arteries, and the distance of the arteries from surface coils. All current MR methods for imaging the coronary arteries use an ECG-triggered segmented three-dimensional data acquisition. Several phase-encoding steps are acquired during each heartbeat, and cumulative data acquisition over several consecutive heartbeats encompasses one plane of k-space. This process is repeated until the entire three-dimensional k-space is covered.

Three-dimensional SSFP imaging is the preferred method for evaluation of the coronary arteries [70], which can be performed during either breath holding or free breathing. Frequency-selective fat-suppression techniques are required in coronary MR angiography to prepare the magnetization to approach a steady state, and reduce fat signal arising from fatty tissue surrounding the coronary arteries [48].

Since both macroscopic field distortions and the chemical shift difference between water and fat signals are increased in similar ways at higher magnetic fields, shimming works equally effective at 3T in most body regions, as known from examinations at 1.5T. More importantly, fat suppression at 3T and the lack of chemical shift artifacts allow investigators to use a relatively lower readout

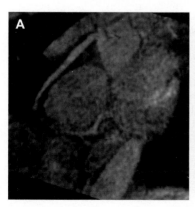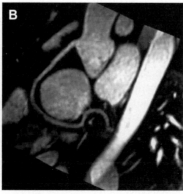

Fig. 7. Reformatted RCA images from two whole-heart acquisition at 3T with *T2*-prepared fast low angle shot (FLASH) (*A*) (no contrast agent given) and inversion-prepared FLASH (*B*) with slow infusion of contrast agent. Note the markedly improved depiction of the coronary artery with contrast-agent administration (*Courtesy of* X. Bi, and D. Li, Chicago, IL).

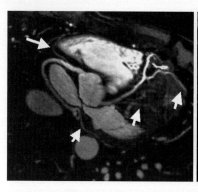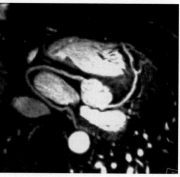

Fig. 8. Whole-heart coronary artery images acquired from two healthy volunteers at 3T. Note that the left and right coronary arteries are sharply depicted and the distal segments and small branches are visible, as indicated by arrows (*Courtesy of* X. Bi, and D. Li, Chicago, IL).

bandwidth, contributing to potentially higher achievable SNR at high magnetic field.

These SNR improvements, together with the enhanced CNR between the blood pool and the myocardium, may provide benefits for clinical coronary MR angiography. With introduction of multicoil technology and a multichannel 3T MR system, and more efficient support of parallel acquisition techniques, such as sensitivity encoding for MR imaging (SENSE) and simultaneous acquisition of spatial harmonics (SMASH), coronary artery MR imaging has become a more pronounced diagnostic tool. Significant improvement in terms of image quality, volume coverage (whole heart), spatial resolution, and acquisition time has been reported on 3T coronary MR angiography using either a single breath-hold technique [71,72] or a navigator-gated free-breathing acquisition (Figs. 7 and 8) [73,74].

Summary

Cardiac MR imaging is evolving rapidly and has matured to the point where it is now widely accepted as a powerful diagnostic tool with significant clinical and research applications. Although the majority of cardiac MR applications seems to be feasible at 3T, with performance and image quality at least similar to or higher in comparison with 1.5T, SAR limitations and susceptibility effects remain a primary concern, with potential challenges ahead. The integration of parallel imaging with 3T, and the existing mutual beneficial effects, may be the most essential contributing factor of high magnetic field to enhance cardiovascular MR applications, paving the way for further development of novel cardiac MR imaging techniques. It is likely that cardiac MR imaging at 3T will meet the challenge through continued developments in machine hardware, pulse sequences, motion compensation, and the use of novel contrast agents.

References

[1] Finn JP, Nael K, Deshpande V, et al. Cardiac MR imaging: state of the technology. Radiology 2006;241(2):338–54.

[2] Edelman RR. Contrast-enhanced MR imaging of the heart: overview of the literature. Radiology 2004;232(3):653–68.

[3] Lima JA, Desai MY. Cardiovascular magnetic resonance imaging: current and emerging applications. J Am Coll Cardiol 2004;44(6):1164–71.

[4] Pennell DJ, Sechtem UP, Higgins CB, et al. Clinical indications for cardiovascular magnetic resonance (CMR): Consensus Panel report. Eur Heart J 2004;25(21):1940–65.

[5] Pruessmann KP, Weiger M, Scheidegger MB, et al. SENSE: sensitivity encoding for fast MRI. Magn Reson Med 1999;42(5):952–62.

[6] Sodickson DK, Manning WJ. Simultaneous acquisition of spatial harmonics (SMASH): fast imaging with radiofrequency coil arrays. Magn Reson Med 1997;38(4):591–603.

[7] Griswold MA, Jakob PM, Heidemann RM, et al. Generalized autocalibrating partially parallel acquisitions (GRAPPA). Magn Reson Med 2002;47(6):1202–10.

[8] Bundy J, Simonetti O, Laub G, et al. TrueFISP imaging of the heart. In: ISMRM. 1999.

[9] Deimling M, Heid O. Magnetization prepared trueFISP imaging. In: SMR. 1994.

[10] Shors SM, Cotts WG, Pavlovic-Surjancev B, et al. Heart failure: evaluation of cardiopulmonary transit times with time-resolved MR angiography. Radiology 2003;229(3):743–8.

[11] Shors SM, Fung CW, Francois CJ, et al. Accurate quantification of right ventricular mass at MR imaging by using cine true fast imaging with steady-state precession: study in dogs. Radiology 2004;230(2):383–8.

[12] Wintersperger BJ, Bauner K, Reeder SB, et al. Cardiac steady-state free precession CINE magnetic resonance imaging at 3.0 tesla: impact of parallel imaging acceleration on volumetric accuracy and signal parameters. Invest Radiol 2006;41(2):141–7.

[13] Nael K, Ruehm SG, Michaely HJ, et al. High spatial-resolution CE-MRA of the carotid circulation

with parallel imaging: comparison of image quality between 2 different acceleration factors at 3.0 Tesla. Invest Radiol 2006;41(4):391–9.

[14] Fenchel M, Deshpande VS, Nael K, et al. Cardiac cine imaging at 3 Tesla: initial experience with a 32-element body-array coil. Invest Radiol 2006;41(8):601–8.

[15] Wen H, Denison TJ, Singerman RW, et al. The intrinsic signal-to-noise ratio in human cardiac imaging at 1.5, 3, and 4 T. J Magn Reson 1997; 125(1):65–71.

[16] Nael K, Saleh R, Lee MH, et al. High-Spatial-Resolution Contrast-Enhanced MR Angiography of Abdominal Arteries with Parallel Acquisition at 3.0 T: Initial Experience in 32 patients. AJR Am J Roentgenol 2006;187:1–15.

[17] Robitaille PM, Abduljalil AM, Kangarlu A. Ultra high resolution imaging of the human head at 8 tesla: 2 K x 2 K for Y2 K. J Comput Assist Tomogr 2000;24(1):2–8.

[18] Wiesinger F, Boesiger P, Pruessmann KP. Electrodynamics and ultimate SNR in parallel MR imaging. Magn Reson Med 2004;52(2):376–90.

[19] Ohliger MA, Grant AK, Sodickson DK. Ultimate intrinsic signal-to-noise ratio for parallel MRI: electromagnetic field considerations. Magn Reson Med 2003;50(5):1018–30.

[20] Bammer R, Schoenberg SO. Current concepts and advances in clinical parallel magnetic resonance imaging. Top Magn Reson Imaging 2004; 15(3):129–58.

[21] Robitaille PM. On RF power and dielectric resonances in UHF MRI. NMR Biomed 1999;12(5): 318–9.

[22] Kangarlu A, Baertlein BA, Lee R, et al. Dielectric resonance phenomena in ultra high field MRI. J Comput Assist Tomogr 1999;23(6):821–31.

[23] Ibrahim TS, Lee R, Abduljalil AM, et al. Dielectric resonances and B(1) field inhomogeneity in UHFMRI: computational analysis and experimental findings. Magn Reson Imaging 2001; 19(2):219–26.

[24] Deshpande VS, Shea SM, Li D. Artifact reduction in true-FISP imaging of the coronary arteries by adjusting imaging frequency. Magn Reson Med 2003;49(5):803–9.

[25] Foxall DL. Frequency-modulated steady-state free precession imaging. Magn Reson Med 2002;48(3):502–8.

[26] Schar M, Kozerke S, Fischer SE, et al. Cardiac SSFP imaging at 3 Tesla. Magn Reson Med 2004;51(4):799–806.

[27] Hennig J, Scheffler K. Hyperechoes. Magn Reson Med 2001;46(1):6–12.

[28] Scheffler K, Heid O, Hennig J. Magnetization preparation during the steady state: fat-saturated 3D TrueFISP. Magn Reson Med 2001;45(6): 1075–80.

[29] Michaely HJ, et al. Analysis of cardiac function—comparison between 1.5 Tesla and 3.0 Tesla cardiac cine magnetic resonance imaging: preliminary experience. Invest Radiol 2006;41(2):133–40.

[30] Gutberlet M, Noeske R, Schwinge K, et al. Comprehensive cardiac magnetic resonance imaging at 3.0 Tesla: feasibility and implications for clinical applications. Invest Radiol 2006;41(2): 154–67.

[31] Fonseca CG, et al. Cardiac Cine MRI at 3.0T: initial experience with gadomer-17 in a swine model. Presented at the 14th Annual ISMRM meeting. Seattle, Washington, 2006.

[32] Higgins CB. MRI of heart disease. Int J Card Imaging 1987;2(4):259–65.

[33] Higgins CB, Stark D, McNamara M, et al. Multiplane magnetic resonance imaging of the heart and major vessels: studies in normal volunteers. AJR Am J Roentgenol 1984;142(4):661–7.

[34] Lieberman JM, Botti RE, Nelson AD. Magnetic resonance imaging of the heart. Radiol Clin North Am 1984;22(4):847–58.

[35] Boxerman JL, Mosher TJ, McVeigh ER, et al. Advanced MR imaging techniques for evaluation of the heart and great vessels. Radiographics 1998;18(3):543–64.

[36] Edelman RR, Chien D, Kim D. Fast selective black blood MR imaging. Radiology 1991; 181(3):655–60.

[37] Simonetti OP, Finn JP, White RD, et al. "Black blood" T2-weighted inversion-recovery MR imaging of the heart. Radiology 1996;199(1): 49–57.

[38] Bluemke DA, Krupinski EA, Ovitt T, et al. MR Imaging of arrhythmogenic right ventricular cardiomyopathy: morphologic findings and interobserver reliability. Cardiology 2003;99(3): 153–62.

[39] Bomma C, et al. Misdiagnosis of arrhythmogenic right ventricular dysplasia/cardiomyopathy. J Cardiovasc Electrophysiol 2004;15(3):300–6.

[40] Busse RF. Reduced RF power without blurring: correcting for modulation of refocusing flip angle in FSE sequences. Magn Reson Med 2004; 51(5):1031–7.

[41] Sodickson DK, Hardy CJ, Zhu Y, et al. Rapid volumetric MRI using parallel imaging with order-of-magnitude accelerations and a 32-element RF coil array: feasibility and implications. Acad Radiol 2005;12(5):626–35.

[42] Zhu Y, Hardy CJ, Sodickson DK, et al. Highly parallel volumetric imaging with a 32-element RF coil array. Magn Reson Med 2004;52(4): 869–77.

[43] Glover GH, Pelc NJ. A rapid-gated cine MRI technique. Magn Reson Annu 1988;299–333.

[44] Sechtem U, Pflugfelder PW, Cassidy MM, et al. Mitral or aortic regurgitation: quantification of regurgitant volumes with cine MR imaging. Radiology 1988;167(2):425–30.

[45] Carr JC, Simonetti O, Bundy J, et al. Cine MR angiography of the heart with segmented true fast imaging with steady-state precession. Radiology 2001;219(3):828–34.

[46] Miller S, Simonetti OP, Carr J, Kramer U, Finn JP. MR Imaging of the heart with cine true fast

imaging with steady-state precession: influence of spatial and temporal resolutions on left ventricular functional parameters. Radiology 2002; 223(1):263–9.

[47] Noeske R, Seifert F, Rhein KH, Rinneberg H. Human cardiac imaging at 3 T using phased array coils. Magn Reson Med 2000;44(6):978–82.

[48] Deshpande VS, Chung YC, Zhang Q, Shea SM, Li D. Reduction of transient signal oscillations in true-FISP using a linear flip angle series magnetization preparation. Magn Reson Med 2003; 49(1):151–7.

[49] Atalay MK, Poncelet BP, Kantor HL, Brady TJ, Weisskoff RM. Cardiac susceptibility artifacts arising from the heart-lung interface. Magn Reson Med 2001;45(2):341–5.

[50] Zerhouni EA, Parish DM, Rogers WJ, Yang A, Shapiro EP. Human heart tagging with MR imaging–a method for noninvasive assessment of myocardial motion. Radiology 1988;169(1): 59–63.

[51] Kramer U, Deshpande V, Fenchel M, et al. [Cardiac MR tagging: optimization of sequence parameters and comparison at 1.5 T and 3.0 T in a volunteer study]. Rofo 2006;178(5):515–24.

[52] Atkinson DJ, Burstein D, Edelman RR. First-pass cardiac perfusion: evaluation with ultrafast MR imaging. Radiology 1990;174(3 Pt 1): 757–62.

[53] Burstein D, Taratuta E, Manning WJ. Factors in myocardial "perfusion" imaging with ultrafast MRI and Gd-DTPA administration. Magn Reson Med 1991;20(2):299–305.

[54] Slavin GS, Wolff SD, Gupta SN, Foo TK. First-pass myocardial perfusion MR imaging with interleaved notched saturation: feasibility study. Radiology 2001;219(1):258–63.

[55] Al-Saadi N, Nagel E, Gross M, et al. Noninvasive detection of myocardial ischemia from perfusion reserve based on cardiovascular magnetic resonance. Circulation 2000;101(12):1379–83.

[56] Chiu CW, So NM, Lam WW, et al. Combined first-pass perfusion and viability study at MR imaging in patients with non-ST segment-elevation acute coronary syndromes: feasibility study. Radiology 2003;226(3):717–22.

[57] Di Bella EV, Parker DL, Sinusas AJ. On the dark rim artifact in dynamic contrast-enhanced MRI myocardial perfusion studies. Magn Reson Med 2005;54(5):1295–9.

[58] Dale BM, Jesberger JA, Lewin JS, et al. Determining and optimizing the precision of quantitative measurements of perfusion from dynamic contrast enhanced MRI. J Magn Reson Imaging 2003;18(5):575–84.

[59] Jerosch-Herold M, Swingen C, Seethamraju RT. Myocardial blood flow quantification with MRI by model-independent deconvolution. Med Phys 2002;29(5):886–97.

[60] Araoz PA, Glockner JF, McGee KP, et al. 3 Tesla MR imaging provides improved contrast in first-pass myocardial perfusion imaging over a range of gadolinium doses. J Cardiovasc Magn Reson 2005;7(3):559–64.

[61] Kim D, Axel L. Multislice, dual-imaging sequence for increasing the dynamic range of the contrast-enhanced blood signal and CNR of myocardial enhancement at 3T. J Magn Reson Imaging 2006;23(1):81–6.

[62] Kim RJ, Wu E, Rafael A, et al. The use of contrast-enhanced magnetic resonance imaging to identify reversible myocardial dysfunction. N Engl J Med 2000;343(20):1445–53.

[63] Klein C, Nekolla SG, Bengel FM, et al. Assessment of myocardial viability with contrast-enhanced magnetic resonance imaging: comparison with positron emission tomography. Circulation 2002;105(2):162–7.

[64] Wagner A, Mahrholdt H, Holly TA, et al. Contrast-enhanced MRI and routine single photon emission computed tomography (SPECT) perfusion imaging for detection of subendocardial myocardial infarcts: an imaging study. Lancet 2003;361(9355):374–9.

[65] Simonetti OP, Kim RJ, Fieno DS, et al. An improved MR imaging technique for the visualization of myocardial infarction. Radiology 2001; 218(1):215–23.

[66] Shea SM, Deshpande VS, Chung YC, et al. Three-dimensional true-FISP imaging of the coronary arteries: improved contrast with T2-preparation. J Magn Reson Imaging 2002;15(5):597–602.

[67] Scheffler K, Hennig J. T(1) quantification with inversion recovery TrueFISP. Magn Reson Med 2001;45(4):720–3.

[68] Kellman P, Arai AE, McVeigh ER, et al. Phase-sensitive inversion recovery for detecting myocardial infarction using gadolinium-delayed hyperenhancement. Magn Reson Med 2002;47(2): 372–83.

[69] Deshpande VS, Shea SM, Laub G, et al. 3D magnetization-prepared true-FISP: a new technique for imaging coronary arteries. Magn Reson Med 2001;46(3):494–502.

[70] Niendorf T, Hardy CJ, Giaquinto RO, et al. Toward single breath-hold whole-heart coverage coronary MRA using highly accelerated parallel imaging with a 32-channel MR system. Magn Reson Med 2006;56(1):167–76.

[71] Bi X, Deshpande V, Simonetti O, et al. Three-dimensional breathhold SSFP coronary MRA: a comparison between 1.5T and 3.0T. J Magn Reson Imaging 2005;22(2):206–12.

[72] Huber ME, Kozerke S, Pruessmann KP, et al. Sensitivity-encoded coronary MRA at 3T. Magn Reson Med 2004;52(2):221–7.

[73] Weber OM, Martin AJ, Higgins CB. Whole-heart steady-state free precession coronary artery magnetic resonance angiography. Magn Reson Med 2003;50(6):1223–8.

[74] Weber OM, Martin AJ, Higgins CB. Whole-heart steady-state free precession coronary artery magnetic resonance angiography. Magn Reson Med 2003;50(6):1223–8.

MAGNETIC
RESONANCE
IMAGING CLINICS

ELSEVIER
SAUNDERS

Magn Reson Imaging Clin N Am 15 (2007) 301–314

Abdominal and Pelvic MR Angiography

Henrik J. Michaely, MD[a,b,*], Ulrike I. Attenberger, MD[b],
Harald Kramer, MD[b], Kambiz Nael, MD[c], Maximilian F. Reiser, MD[b],
Stefan O. Schoenberg, MD[a,b]

- Imaging protocol for abdominal MR angiography
- Contrast agents for abdominal MR angiography
- Clinical application
- Future developments
- Summary
- References

Magnetic resonance angiography (MRA) of the abdominal and pelvic vessels has evolved into the diagnostic modality of choice for various clinical indications ranging from suspected aortic dissection over portal vein diseases to renovascular diseases [1,2]. Imaging of the renal arteries in hypertensive patients to rule out renal artery stenosis is by far the most common indication for abdominal MRA followed by diseases of the aorta and diseases of the mesenteric vessels (Figs. 1 and 2). MRA of the abdominal vessels is also performed as parts of peripheral run-off studies and part of whole-body MRA in patients with diabetes or generalized atherosclerosis (Fig. 3) [3].

The beauty of MRA lies in the combination of three-dimensional noninvasive imaging with CL257administration of only small amounts of well-tolerated contrast agents. With current 1.5T MR-scanners, the optimally achievable acquired spatial resolution is 1 mm [3] voxel size acquired in approximately 25 to 30 seconds [3]. However, compared with the inplane spatial resolution of 0.3 mm [2] of digital subtraction angiography (DSA), the spatial resolution of MRA is inferior [4]. From previous theoretical calculations of the required spatial resolution of MRA it was concluded that at least three pixels should constitute the luminal diameter [5], which implies an acquired spatial resolution of at least 1.5 mm for the proximal renal arteries. According to these calculations, a higher spatial resolution would be required for the distal renal arteries. Equally important for the depiction of smaller vessels such as the distal renal arteries is to acquire the MRA data sufficiently fast to avoid motion artifacts and image blurring. Vasbinder and colleagues [6] addressed the issue of distal renal artery motion during breath-hold MRA. They found that the distal parts of the renal vessels are always subject to random diaphragmatic motion even during breathhold. This was underlined by an interobserver study using two different factors of parallel imaging for renal MRA. The group with the higher parallel imaging acceleration factor and hence with

This work was supported in part by the Verein MagnetresonanzForschung e.V.
[a] Institute of Clinical Radiology, University Hospital Mannheim, Medical Faculty Mannheim–University of Heidelberg, Theodor-Kutzer-Ufer 1-3, 68167 Mannheim, Germany
[b] Institute of Clinical Radiology, University of Munich–Grosshadern Campus, Munich, Germany
[c] Department of Cardiovascular Radiology, University of California, Los Angeles, CA, USA
* Corresponding author. Institute of Clinical Radiology, University Hospital Mannheim, Medical Faculty Mann-heim, University of Heidelberg, Theodor-Kutzer-Ufer 1-3, 68167 Mannheim, Germany.
E-mail address: henrik.michaely@rad.ma.uni-heidelberg.de (H.J. Michaely).

1064-9689/07/$ – see front matter © 2007 Elsevier Inc. All rights reserved.
mri.theclinics.com

doi:10.1016/j.mric.2007.06.001

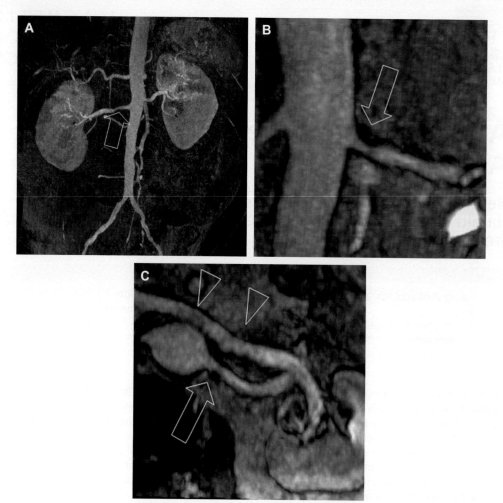

Fig. 1. (*A*) 30-mm thin maximum intensity projection (MIP) of a 3T renal MRA exam demonstrating a intermediate RAS of the right renal artery (*arrow*) with poststenotic dilatation. (*B*) A 10-mm thin coronal MIP acquired at 3T during the steady state after gadofosvest injection. An intermediate-grade renal artery stenosis is visible (*arrow*). (*C*) In the 10-mm thin axial MIP of the same patient, the stenotic segment can be clearly demonstrated (*arrow*). The venous enhancement (*arrowheads*) is not disturbing.

the faster MRA acquisition showed significantly better image quality of the distal parts of the renal arteries than the group with the longer lasting MRA acquisition [7]. In addition, the use of isotropic voxels is a third requirement for high-quality MRA. Isotropic voxels allow for lossless reformats, which is important in assessing complex vascular structures such as bypasses or normal anatomic variants. Isotropic voxels are also a prerequisite to assess the area stenosis in the cross-sectional view instead of assessing the degree of stenosis in the diameter view. This approach was found to be more accurate than the commonly used diameter stenosis [8] and the results showed a strong correlation to intravascular ultrasound. In addition, the slab of the MRA needs to be sufficiently thick to include the entire abdominal aorta and its major branches.

A high spatial resolution, fast acquisition with sufficient volume coverage, and good image contrast are all dependent on sufficiently available signal-to-noise ratio (SNR). Because of the lower SNR at 1.5T, abdominal MRA is inherently confined to a lower spatial resolution than at 3T. Imaging at 3T provides a theoretically doubled SNR [9,10], an improved background suppression as a consequence of the prolonged T1-times of most tissues [9,11], and an increased contrast agent effectiveness [12]. Therefore 3T imaging is proclaimed as the "field strength of choice" for MRA by many authors.

Imaging protocol for abdominal MR angiography

Abdominal and pelvic MRA should be embedded in a comprehensive imaging protocol consisting

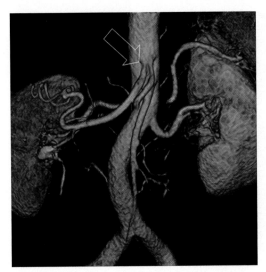

Fig. 2. A 30-mm thin coronal volume-rendered image acquired at 3T demonstrating a separate origin of the hepatic artery from the aorta (*arrow*). The high spatial resolution of this MRA acquisition facilitates exact demarcation of the different vessels.

of localizers, morphologic sequences, and the MRA. The MRA sequence should be acquired at least three times: one sequence before the administration of the contrast agent bolus, an arterial-dominant phase, and a venous-portal phase. An additional third phase post–contrast administration can be of value when a venous pathology is the main focus of the examination (Fig. 4). Additional functional measurements such as phase-contrast flow measurements of the renal arteries [13] or dynamic contrast-enhanced renal perfusion measurements [14] increase the diagnostic accuracy and the diagnostic level of confidence. They are of particular value in patients with stents in whom an in-stent re-stenosis cannot be excluded on morphologic images because of susceptibility artifacts, particularly as the susceptibility artifacts are more pronounced at 3T [15]. In the case of abdominal MRA, the slab should cover the entire abdominal aorta from the diaphragm down to the external iliac arteries. This is of concern as aberrant renal vessels may branch off from the entire aorta and from the iliac arteries. The slab thickness should include the vessels of interest and is usually between 8 and 15 cm thick depending on the selected partition thickness and the number of partitions. A coronal slice orientation is normally preferred as the celiac axis and its branches, the superior and inferior mesenteric arteries, the renal arteries, the entire aorta, and the iliac vessels can be imaged. A sagittal slab can be chosen if the exam is focused on the aorta (Fig. 5). Choosing a sagittal slab orientation allows

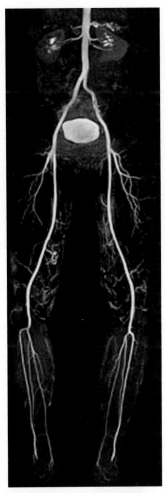

Fig. 3. Fused MIP image of a peripheral run-off study at 3T. Because of the moving table technique, the spatial resolution of this run-off study ($1.2 \times 1.2 \times 1.2$ mm^3) is slightly inferior to that of a dedicated renal MRA exam ($0.9 \times 0.8 \times 0.9$ mm^3). An accessory left renal artery can be appreciated.

for a smaller field of view with the consequence of a higher spatial resolution. With a coronal slab, a phase (left $\rightarrow$ right phase-encoding) field of view between 380 mm and 500 mm has to be chosen to avoid aliasing. If a short imaging protocol is used, the patient can be positioned with his or her arms over the head to minimize the phase field of view. Compared with 1.5T, the specific parameters of repetition time (TR), echo time (TE), flip angle, and bandwidth (BW) need to be adopted specifically to optimize the image acquisition and quality at 3T. As the T1-times of the blood are minimized during the first pass of the contrast agent, the TR should be chosen as small as possible for a heavily T1-weighted image with little background signal. At 3T the readout BW can be increased by 40% to

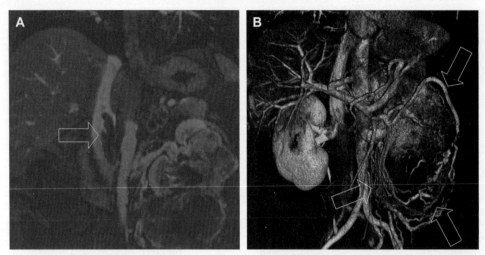

Fig. 4. (*A*) Coronal source image of the venous phase of a 3T MRA demonstrating a left renal tumor with invasion into the renal pelvis and with tumor thrombus in the inferior vena cava (*arrow*). (*B*) In the volume-rendered view of the same venous phase, multiple feeding tumor vessels become apparent (*arrows*).

100% to minimize the TR without deteriorating image quality substantially [16]. Typically a TR of 3.0 ms to 3.5 ms can be achieved. However, short TRs may lead to a potential overstimulation of peripheral nerves so that the inbuilt stimulation monitor may automatically increase the TR to a noncritical level. As the susceptibility increases with the square of the field strength, it is prudent to minimize the TE as well. At 3T, fat and water protons are in-phase at 2.2 ms and 4.4 ms and out-of-phase at 1.1 ms and 3.3 ms. Therefore, with the typically used TE of 1 ms to 1.4 ms more chemical shift artifacts along the vessel border can be seen at 3T than at 1.5T. Whether this particular characteristic of 3T imaging is interfering with image interpretation remains unclear at this time. The increased chemical

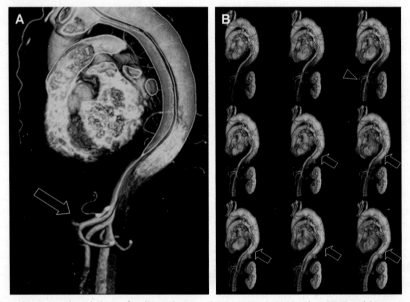

Fig. 5. (*A*) Thin volume-rendered view of a dissecting aortic aneurysm acquired at 3T. For this exam a sagittal slab with 1-mm isotropic resolution and parallel imaging acceleration factor 3 was chosen for a total acquisiton time of 20 seconds. The main abdominal branches of the aorta originate from the true, thin lumen. (*B*) In the time-resolved MRA of the same patient there is still remaining contrast agent in the false lumen. Again, the early enhancment of the main abdominal branches is seen (*arrowhead*), while the false, large lumen enhances very slowly (*arrows*).

shift artifacts may however increase the background suppression. Fast gradient-echo sequences as used for MRA will lead to a better background suppression at 3T as the longitudinal relaxation is slower because of the increased T1 times at higher field strengths [11]. The kidney and liver, for example, reveal 9% to 38% higher T1-relaxation times while the T1-relaxation time of subcutaneous fat is increased by 11% [11]. Probably the most important parameter in MRA at 3T is the parallel imaging (PI) acceleration factor. PI techniques such as GRAPPA [17] and SENSE [18] allow for increased spatial resolution or shortened scan time. Currently at 1.5T, parallel imaging technique (PAT) factors of 2 or rarely 3 are being used [3,8]. Further increasing the PAT factors—and hence increasing the spatial resolution—is ultimately limited by SNR as the SNR is inversely proportional to the square root of the PI acceleration factor. At 3T, parallel imaging acceleration factors of 3 or higher are feasible [16]. PAT factors greater than 3 are particularly applicable when parallel acceleration is chosen for the phase-encoding and the partition-encoding direction [19]. In the case of two-dimensional PI, the acceleration factors in phase-encoding and partition-encoding direction have to be multiplied to yield the overall acceleration factor. Two-dimensional PI with higher PAT factors is superior to PAT in one direction as the coil sensitivity profiles can be differentiated better over an entire three-dimensional volume leading to reconstruction artifacts. Studies on the image quality of abdominal vessels report a better image quality with PI [7,20]. So, overall, abdominal MRA at 3T profits strongly from PI with acceleration factors of 3 to 4 while the SNR/contrast to noise ratio (CNR) is still sufficient.

PI is also a suitable technique for minimizing the energy deposition in the patient who is strictly limited. While the SNR is approximately doubled at 3T, the specific absorption rate (SAR) is increased by a factor of four with the transition from 1.5T to 3T [9]. Therefore, there is a strong need to minimize the number of applied radiofrequency pulses and to minimize the flip angle to stay within the SAR limit. Theoretically, a PAT factor of 4 compensates for the increase in SAR at 3T. However in practice, limiting factors such as insufficient coil design may disprove the above equation.

Contrast agents for abdominal MR angiography

At 1.5T, MRA exams are typically performed after the bolus injection of 0.2 mmol/kg body weight or even 0.3 mmol/kg body weight of standard extracellular contrast agents (Gd-DTPA, Mangevist, Bayer Schering Pharma, Berlin, Germany; Gadodiamide,

Omniscan, GE Healthcare, Little Chalfort, UK; Gd-DOTA, Dotarem, Guerbet, Paris, France; or Gadoteridol, Prohance, Bracco, Milan, Italy). Because of the longer acquisition times of MRA sequences at 1.5T, an injection rate of 1.5 to 2.0 mL/s is typically chosen. With a decreasing voxel size, higher factors of parallel imaging, and hence a decreasing SNR, the use of dedicated contrast agents for state-of-the-art MRA seems useful. In Europe three "high-end" contrast agents are commercially available. They are either characterized by a 1-molar formulation (gadobutrol, Gadovist, Bayer Schering Pharma), a slight protein interaction with a 20% to 30% higher relaxivity than standard extracellular contrast agents (Gd-BOPTA, Multihance, Bracco) or a strong protein binding (gadofosveset [formerly MS-325], Vasovist, Bayer Schering Pharma), which reveals an up to fourfold higher relaxivity than standard extracellular contrast agents (Fig. 6) [12]. Despite their different pharmacokinetic properties, they are all suitable agents for MRA as they provide better enhancement than standard extracellular contrast agents [21–26]. The increased CNR that can be seen with these substances is thought to be caused by the better bolus geometry in case of the 1-molar agent and because of the higher relaxivity during the first pass in the case of protein-binding agents. In addition, gadofosveset allows for an extended imaging window of up to 1 hour postinjection [27]. It can be used for first-pass MRA like a conventional extracellular contrast agent and allows for repetitious MRA exams in the steady state. One possible application is to acquire the first-pass MRA as a time-resolved study to display the blood flow hemodynamics and to measure the renal perfusion. In the high-resolution steady state exam the renal arteries can then be examined with high spatial resolution (Fig. 7). Other potential applications comprise venous imaging with high SNR or extended anatomic coverage with MRA of other vascular territories during the steady state.

As the relaxivity of most contrast agents is decreased by less than 20% with the transition from 1.5T to 3T (eg, gadobutrol from $R1 = 5.2$ L mmol^{-1} s^{-1} at 1.5T to $R1 = 5.0$ L mmol^{-1} s^{-1} at 3T; Gd-DTPA from $R1 = 4.1$ L mmol^{-1} s^{-1} at 1.5T to $R1 = 3.7$ L mmol^{-1} s^{-1} at 3T) the relative contrast agent efficacy is increased at 3T. Recent studies therefore report an unchanged or even improved image quality of 3T MRA with reduced administered amount of contrast agent (Fig. 8) [28–30]. Depending on the study design, the amount of contrast agent was reduced by 25% to 50% to an overall dose of 0.1 mmol/kg body weight. Reduction of the administered amount of contrast agent is economically desirable, but particularly in patients with suspected renal disease it is of value from a safety point

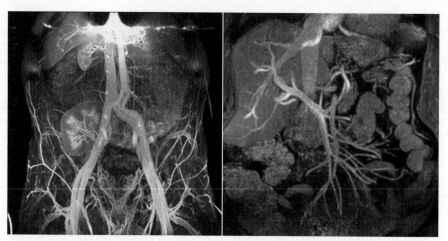

Fig. 6. Steady-state images acquired at 3T 15 minutes after the injection of gadofosvest. The lobar and segmental branches of the transplant renal artery are equally well enhanced as the portal-venous system.

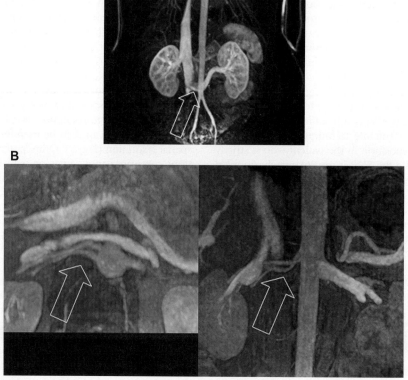

Fig. 7. (*A*) A 30-mm thin MIP of a single frame of a time-resolved echo-shared angiographic technique (TREAT) sequence after the bolus injection of 0.03 mmol/kg BW gadofosvest demonstrating an aberrant course of the left renal vein (*arrow*). (*B*) Ten-mm thin coronal and transverse MIPs of a different patient acquired in the steady state with submillimeter high–spatial resolution at 3T clearly show two right renal arteries (*arrows*).

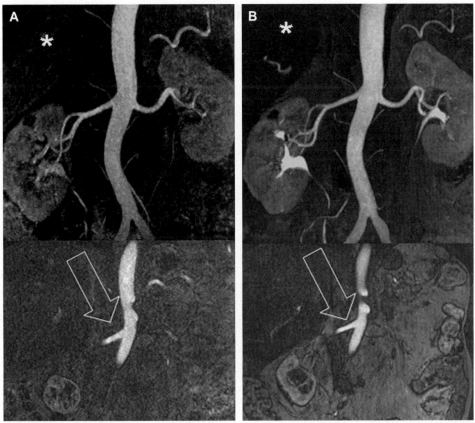

Fig. 8. (*A*) A 30-mm thin MIP and source image (1.5T, 1.0 × 0.8 × 1.0 mm³) acquired after the injection of 0.2 mmol/kg gadobutrol. (*B*) A 30-mm thin MIP and source image (3T, 0.9 × 0.8 × 0.9 mm³) of the same patient acquired after the injection of 0.1 mmol/kg Gd-BOPTA. Even with a bissected amount of gadolinium at 3T the image quality and the depiction of the (distal) renal arteries (*arrows*) seems superior at 3T. Note the reduced background noise (*star*).

of view. Patients with heavily decreased renal function (glomerular filtration rate < 30 mL/min/ 1.72 m²) are at particular risk for developing neph- rogenic systemic fibrosis (NSF), a rare but poten- tially deadly disease that seems to be linked to the prior administration of certain Gd-chelates [31]. At this time (April 2007), proven cases of NSF have only been reported with gadodiamide, which ac- counts for most cases, and with Gd-DTPA, which ac- counts for a smaller portion of cases. Particularly higher doses (0.2 mmol/kg of body weight (BW) and higher) of gadodiamide in patients with chronic renal failure and with previous proinflammatory events seem to increase the relative risk of develop- ing NSF significantly [32,33]. If a contrast-enhanced MRA is clinically warranted in high-risk patients it seems appropriate to perform the exam with a mini- mal dose of contrast agents. Imaging at 3T with a 0.1-M dose of contrast agents is one potential solu- tion where a good spatial resolution and SNR can be achieved with a minimal amount of contrast

agent only [29]. One future solution could be the use of ultra small particles of iron oxide contrast agents such as SHU 555C (Bayer Schering Pharma). These agents are suitable for MRA and also allow for a long imaging window of several hours as they are cleared of the blood slowly. In contrast to Gd-based paramagnetic agents, their relaxivity seems to be less affected by higher field strengths. However, none of these agents has been approved for patient use in the United States, Europe, or Japan.

Clinical application

Renal artery stenosis (RAS) is the most common cause of secondary hypertension [34,35] with a prevalence of approximately 4% in Western coun- tries [36]. The prevalence of atherosclerotic RAS in- creases with age and concomitant diseases such as hypertension, diabetes mellitus, or coronary artery disease and can reach 47% [37–41]. RAS will lead to ischemic nephropathy with subsequent end-stage renal disease (ESRD) [34] if not detected and treated properly. RAS is estimated to account for 10% to 40% of ESRD [42] in patients without identified primary renal disease such as glomerulo-nephritis or autosomal dominant polycystic kidney disease. Among all patients with RAS, atherosclerotic RAS can be found in 90% of patients with RAS while fibromuscular dysplasia (FMD) accounts for the remaining 10% of cases [34,41,43]. FMD mainly affects younger female patients, whereas atherosclerotic RAS is a disease of elderly patients.

Detection and characterization of RAS is problematic in two ways. First, there is a considerable overlap of different renal disease complexes including atherosclerotic vascular disease, primary hypertension, and renal parenchymal disease [34]. Secondary hypertension may be the consequence of renal artery stenosis but in a patient with concomitant renoparenchymal disease the initial reason for the hypertension often cannot be determined based on morphologic imaging only. Second, the accuracy of the currently used diagnostic tests varies significantly. Ultrasound is heavily user-dependent and the reported studies on MRA are nonconclusive. Initial studies and meta-studies on the accuracy of detecting and grading RAS with MRA were extremely positive [44–47], while a more recent meta-study found a sensitivity/specificity of only 62%/84% for the correct grading of RAS with MRA [48]. The poor results of this meta-study can be contributed to several factors. In contrast to the positive initial studies, a retrospective approach was chosen and also patients suffering from FMD were included. Because of subtle changes and the distal location of the FMD lesions, they may have been missed on the 1.5T and 1.0-T MRA exams with relatively low spatial resolution.

3T MRA offers several advantages that are beneficial for imaging the renal arteries and for differentiating between renovascular and renoparenchymal disease. As explained above, the higher SNR at 3T can be directly translated into a higher spatial resolution and shorter acquisition times, which are two prerequisites for successful depiction of FMD and distal RAS (Fig. 9) [16]. This has also been confirmed by initial clinical studies with correlation to invasive angiography [49]; however, studies with a larger number of patients have not been published at this time. Functional imaging studies such as first-pass renal perfusion studies and blood-oxygen level dependent imaging (BOLD), which can be helpful in differentiating renovascular disease from renoparenchymal disease, also directly benefit from the higher field strengths [50,51]. Imaging with high spatial resolution and isotropic voxels, which is facilitated by the higher SNR at 3T, is a prerequisite for lossless postprocessing including the calculation of curved multiplanar reformats and cross-sectional views such as the determination of the area stenosis. The area stenosis correlates better with DSA than the diameter stenosis [8] and leads to a better interobserver agreement,

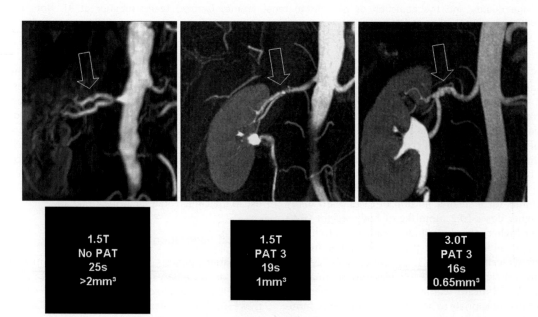

Fig. 9. Thin MIPs of three different patients with proven FMD. At 1.5T the changes are not visible or can only be barely seen. At 3T the typical string of bead appearance can be seen. The boxes below the MIP images represent the decreasing voxel size with the key parameters field strength, parallel imaging techniques (PAT), voxel size, and acquistion time. (*Left MIP image courtesy of* Martin Prince, New York, NY.)

which is particularly pronounced for intermediate-grade RAS (Fig. 10). In previous studies, high-grade stenoses and occlusions were almost always correctly graded while intermediate-grade stenoses were always a source of error. Apart from the detection of FMD and the correct grading of RAS, high spatial resolution is mandatory in the evaluation of potential living kidney donors. To avoid transplant dysfunction, all renal arteries—including small accessory arteries often supplying the uretero-pelvic junction—have to be displayed to be included in the transplantation. As accessory arteries may originate from the entire aorta or the iliac arteries, a large field of view is indicated in patients who are evaluated as potential living kidney donors. In these patients, multiphasic exams are of particular interest as the venous anatomy has to be reported equally well. Intravascular contrast agents or those with a slight protein interaction do better at this (Fig. 7). Also in patients post–renal transplant and with suspected graft dysfunction, multiphasic MRA exams are indicated to rule out renal artery stenosis, renal vein thrombosis, and iliac artery dissection of aneurysm, which are common complications of the perioperative time (Fig. 11) [52].

Imaging of the aorta can be performed in a similar way to renal imaging with a sagittal orientation of the imaging volume rather than coronal. In patients with suspected dissection or occlusion of the abdominal aorta, multiphasic or time-resolved MRA exams should be added to the examination

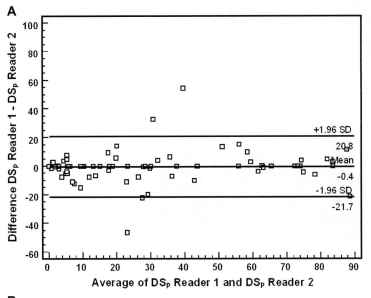

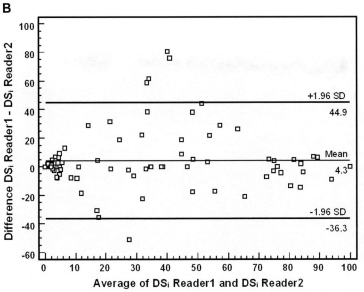

Fig. 10. These Bland-Altman plots demonstrate the improvement in interobserver agreement for the grading of renal artery stenoses if the area stenosis is used (*B*) instead of the diameter stenosis (*A*). (*Reprinted from* Schoenberg SO, Rieger J, Weber CH, et al. High-spatial-resolution MR angiography of renal arteries with integrated parallel acquisitions: comparison with digital subtraction angiography and US. Radiology 2005; 235:687; with permission.)

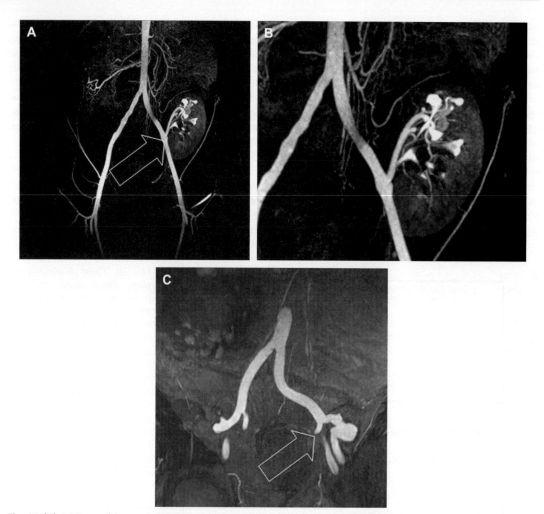

Fig. 11. (*A*) A 30-mm thin coronal MIP image acquired at 3T with submillimeter spatial resolution (0.9 × 0.8 × 0.9 mm^3) after the injection of 0.1 mmol/kg Gd-chelates in a patient with suspected renal transplant artery stenosis (*arrow*). (*B*) The close-up view of the renal artery demonstrates a homogeneously enhanced vessel with nonsuspicous lobar branches. No vascular pathology could be observed. (*C*) A 30-mm thin oblique MIP (3T, submilimeter spatial resolution, 0.1 mmol/kg Gd-chelates) demonstrating a postoperative aneurysm of the left external iliac artery (*arrow*).

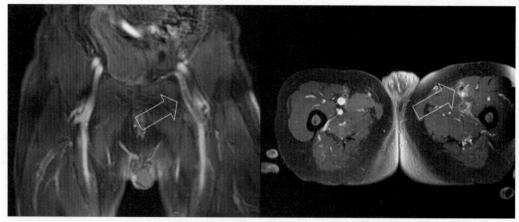

Fig. 12. Coronal and transverse source images acquried at 3T during the steady state after the injection of gadofosvest demonstrating a thrombosis of the left superficial femoral artery (*arrows*).

protocol [53]. This allows for characterization of the blood flow in the true and false lumen and assessment of the perfusion of the kidneys. Initial studies on the detection of endoleaks favored the application of intravascular contrast agents with delayed images on which a slow blood flow into the aneurysm could be demonstrated [54].

With the introduction of the new intravascular contrast agent, gadofosveset, venous imaging has been largely facilitated. Venous studies can now be easily acquired in the steady state after the injection of gadofosveset without compromises in image quality (Fig. 12) [55]. If the intravascular contrast agent is not available, contrast agents with slight protein interaction such as Gd-BOPTA or higher concentration like gadobutrol can serve as suitable alternative. The imaging window is however limited so that the acquisition of the venous MRA should take place immediately after the arterial phase (Fig. 4).

Future developments

MRA has always been a driving force behind the development of MR techniques. New technical innovations on the horizon of MRA are already in sight and have been used in initial studies. Among the very promising techniques is the so-called off-resonance contrast angiography (ORCA) [56]. ORCA contrast depends not on T1 but on

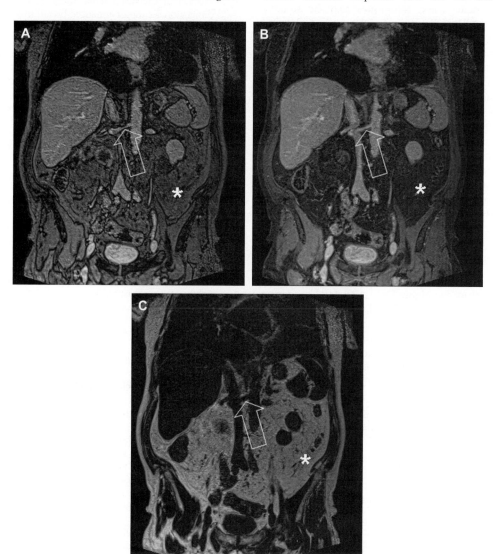

Fig. 13. View of 1.2-mm thin source images of 3T steady state MRA with Dixon fat suppression demonstrating the in-phase reconstruction (*A*), the water-only reconstruction (*B*), and the fat-only reconstruction (*C*). The right renal artery (*arrow*) can be best visualized on the water-only reconstruction where the fat signal is completely eliminated (*star*). In the fat-only image the vessels cannot be evaluated.

Gd-induced shifts in intravascular resonance frequency because of the bulk magnetic susceptibility effects of Gadolinium and seems to provide good background suppression without image subtraction. Edelman and colleagues [57] also presented the idea of a scoutless abdominal MRA exam based on nonselective RF-excitation with two-dimensional acceleration that yielded a 30% decrease in imaging time without a significant loss in SNR. Other very promising and already commercially available techniques are the Dixon-based fat-saturation techniques, which require longer imaging times of reconstruction of fat-only and water-only images [58,59]. Particularly for intravascular contrast agents with sufficient imaging time in the steady state, these techniques may be suitable (Fig. 13). The full potential of the intravascular contrast agent that has been commercially available in Europe since April 2006 has not been tapped so far. Dedicated MRA sequences with respiratory gating and EKG gating seem promising for imaging in the steady state as they allow extended imaging times and hence higher SNR and a higher spatial resolution. Proof-of-concept studies have already been performed in an animal model but no clinical studies have been published so far [60]. Similarly, proof-of-concept animal studies for the detection of gastrointestinal (GI) bleeding with intravascular contrast agents have been published [61] without any clinical follow-up studies in humans.

Summary

MRA of the abdominal and pelvic vessels greatly profits from the higher SNR at 3T. MRA sequences that are adapted to 3T allow for higher spatial resolution, shorter acquisition times, and reduced amount of administered contrast agent. Particularly the combination of parallel imaging and 3T is beneficial in increasing image quality and minimizing 3T-specific problems such as the increased SAR. Initial clinical studies, which were performed on a small level, show promising results for the accuracy of the detection of vascular disease. The advent of new intravascular contrast agents such as gadofosveset will additionally broaden the spectrum of potential MRA applications toward more comprehensive exams. Overall it seems that the physical benefits of 3T can be translated into an improved MRA exam.

References

[1] Leiner T. Magnetic resonance angiography of abdominal and lower extremity vasculature. Top Magn Reson Imaging 2005;16:21–66.

[2] Schoenberg SO, Rieger J, Nittka M, et al. Renal MR angiography: current debates and developments in imaging of renal artery stenosis. Semin Ultrasound CT MR 2003;24:255–67.

[3] Michaely HJ, Dietrich O, Nael K, et al. MRA of abdominal vessels: technical advances. Eur Radiol 2006;16:1637–50.

[4] Vosshenrich R, Fischer U. Contrast-enhanced MR angiography of abdominal vessels: is there still a role for angiography? Eur Radiol 2002;12:218–30.

[5] Hoogeveen RM, Bakker CJ, Viergever MA. Limits to the accuracy of vessel diameter measurement in MR angiography. J Magn Reson Imaging 1998;8:1228–35.

[6] Vasbinder GBC, Maki JH, Nijenhuis RJ, et al. Motion of the distal renal artery during three-dimensional contrast-enhanced breath-hold MRA. J Magn Reson Imaging 2002;16:685–96.

[7] Michaely HJ, Herrmann KA, Kramer H, et al. High-resolution renal MRA: comparison of image quality and vessel depiction with different parallel imaging acceleration factors. J Magn Reson Imaging 2006;24:95–100.

[8] Schoenberg SO, Rieger J, Weber CH, et al. High-spatial-resolution MR angiography of renal arteries with integrated parallel acquisitions: comparison with digital subtraction angiography and US. Radiology 2005;235:687–98.

[9] Campeau NG, Huston J 3rd, Bernstein MA, et al. Magnetic resonance angiography at 3.0 Tesla: initial clinical experience. Top Magn Reson Imaging 2001;12:183–204.

[10] Merkle EM, Dale BM, Paulson EK. Abdominal MR imaging at 3T. Magn Reson Imaging Clin N Am 2006;14:17–26.

[11] de Bazelaire CM, Duhamel GD, Rofsky NM, et al. MR imaging relaxation times of abdominal and pelvic tissues measured in vivo at 3.0 T: preliminary results. Radiology 2004;230:652–9.

[12] Rohrer M, Bauer H, Mintorovitch J, et al. Comparison of magnetic properties of MRI contrast media solutions at different magnetic field strengths. Invest Radiol 2005;40:715–24.

[13] Schoenberg SO, Knopp MV, Londy F, et al. Morphologic and functional magnetic resonance imaging of renal artery stenosis: a multireader tricenter study. J Am Soc Nephrol 2002;13:158–69.

[14] Michaely HJ, Schoenberg SO, Oesingmann N, et al. Renal artery stenosis: functional assessment with dynamic mr perfusion measurements–feasibility study. Radiology 2006;238:586–96.

[15] Merkle EM, Dale BM. Abdominal MRI at 3.0 T: the basics revisited. AJR Am J Roentgenol 2006;186:1524–32.

[16] Michaely HJ, Nael K, Schoenberg SO, et al. The feasibility of spatial high-resolution magnetic resonance angiography (MRA) of the renal arteries at 3.0 T. Rofo 2005;177:800–4.

[17] Griswold MA, Jakob PM, Heidemann RM, et al. Generalized autocalibrating partially parallel

acquisitions (GRAPPA). Magn Reson Med 2002; 47:1202–10.

[18] Pruessmann KP, Weiger M, Scheidegger MB, et al. SENSE: sensitivity encoding for fast MRI. Magn Reson Med 1999;42:952–62.

[19] Fenchel M, Nael K, Deshpande VS, et al. Renal magnetic resonance angiography at 3.0 Tesla using a 32-element phased-array coil system and parallel imaging in 2 directions. Invest Radiol 2006;41:697–703.

[20] Ho LM, Merkle EM, Paulson EK, et al. Contrast-enhanced hepatic magnetic resonance angiography at 3 T: does parallel imaging improve image quality? J Comput Assist Tomogr 2007;31: 177–80.

[21] Huppertz A, Rohrer M. Gadobutrol, a highly concentrated MR-imaging contrast agent: its physicochemical characteristics and the basis for its use in contrast-enhanced MR angiography and perfusion imaging. Eur Radiol 2004; 14(Suppl 5):M12–8.

[22] Tombach B, Heindel W. Value of 1.0-M gadolinium chelates: review of preclinical and clinical data on gadobutrol. Eur Radiol 2002;12: 1550–6.

[23] Goyen M, Herborn CU, Vogt FM, et al. Using a 1 M Gd-chelate (gadobutrol) for total-body three-dimensional MR angiography: preliminary experience. J Magn Reson Imaging 2003;17: 565–71.

[24] Herborn CU, Lauenstein TC, Ruehm SG, et al. Intraindividual comparison of gadopentetate dimeglumine, gadobenate dimeglumine, and gadobutrol for pelvic 3D magnetic resonance angiography. Invest Radiol 2003;38:27–33.

[25] Wikstrom J, Wasser MN, Pattynama PM, et al. Gadobenate dimeglumine-enhanced magnetic resonance angiography of the pelvic arteries. Invest Radiol 2003;38:504–15.

[26] Goyen M, Debatin JF. Gadobenate dimeglumine (MultiHance) for magnetic resonance angiography: review of the literature. Eur Radiol 2003; 13(Suppl 3):N19–27.

[27] Goyen M, Edelman M, Perreault P, et al. MR angiography of aortoiliac occlusive disease: a phase III study of the safety and effectiveness of the blood-pool contrast agent MS-325. Radiology 2005;236:825–33.

[28] Michaely HJ, Herrmann KA, Nael K, et al. Functional renal imaging: nonvascular renal disease. Abdom Imaging 2007;32:1–16.

[29] Michaely HJ, Kramer H, Lodemann KP, et al. Renal MRA at 3.0T with 0.1 mmol/kg gadolinium—interindividual comparision to renal MRA at 1.5 T with full dose of gadolinium. Presented at the Annual Conference of the International Society for Magnetic Resonance in Medicine. Berlin (Germany), 2007.

[30] Herborn C, Watkins D, Runge V, et al. Effect of dose bisection at 3.0T on contrast-enhanced magnetic resonance angiography of the renal arteries. In Proceedings 13th Scientific Meeting,

International Society for Magnetic Resonance in Medicine. Seattle (WA);2006. p. 512.

[31] Grobner T. Gadolinium–a specific trigger for the development of nephrogenic fibrosing dermopathy and nephrogenic systemic fibrosis? Nephrol Dial Transplant 2006;21:1104–8.

[32] Sadowski EA, Bennett LK, Chan MR, et al. Nephrogenic systemic fibrosis: risk factors and incidence estimation. Radiology 2007;243:148–57.

[33] Broome DR, Girguls MS, Baron PW. Gadodlamide-associated nephrogenic systemic fibrosis: why radiologists should be concerned. AJR AM J Roontgenol 2007;188:586–92.

[34] Safian RD, Textor SC. Renal-artery stenosis. N Engl J Med 2001;344:431–42.

[35] Klatte EC, Worrell JA, Forster JH, et al. Diagnostic criteria of bilateral renovascular hypertension. Radiology 1971;101:301–4.

[36] Sawicki PT, Kaiser S, Heinemann L, et al. Prevalence of renal artery stenosis in diabetes mellitus—an autopsy study. J Intern Med 1991;229: 489–92.

[37] Rihal CS, Textor SC, Breen JF, et al. Incidental renal artery stenosis among a prospective cohort of hypertensive patients undergoing coronary angiography. Mayo Clin Proc 2002;77:309–16.

[38] Harding MB, Smith LR, Himmelstein SI, et al. Renal artery stenosis: prevalence and associated risk factors in patients undergoing routine cardiac catheterization. J Am Soc Nephrol 1992;2:608–16.

[39] Olin JW, Melia M, Young JR, et al. Prevalence of atherosclerotic renal artery stenosis in patients with atherosclerosis elsewhere. Am J Med 1990; 88:46N–51N.

[40] Wachtell K, Ibsen H, Olsen MH, et al. Prevalence of renal artery stenosis in patients with peripheral vascular disease and hypertension. J Hum Hypertens 1996;10:83–5.

[41] Textor SC. Epidemiology and clinical presentation. Semin Nephrol 2000;20:426–31.

[42] Scoble JE, Hamilton G. Atherosclerotic renovascular disease. BMJ 1990;300:1670–1.

[43] Slovut DP, Olin JW. Fibromuscular dysplasia. N Engl J Med 2004;350:1862–71.

[44] Thornton J, O'Callaghan J, Walshe J, et al. Comparison of digital subtraction angiography with gadolinium-enhanced magnetic resonance angiography in the diagnosis of renal artery stenosis. Eur Radiol 1999;9:930–4.

[45] Leung DA, Hoffmann U, Pfammatter T, et al. Magnetic resonance angiography versus duplex sonography for diagnosing renovascular disease. Hypertension 1999;33:726–31.

[46] Wasser MN, Westenberg J, van der Hulst VP, et al. Hemodynamic significance of renal artery stenosis: digital subtraction angiography versus systolically gated three-dimensional phase-contrast MR angiography. Radiology 1997;202:333.

[47] Tan KT, van Beek EJ, Brown PW, et al. Magnetic resonance angiography for the diagnosis of renal artery stenosis: a meta-analysis. Clin Radiol 2002;57:617.

[48] Vasbinder GB, Nelemans PJ, Kessels AG, et al. Accuracy of computed tomographic angiography and magnetic resonance angiography for diagnosing renal artery stenosis. Ann Intern Med 2004;141:674.

[49] Kramer U, Nael K, Laub G, et al. High-resolution magnetic resonance angiography of the renal arteries using parallel imaging acquisition techniques at 3.0 T: initial experience. Invest Radiol 2006;41:125.

[50] Li LP, Vu AT, Li BS, et al. Evaluation of intrarenal oxygenation by BOLD MRI at 3.0 T. J Magn Reson Imaging 2004;20:901.

[51] Michaely HJ, Kramer H, Oesingmann N, et al. Intraindividual comparison of MR-renal perfusion imaging at 1.5 T and 3.0 T. Invest Radiol 2007; 42:406.

[52] Michaely HJ, Schoenberg SO, Rieger JR, et al. MR angiography in patients with renal disease. Magn Reson Imaging Clin N Am 2005;13:131.

[53] Schoenberg SO, Wunsch C, Knopp MV, et al. Abdominal aortic aneurysm. Detection of multilevel vascular pathology by time-resolved multiphase 3D gadolinium MR angiography: initial report. Invest Radiol 1999;34:648.

[54] Cornelissen SA, Prokop M, Adriaensen ME, et al. Visualizing slow-flow endoleak after endovascular abdominal aortic aneurysm repair with the new blood pool agent Vasovist. In Proceedings

of the International Society for Magnetic Resonance in Medicine, Berlin (Germany).

[55] Ruehm SG. MR venography. Eur Radiol 2003;13: 229.

[56] Edelman RR, Storey P, Dunkle E, et al. Gadolinium-enhanced off-resonance contrast angiography. Magn Reson Med 2007;57:475.

[57] Edelman R, Li W, Dunkle E, et al. Scoutless abdominal angiography at 3 Tesla with two-dimensional acceleration. In Proceedings 13th Scientific Meeting, International Society for Magnetic Resonance in Medicine. Seattle (WA), p. 1930.

[58] Reeder SB, Hargreaves BA, Yu H, et al. Homodyne reconstruction and IDEAL water-fat decomposition. Magn Reson Med 2005;54:586.

[59] Reeder SB, McKenzie CA, Pineda AR, et al. Water-fat separation with IDEAL gradient-echo imaging. J Magn Reson Imaging 2007;25:644.

[60] Spuentrup E, Buecker A, Meyer J, et al. Navigator-gated free-breathing 3D balanced FFE projection renal MRA: comparison with contrast-enhanced breath-hold 3D MRA in a swine model. Magn Reson Med 2002;48:739.

[61] Hilfiker PR, Weishaupt D, Kacl GM, et al. Comparison of three dimensional magnetic resonance imaging in conjunction with a blood pool contrast agent and nuclear scintigraphy for the detection of experimentally induced gastrointestinal bleeding. Gut 1999;45:581.

ELSEVIER
SAUNDERS

MAGNETIC
RESONANCE
IMAGING CLINICS

Magn Reson Imaging Clin N Am 15 (2007) 315–320

Breast MR Imaging at 3T

Christiane K. Kuhl, MD

- Clinical role of breast MR imaging
- The temporal versus spatial dilemma of dynamic breast MR imaging
- The different technical approaches to breast MR imaging
- Why move to 3T?
- Physics effects of 3T and how they affect breast imaging
- What is the current level of evidence regarding high-field breast MR imaging?
- References

Clinical role of breast MR imaging

Breast MR imaging is evolving as the most sensitive imaging method for diagnosing invasive or preinvasive, primary and recurrent breast cancer [1,2]. It becomes increasingly clear that MR imaging, because of its higher sensitivity compared with mammography and breast ultrasound, should not be used only as a second-line imaging modality (ie, to clarify equivocal mammographic or sonographic findings), but as a primary imaging tool for screening women at increased risk for breast cancer and for staging women who have biopsy-proven cancer and who are candidates for breast-conserving surgery. Several studies investigated the diagnostic accuracy of MR imaging compared with that of mammography (and also ultrasound) for screening women at increased familial risk; all studies are concordant that MR imaging doubles or even triples the sensitivity with which familial breast cancer is identified. Regarding preoperative staging of breast cancer, a series of studies investigated the added value of MR imaging compared with mammography and ultrasound. MR imaging is the most accurate modality to depict the actual size of a breast cancer, including its intraductal component. Because breast cancer is one of the few cancer types that are usually operated on with curative intention, achieving clear, tumor-free margins is important. MR imaging is best in providing a road map for the surgeon. In addition, all published studies are concordant that MR imaging is able to detect additional mammographically and sonographically occult multicentric breast cancer (ie, breast cancers that arise in a different quadrant from the index cancer) in the same and also in the opposite breast. Last, the exceedingly high negative predictive value of MR imaging enables the radiologist to confidently exclude the presence of breast cancer, which is helpful to avoid a preventive mastectomy (a procedure many women diagnosed with breast cancer undergo for fear of recurrent or contralateral breast cancer).

In addition to providing information on cross-sectional morphology of breast tumors, MR imaging, unlike mammography or breast ultrasound, also provides functional information. This functional information indicates cancer perfusion, metabolic activity, and cellular turnover. Contrast enhancement kinetics and spectral fingerprint on 1H MR spectroscopy can be used as surrogate markers for a given cancer's biologic aggressiveness. This can be exploited in several ways: for differential diagnosis of malignant versus benign tumors, to indicate the metastatic potential of a given cancer (as another prognostic marker, in addition to more established markers, such as TNM stage, grading, receptor status, HER-2 neu status), to indicate the likelihood with which a given cancer will respond to systemic treatment (a so-called "predictive

Department of Radiology, University of Bonn, Sigmund-Freud-Str., 25, 53105 Bonn, Germany
E-mail address: kuhl@uni-bonn.de

marker"), and to monitor the actual response to systemic treatment [2].

The temporal versus spatial dilemma of dynamic breast MR imaging

Contrast-enhanced breast MR imaging is technically demanding because both breasts must be imaged repeatedly (dynamic contrast-enhanced MR imaging) within a short period of time with high spatial resolution [1]. The need for a high spatial resolution is easy to understand; diagnosis of breast cancer and its distinction from benign tumors is achieved mainly by depicting a cancer's typical morphology, margins, and internal architecture. The spicules of breast cancers are usually smaller than 1 mm in diameter, which is why a coarse spatial resolution fails to resolve these important architectural details. All other breast imaging techniques (such as mammography and ultrasound) use the highest possible spatial resolution to help identify these important features; the same should be attempted for breast MR imaging. In-plane spatial resolution should be smaller than 1 mm, better at approximately 0.5 mm. Through-plane resolution (section thickness) is less crucial; it should be less than 3 mm.

Although it is intuitively plausible that a high spatial resolution is required for breast MR imaging, the requirements regarding acquisition speed (temporal resolution) are less self-explanatory. The reason for a high acquisition speed is indeed twofold. First, early arterial phase imaging is important to attain a sufficient contrast resolution, which is as important for the analysis of morphology as is spatial resolution. Second, fast, dynamic imaging is helpful because it enables the assessment of enhancement kinetics, functional information that can be exploited as an independent diagnostic criterion in addition to tumor morphology.

Breast cancers (much less often benign tumors) exhibit only a transient enhancement, a pattern referred to as washout time course. After contrast injection, a cancer exhibits fast and strong enhancement. This early enhancement is achieved within the first 60 to 120 seconds after injection. Thereafter, a more or less rapid and more or less complete signal intensity loss occurs. This washout pattern is specific for breast cancers; if an enhancing mass exhibits this time course, it is considered suspicious for breast cancer, even if its morphology may appear benign. Accordingly, dynamic imaging, ideally with a temporal resolution of 60 seconds per acquisition (always less than 120 seconds per acquisition), is useful to help identify a washout time course as an independent predictor of malignancy.

So although the washout pattern of cancers can be considered helpful because it provides diagnostic information, it can also be considered detrimental because it is the reason for the temporal versus spatial dilemma that we face in breast MR imaging. The problem is that because of the signal intensity loss of cancers in the post-initial period, the contrast (ie, the signal intensity difference) between an enhancing cancer and the surrounding fibroglandular tissue (FGT) fades rapidly during the dynamic series. The FGT itself exhibits enhancement, as do all other glands of the human body. The enhancement of the normal FGT is more or less fast and always progressive. About 3 to 4 minutes after injection (depending on the amount of residual FGT, the degree of enhancement in that residual FGT, and the presence and extent of a washout time course in the cancer), the contrast between the cancer and the surrounding normal FGT can be cancelled out. Accordingly, there is only a narrow time window during which the acquisition of images is possible with high cancer-to-FGT contrast. Delayed, high spatial resolution imaging is therefore not very useful. It especially fails to depict cancers with sufficient contrast resolution. Only tumors with persistent enhancement (such as fibroadenomas) are seen well on delayed postcontrast images.

The different technical approaches to breast MR imaging

Breast MR imaging comes in two different versions: bilateral axial dynamic subtracted technique and primarily unilateral semi- or nondynamic, sagittal, actively fat-suppressed technique. The bilateral axial dynamic subtracted version has been the traditional breast MR imaging technique used in Europe [3,4]. The unilateral sagittal, actively fat-suppressed technique was most popular in the United States. The reason for the different techniques was mainly because of different vendor prevalence. In the early days of breast MR imaging, some vendors did not offer a bilateral breast coil. Making virtue out of necessity, the unilateral sagittal technique was useful because the small field of view (FOV) for unilateral sagittal imaging translated into a high spatial resolution, even with only small acquisition matrices. Because field homogeneity is less of a problem with small FOVs, fat suppression could be used. Because this was not attainable in a dynamic mode, nondynamic techniques were preferred. In Europe, the two most popular vendors offered bilateral breast coils. Accordingly, bilateral axial imaging was used. Because a large FOV is required to cover both breasts in the axial view, field inhomogeneities precluded the use of active fat suppression. Because the bilateral acquisition resulted in a relatively poor spatial resolution, contrast-enhancement kinetics were mainly used for differential diagnosis. This dynamic approach, in turn, would also conflict with active fat suppression, because active fat suppression was time consuming.

Today these two different camps are less strictly separated, mainly because of the technical progress that has been made over the last two decades. But even today, most United States radiologists stick to the sagittal acquisition and use active fat suppression and often additional subtraction of fat-suppressed images. Although the sagittal view is an intuitive way to look at breast images (in particular for breast surgeons), this approach has some substantial disadvantages. If bilateral sagittal imaging is attempted, this requires at least double the number of sections compared with what is required for bilateral axial MR imaging. Even with the use of parallel image acquisition, this is difficult to reconcile with the requirement of fast imaging. In addition, parallel imaging is associated with some 30% signal-to-noise ratio (SNR) loss. This SNR loss adds to the already high image noise, which in turn is caused by the need to use high image matrices with only one single signal average (number of signal averages and number of excitations). Active fat suppression further reduces the image SNR because fatty tissue is the most important contributor of proton signal in the breast. Accordingly, the resulting images may offer only borderline signal to noise, particularly if they are subtracted.

Another downside to sagittal imaging is that a direct side-by-side comparison of both breasts is difficult (or only feasible with reconstructed images, which in turn exhibit only a low resolution). Because symmetry (or lack thereof) is an important criterion for the categorization of non-masslike enhancement, this substantially increases the difficulty caused by this frequent diagnostic problem.

Although active fat suppression is now achievable virtually without time penalty, it not only reduces image SNR but it can also be disadvantageous for differential diagnosis. Fatty tissue signal inside an enhancing lesion has a high negative predictive value: a lesion with fat signal inside is virtually always benign. This information is lost. More importantly, fatty tissue is the only contrast material that is available in mammography. It provides important architectural information—information mammographers have been using for the last 40 years. This information is important for differential diagnosis, particularly to identify breast cancers that exhibit less-than-typical enhancement but are visible because of the architectural distortions they cause. All this information is lost if only fat-suppressed imaging is used.

Accordingly, at 1.5T, we stick to a non–fat-suppressed protocol, in the axial orientation, use subtraction (to highlight enhancing structures), and then use the nonsubtracted T1 pre- and postcontrast source images for further interpretation. With axial bilateral non–fat-suppressed imaging, the same in- and through-plane resolution is achieved within shorter acquisition times when compared with sagittal bilateral acquisitions; unlike bilateral sagittal imaging this is achievable without parallel imaging, and, in particular, with substantially higher image SNR. Because image blurring and phase errors cause unsharp contours of fine anatomic structures on non–fat-suppressed three-dimensional (3D) gradient echo images, we strongly recommend to use (multislice) two-dimensional (2D) gradient echo at 1.5T. Our recommended protocol is thus axial orientation, field of view to cover both breasts (typically 320 mm), 2D multislice gradient echo with shortest possible repetition time (TR), in-phase echo time, high flip angle, full Fourier imaging, no parallel acquisition, full non-interpolated 512×512 acquisition matrix, less than 3-mm section thickness, at an acquisition time of 100 seconds per dynamic scan. We would like to do the same at 3T, but for reasons mentioned in the following, this is probably not practicable.

Why move to 3T?

In general, the situation in dynamic breast MR imaging is comparable to the arena of contrast-enhanced MR angiography. In both arenas, large anatomic areas have to be covered, but still fine anatomic details have to be resolved. In breast MR imaging, as in contrast-enhanced angiography, image acquisition has to be synchronized with the peak arterial (in breast MR imaging: cancer) enhancement and has to be completed before venous (in breast MR imaging: fibroglandular) enhancement occurs. If the acquisition of the postcontrast images in breast MR imaging is delayed it is possible that the cancer-to-FGT contrast is reduced or even cancelled out by the time the contrast-determining lines of k-space are read. With time-consuming acquisition strategies used to acquire images with very high spatial resolution, one may run the risk of missing breast cancers with strong washout, particularly if a cancer is situated amidst strongly enhancing breast parenchyma.

It is clear that the temporal versus spatial dilemma of contrast-enhanced angiography and contrast-enhanced dynamic breast MR imaging will profit from the higher SNR that should be expected from imaging at higher magnetic fields.

Physics effects of 3T and how they affect breast imaging

Higher magnetic fields go along with physics changes that are in part beneficial, but in part also detrimental for breast MR imaging. The higher SNR is clearly advantageous. Yet in most clinical scenarios, the full 3T SNR advantage is not available and a doubled SNR is not to be expected. This is because some of the high-field–inherent physics effects have to be compensated for by techniques that, in turn, take SNR. Accordingly, the SNR advantage will be offset, at least in part.

The *in-phase echo time* is shorter at 3T (it is 2.3 milliseconds compared with 4.6 milliseconds at 1.5T). This situation may be advantageous because the shorter echo time can help compensate for the stronger susceptibility effects at 3T. The downside is, however, that even a small phase deviation of 1.15 milliseconds is sufficient to establish opposed phase echo times, a setting that is to be avoided for breast imaging, including actively fat-suppressed approaches.

The *longer T1 relaxation times* at 3T should, in principle, require a prolongation of the repetition time. This prolongation, however, would reduce the temporal resolution, which is not acceptable. If the TR is kept at the same levels as it is at 1.5T, some of the 3T SNR advantage is lost.

The *flip angles* may have to be reduced at 3T because radiofrequency (RF) deposition increases exponentially with increasing flip angle. Although this may not be important for 3D acquisition strategies, it does cause problems for 2D protocols.

The *broader separation of fat and water resonance frequencies* should facilitate fat suppression at 3T, and should also improve spectroscopic resolution. In clinical practice, the stronger susceptibility effects at 3T also lead to a line broadening of the respective peaks, which means that the peaks may overlap to the same extent as they do at 1.5T.

The *exponential increase of RF absorption* at 3T versus 1.5T brings about multiple problems. SAR regulations would not allow a dynamic acquisition that comes at least close to what is usually achieved at 1.5T. Accordingly, parallel imaging must be used to reduce the number of RF pulses needed for image generation. Because parallel imaging takes SNR (to a variable degree, but inevitably), some 3T SNR will again be lost.

Dielectric effects may contribute to an inhomogeneous RF propagation in tissue. For breast MR imaging, it seems that the concentric signal intensity losses that are known (eg, from abdominal high-field MR imaging) are not to be expected. Another, more insidious artifact may occur, however. Possibly (albeit not definitely) because of dielectric effects, substantial *B1 field heterogeneities* have been documented to occur for high-field breast MR imaging [5]. This means that the actual flip angle will be lower than prescribed in some parts of the image. In other words, within the field of view (ie, within the same image) spatial variations of the flip angles may occur and thus spatial variations of the T1 contrast, which translates into a spatially variable effect (in observable signal intensity increase) of a given amount of contrast material. For 3D dynamic protocols, even with a somewhat reduced flip angle, the resulting enhancement (signal intensity increase) is still high enough to yield a strong signal in subtracted images. For 2D dynamic protocols (like the ones that are in use for 1.5T imaging), however, the flip angle variations may cause substantially reduced signal intensity increase and may conceivably even lead to seemingly non-enhancing breast cancers. In a paper published by our group [6], the contrast enhancement observed at 3T was consistently lower than the enhancement obtained for the same lesions at 1.5T. In summary, for the time being, 2D and 3D protocols may go along with reduced enhancement compared with 1.5T. For 2D, the risk for reduced enhancement is significant, which is why this technique should be avoided at 3T. Because non–fat-suppressed 3D gradient echo imaging can be associated with substantial blurring and artifacts already at 1.5T, and even more so at 3T, it seems that for the time being, breast imaging at 3T may only be feasible with an active fat-suppression protocol (Fig. 1). The European approach (ie, contrast-enhanced breast MR imaging with axial, large field-of-view, dynamic subtracted imaging) may not be suitable for high-field breast MR imaging.

What is the current level of evidence regarding high-field breast MR imaging?

Despite the similar challenges and high-field–associated opportunities of contrast-enhanced angiography and contrast-enhanced breast MR imaging, a huge disparity becomes obvious when one simply compares the number of publications that deal with the respective topics. A rapidly growing body of evidence is available for contrast-enhanced angiography at 3T of virtually all body areas, in sharp contrast to the absolute paucity of papers that deal with high-field breast MR imaging. At the time this article was written, a total of two studies had been published on high-field breast MR imaging in peer-reviewed journals. One, by the Stanford group [7], deals with T1 relaxation time measurements in healthy volunteers. The other one, by our group [6], is a study on 37 patients with a total of 53 contrast-enhancing lesions who underwent

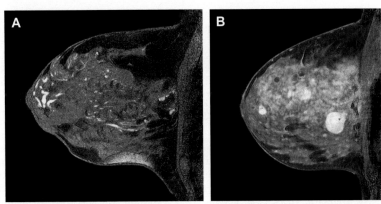

Fig. 1. High spatial-resolution imaging at 3T. Sagittal T1-weighted 3D segmented gradient echo imaging with active fat suppression (SPAIR), with an FOV of 250 mm and a true (non-interpolated) imaging matrix of 512 × 480, section thickness 1 mm, 89 sections covering one breast, voxel size: $0.5 \times 0.5 \times 1.0$ mm^3 in a total acquisition time of 2 minutes. Note duct ectasia in 1a and round enhancing mass in 1b, corresponding to a fibroadenoma.

contrast-enhanced breast MR imaging twice, once at 1.5T and once at 3T. The results were encouraging in that a high image quality was achieved at 3T; at ROC analysis, a higher specificity was obtained with 3T. The surprisingly lower enhancement of lesions, probably in part secondary to the B1 field heterogeneities mentioned earlier, may have contributed to the overall higher specificity.

It is difficult to set up studies with intraindividual comparison, particularly in the field of breast MR imaging, in which the two studies have to be done on two separate days to avoid confounding factors due to pre-existing tissue contrast material. However, a intraindividual comparison is clearly indispensable to investigate the added value of a higher magnetic field, however, especially regarding breast MR imaging. The variations of contrast material enhancement of benign and malignant lesions from one patient to another are huge. If no intraindividual comparison is possible, between-patient variations of contrast enhancement override any existing field-related effects, or mimic absent field-related benefits. Accordingly, studies that are to explore the benefit of high-field breast MR imaging have to offer each patient's 1.5T results as internal reference. Two breast MR imaging studies on two separate days are, however, difficult to fit into the short preoperative time period that is available in patients who have known breast cancer and who are awaiting surgery. This difficulty may be one reason for the low numbers of studies on the issue of high-field breast MR imaging. Another reason may be technical difficulties mentioned earlier.

For all functional breast MR imaging techniques, the additional SNR afforded by higher magnetic fields may indeed be useful. There is initial experience available (still in the anecdotal range) that

apparent diffusion coefficients (ADC) of benign and malignant breast tissues differ, with malignant lesions exhibiting restricted diffusion (ie, lower ADC values), possibly because of their increased cellularity. Whether or not this can be used to further improve differential diagnosis remains to be seen. Similar to diffusion weighted imaging, proton MR spectroscopy has been used to improve the differential diagnosis of breast cancer and benign changes [8–13]. The detectability of a choline peak seems to be an important independent marker of breast cancer, offering a high specificity but only a limited sensitivity; few benign tumors exhibit a choline peak, yet some breast cancers, in particular the intraductal cancers, are choline-negative also. A possible reason may be the limited spatial resolution with which MR spectroscopy is performed at 1.5T. To maintain an acceptable SNR, voxels (ie, the tissue volume from which the spectral signals is obtained) need to be relatively large. Partial averaging with normal fibroglandular tissue inevitably occurs, particularly in small cancers and in ductal carcinoma in situ (DCIS). With the higher SNR that is offered by high-field systems, spectroscopy voxel sizes may be chosen smaller, which will likely help improve the detectability of choline in small lesions and DCIS.

References

[1] Kuhl C. The current status of breast MR imaging. Part I. Choice of technique, image interpretation, diagnostic accuracy, and transfer to clinical practice. Radiology 2007;244:356–78.

[2] Kuhl CK. The current status of breast MR imaging. Part II. Clinical applications. Radiology 2007;244:672–91.

[3] Kuhl CK, Schild HH. Dynamic image interpretation of MRI of the breast. J Magn Reson Imaging 2000;12:965–74.

[4] Kuhl CK, Schild HH, Morakkabati N. Dynamic bilateral contrast-enhanced MR imaging of the breast: trade-off between spatial and temporal resolution. Radiology 2005;236:789–800.

[5] Kuhl CK, Kooijman H, Gieseke J, et al. Effect of B1 Inhomogeneity on breast MR imaging at 3.0 T. Radiology 2007;244:929–30.

[6] Kuhl CK, Jost P, Morakkabati N, et al. Contrast-enhanced MR imaging of the breast at 3.0 and 1.5 T in the same patients: initial experience. Radiology 2006;239:666–76.

[7] Rakow-Penner R, Daniel B, Yu H, et al. Relaxation times of breast tissue at 1.5T and 3T measured using IDEAL. J Magn Reson Imaging 2006;87–91.

[8] Bolan PJ, Nelson MT, Yee D, et al. Imaging in breast cancer: magnetic resonance spectroscopy. Breast Cancer Res 2005;7:149–52 [Epub 2005 May 12].

[9] Thomas MA, Wyckoff N, Yue K, et al. Two-dimensional MR spectroscopic characterization of breast cancer in vivo. Technol Cancer Res Treat 2005;4:99–106.

[10] Jacobs MA, Barker PB, Argani P, et al. Combined dynamic contrast enhanced breast MR and proton spectroscopic imaging: a feasibility study. J Magn Reson Imaging 2005;21:23–8.

[11] Jacobs MA, Barker PB, Bottomley PA, et al. Proton magnetic resonance spectroscopic imaging of human breast cancer: a preliminary study. J Magn Reson Imaging 2004;19:68–75.

[12] Roebuck JR, Cecil KM, Schnall MD, et al. Human breast lesions: characterization with proton MR spectroscopy. Radiology 1998;209:269–75.

[13] Cecil KM, Schnall MD, Siegelman ES, et al. The evaluation of human breast lesions with magnetic resonance imaging and proton magnetic resonance spectroscopy. Breast Cancer Res Treat 2001;68:45–54.

MAGNETIC
RESONANCE
IMAGING CLINICS

Magn Reson Imaging Clin N Am 15 (2007) 321–347

ELSEVIER
SAUNDERS

Liver MR Imaging: 1.5T versus 3T

Miguel Ramalho, MD, Ersan Altun, MD, Vasco Herédia, MD,
Mauricio Zapparoli, MD, Richard Semelka, MD*

- State of the art at 1.5T
- State of the art at 3T
- Diffuse liver diseases
  Fatty liver
  Hemochromatosis
  Chronic hepatitis and cirrhosis
- Malignant liver lesions
  Hepatocellular carcinoma
  Metastases

- Benign liver lesions
  Cysts
  Bile duct hamartoma
  Hemangiomas
  Focal nodular hyperplasia
  Adenoma
  Infectious and inflammatory masses
- Summary and outlook
- References

MR imaging is considered the most accurate modality to image the liver for the detection and characterization of focal and diffuse liver disease. The superiority of MR imaging compared with other imaging modalities for liver evaluation has become even more apparent because of substantial improvements in 1.5T magnets, with faster image acquisition and better image quality.

Over the last several years, systems that operate at high magnetic field strength have become more prevalent, particularly at academic and research centers. Following US Food and Drug Administration approval of 3T whole-body systems in 2002, a shift in interest in research development from 1.5T to 3T occurred, with wide clinical use in many institutions.

The major expected advantage of 3T compared with 1.5T is the anticipated gain in signal strength and signal to noise ratio (SNR). Theoretically, this boost in SNR—an almost two-fold signal gain—could be appreciated with improved image quality or reduced examination times. Unfortunately,

several potential disadvantages, such as an increase in imaging artifacts, changes in relaxation kinetics [1,2], and specific absorption rate (SAR) constraints, have to be considered [3,4]. Those limitations bring technical challenges in transferring 1.5T protocols to 3T, principally to abdominal imaging as the result of proper sequence design, incorporating breath-hold issues and large fields of view. Although 3T systems are advantageous for musculoskeletal, neuroimaging, and angiographic applications [5–11], few articles have been published regarding their use for abdominal and, particularly, liver examinations [12–16].

State of the art at 1.5T

Advancements in MR imaging hardware, software, and contrast agents have made a major impact on imaging of the liver. Phased-array surface coil technology significantly improved SNR, and conventional spin-echo pulse sequences have been replaced by faster sequences. Gradient-echo

Department of Radiology, University of North Carolina at Chapel Hill, CB#7510, 101 Manning Drive, Chapel Hill, NC 27599-7510, USA
* Corresponding author.
E-mail address: richsem@med.unc.edu (R. Semelka).

1064-9689/07/$ – see front matter © 2007 Elsevier Inc. All rights reserved.
mri.theclinics.com
doi:10.1016/j.mric.2007.06.003

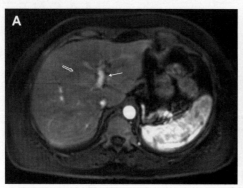
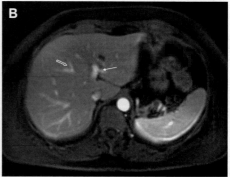

Fig. 1. Transverse T1-weighted 3D GRE postgadolinium sequences at 3T. (*A*) Hepatic arterial–dominant phase demonstrates contrast enhancement of central portal veins (*solid arrow* identifies left portal branch), whereas hepatic veins remain unenhanced (*open arrow*). (*B*) Hepatic venous phase shows enhancement of the entire vascular system. The solid arrow identifies the left portal branch and the open arrow points to the hepatic veins.

(GRE) sequences generally are used for T1-weighted sequences, and echo-train sequences are used for T2-weighted sequences. Introduction of parallel imaging technique has enabled further reduction of acquisition time and improved spatial resolution, although further refinement is necessary to overcome artifact and SNR considerations.

With current technology development, 1.5T is considered the standard of reference for providing optimization of rapid acquisition techniques while maintaining SNR.

Current liver protocol uses short acquisition–time sequences to avoid motion artifacts, mainly respiration, which, in the past, have lessened the reproducibility of MR imaging. A standard protocol uses breathing-independent sequences and breath-hold sequences that minimize motion artifact and spatial misregistration.

At 1.5T, the current standard MR liver protocol includes a T2-weighted sequence, a T1-weighted sequence, and serial postgadolinium GRE sequences. Ima00ging properties, demonstrated by their appearance on T1, T2, and early and late postgadolinium images, allow highly detailed evaluation of diffuse and focal liver abnormalities.

The predominant information provided by T2-weighted sequences is about fluid content, fibrotic tissue, and iron content (reflected by high, low, and very low signal intensity, respectively). Half-Fourier single-shot techniques should be used routinely because they are relatively insensitive to breathing artifacts. These techniques are sequential single-section techniques, in which each slice takes approximately 1 second to acquire, and central *k*-space is acquired in about 20% of that time. Because fatty liver has high signal intensity on echo-train spin-echo sequences, fat suppression generally is applied for at least one set of images (eg, to accentuate the high signal intensity of focal liver lesions on T2-weighted images). Fat suppression also improves visualization of regions bordered by fat, such as subcapsular parenchyma. The major disadvantage of echo-train sequences is that T2 differences between tissues are decreased.

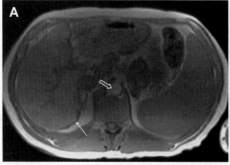
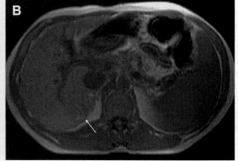

Fig. 2. Transverse T1-weighted SGE in-phase images at 3T (*A*) and 1.5T (*B*) in a man who has liver cirrhosis. A hypointense band (*solid arrow*) at the peripheral edge of the liver, which is due to a chemical shift artifact of the first kind, is more pronounced on the 3T in-phase image. SGE in- and out-of-phase sequences at 3T exhibit more pronounced inflow effects (bright vessel, *open arrow*) than at 1.5T.

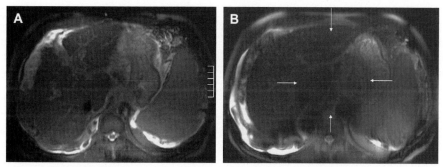

Fig. 3. Transverse T2-weighted SS-ETSE images at 1.5T (*A*) and 3T (*B*) in a man with liver cirrhosis and moderate ascites. Concentric signal loss (*arrows*), which represents standing wave/conductivity effects, is present on the 3T image but is not appreciable at 1.5T. Standing wave/conductivity effects becomes more apparent at higher magnetic field strengths and are more frequent in large patients and patients who have ascites, most frequently compromising T2-weighted sequences.

To compensate for this, a short tau inversion recovery (STIR) sequence can be done. Although image quality generally is fair, TurboSTIR is a short-duration T2-type sequence that can be performed within a breath-hold [17]. At least one T2-weighted sequence in the coronal plane may be of help in evaluating the superior and inferior margins of the liver, particularly the infracardiac portion of the left lobe [18].

Precontrast T1-weighted sequences are extremely important in lesion characterization. Most lesions are mildly or moderately low in signal intensity.

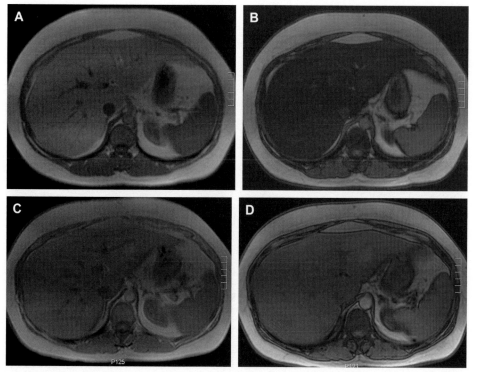

Fig. 4. Fatty liver at 1.5T and 3T. Transverse in-phase (*A, C*) and out-of-phase (*B, D*) SGE T1-weighted images in the same patient at 1.5T (*A, B*) and 3T (*C, D*). The liver is enlarged and demonstrates higher signal intensity than normal on in-phase T1-weighted images. The out-of-phase image shows a decrease in the signal intensity of the liver, better appreciated at 1.5T (*C*), which is consistent with severe fatty deposition. At 3T (*D*), the signal decrease of the liver is not as evident and converges with the signal intensity of the spleen, which is suggestive of mild fatty infiltration. These differences may be related, in part, to different T1 relaxation times at 3T, making small amounts of fat accumulation more difficult to appreciate.

Lesions with high fluid or fibrous tissue content are moderately or substantially low in signal intensity. Hemorrhagic lesions, those with high protein or fat content, and well-differentiated melanoma metastases are high in signal intensity. Fat has high signal intensity on T1-weighted imaging, and the routine use of an additional fat attenuating technique facilitates reliable characterization of fatty lesions. Spoiled gradient-echo (SGE) sequences are important and versatile for studying liver disease, providing T1-weighted imaging in a short amount of time and allowing chemical shift imaging in the same dual echo acquisition with spatially matched slices. The two echo times are chosen so that fat and water peaks are in 180° opposed-phase (2.2 milliseconds) and in-phase (4.4 milliseconds). Opposed-phase (out-of-phase) images are useful to detect small amounts of fat in liver lesions and in hepatic parenchyma. If fat and water are in the same voxel the signal intensity decreases on the out-of-phase sequence, with maximal signal loss occurring when fat and water signals are in equal proportion.

Gadolinium chelate enhancement is performed routinely with three-dimensional (3D) GRE breath-hold sequences (eg, volumetric interpolated breath-hold examination; VIBE). On older systems, although at the expense of thicker sections, two-dimensional (2D) SGE provides good image quality and may show better soft tissue contrast than 3D GRE acquisition.

Fat suppression usually is used to reduce motion artifacts and increase lesion conspicuity. Focal liver lesions that derive their predominant blood supply from hepatic arterial branches and enhance substantially on immediate postgadolinium images are termed "hypervascular" and are visualized best during the hepatic arterial–dominant phase of liver enhancement; hypovascular tumors may be more conspicuous on images obtained 1 minute postcontrast. Moreover, most hypovascular tumors also are seen well on the hepatic arterial–dominant phase. Most diagnostic information can be derived from the hepatic arterial–dominant phase, with correct timing verified by observing contrast enhancement of the central portal veins, whereas hepatic veins remain unenhanced (Fig. 1) [19]. Adequate delay between initiation of contrast injection and initiation of 3D GRE sequence is crucial (15–20 seconds for most patients). This allows visualization of the early enhancement pattern of lesions to aid in

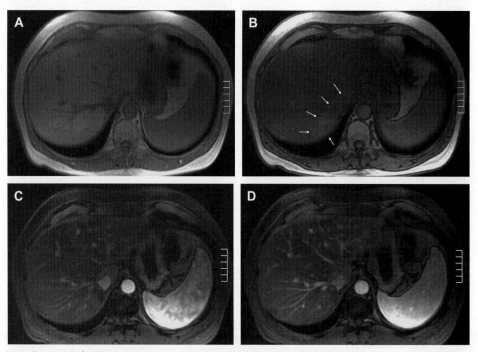

Fig. 5. Fatty liver with focal sparing. Transverse T1-weighted SGE in-phase (*A*) and out-of-phase (*B*) images and immediate (*C*) and 90-second (*D*) fat-suppressed postgadolinium 3D GRE images at 3T. The liver shows high signal intensity on the in-phase image (*A*), with a nonhomogeneous decrease of signal intensity on the out-of-phase image (*B*), lower than the spleen, with a focal high-intensity area in the posterior aspect of segment VII (*arrows*) consistent with severe fatty deposition with focal sparing. Geographic regions of normal liver within fatty liver may mimic the appearance of mass lesions, although liver enhancement is uniform, consistent with simple fatty liver (*C*, *D*).

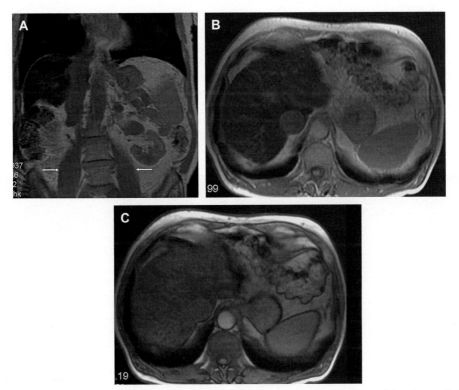

Fig. 6. Coronal T2-weighted SS-ETSE image (*A*) and transverse T1-weighted SGE in-phase (*B*) and out-of-phase (*C*) images at 3T. Coronal images facilitate comparison of signal intensity of the liver and spleen with psoas muscle (*arrows*). The liver is low in signal intensity on T2-weighted (*A*) and T1-weighted SGE in-phase (*B*) images, consistent with substantial iron deposition. The out-of-phase image (*C*) shows higher signal intensity of the liver than the in-phase acquisition because of lesser TE and inherent less T2* decay. The spleen is normal in signal intensity on both sequences, reflecting that iron is not in the RES but accumulated in the hepatocytes, consistent with primary hemochromatosis.

characterization and optimizes the detection of hypervascular lesions. The optimal time for early hepatic venous phase is less critical (45–75 seconds), showing enhancement of the entire vascular system. The early hepatic venous phase maximizes contrast between hypovascular lesions and the liver and can be used to evaluate the contrast washout pattern, which is a useful discriminating feature. Images acquired 1.5 to 10 minutes after contrast injection are in the interstitial phase of

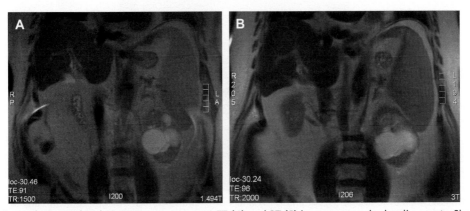

Fig. 7. Coronal T2-weighted SS-ETSE sequences at 1.5T (*A*) and 3T (*B*) in a woman who has liver cysts. Similar TE times at 1.5T (91 milliseconds) and 3T (96 milliseconds) result in lower signal appearance of the liver at 3T, reflecting greater T2* decay, which can simulate iron deposition. It is important to compare the signal intensity of the liver with psoas muscle.

enhancement, which aids in evaluating persistent enhancement of hemangiomas, washout characteristics of liver lesions, or delayed enhancement of fibrotic tissue or tumors, such as cholangiocarcinoma. There is no demonstrated benefit to routinely waiting longer than 5 minutes [20]. 3D GRE imaging provides acquisition of thinner sections than used typically for 2D images, with contiguous slices allowing detection of smaller lesions. Furthermore, there is multiplanar capacity, allowing assessment of liver vascular anatomy [21].

Other classes of contrast agents have been developed for liver MR studies. Liver-specific contrast agents may be classified as reticuloendothelial system (RES) specific or hepatocyte specific. RES-specific contrast agents are superparamagnetic particles of iron oxide (SPIO) that distort local magnetic field, causing signal loss on T2-weighted

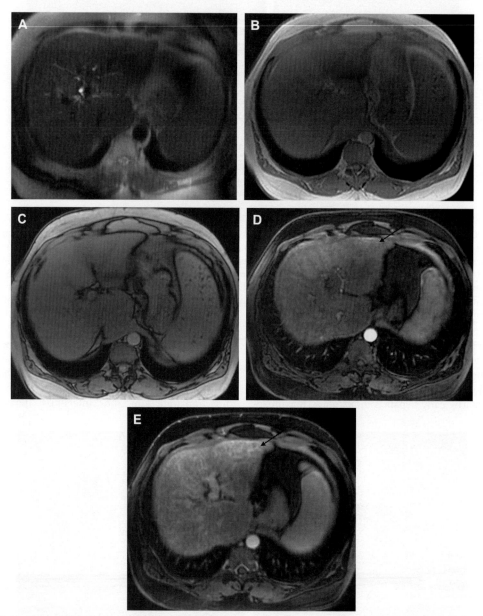

Fig. 8. Transverse SS-ETSE image (*A*); in-phase (*B*) and out-of-phase (*C*) SGE images; and immediate (*D*) and late-phase (*E*) fat-suppressed 3D GRE postgadolinium images at 3T. Fibrosis is not shown well on short-TE out-of-phase SGE images at 3T (*C*), unlike the situation at 1.5T. There is a linear pattern of fibrosis throughout the liver that is appreciated better on immediate (*D*) and late (*E*) postgadolinium sequences, visualized as low-signal linear structures and enhancing linear structures, respectively (*arrow*).

images. These agents are removed from circulation mainly by functioning Kupffer cells, accumulating iron within the intracellular space. Tumors without Kupffer cells and with mild to moderately increased signal on T2-weighted images become more conspicuous relative to the very low signal intensity of liver parenchyma. The only agent in the class that is approved in the United States is SPIO ferumoxides. These agents are not used widely in daily clinical practice. Focal nodular hyperplasia (FNH), hepatocellular adenoma (HCA), and regenerative and dysplastic nodules contain Kupffer cells to a varying degree; their relative signal loss may parallel the signal loss in normal hepatic parenchyma after iron oxide administration [22,23]. Well-differentiated HCCs also may contain Kupffer cells and exhibit contrast uptake. Heterogeneous and diminished uptake of iron oxide by fibrotic tissue in cirrhosis can mimic HCC [23,24]. The long infusion period, lack of dynamic enhancement information, and adverse effects (severe back pain) are other major inconvenient aspects of this agent.

Contrast agents with combined perfusion and tissue-selective properties are of great clinical interest. Two contrast agents that have achieved clinical use and that combine the properties of a non-specific gadolinium-based contrast agent with that of a hepatocyte-specific agent are Gd-BOPTA and Gd-EOB-DTPA (not approved by the US Food and Drug Administration). These chelates are administered as a bolus injection, allowing hemodynamic early perfusional data and late hepatobiliary contrast enhancement. The main difference is the degree of biliary excretion. Approximately 4% of the administered dose of Gd-BOPTA is excreted in the bile, whereas 50% of Gd-EOB-DTPA undergoes biliary excretion, providing sustained enhancement of liver parenchyma approximately 1 to 2 hours and 10 to 20 minutes after injection, respectively. One major indication is the differentiation between FNH, which contains bile ducts, and HCA, which does not [25]. In general, focal lesions that are not bile duct–containing hepatocellular lesions show improved conspicuity by the increase in signal of

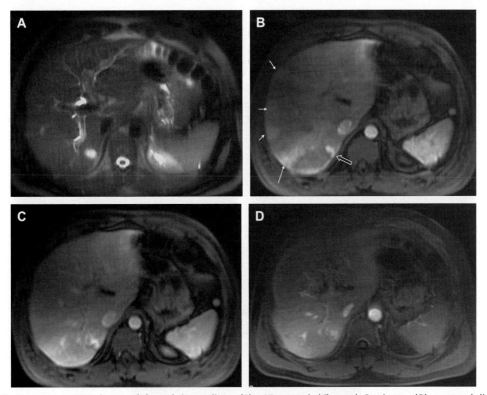

Fig. 9. Transverse STIR image (*A*) and immediate (*B*), 45-second (*C*), and 2-minute (*D*) postgadolinium T1-weighted 3D GRE images at 3T. Chronic liver disease with heterogeneous and patchy enhancement on early-phase image (*B, arrows*) that fades to homogeneity with background liver on 45-second image (*C*) and remains homogeneous on late-phase image (*D*). This finding is consistent with acute-on-chronic hepatitis. Note a small hemangioma in the posterior aspect of the right hepatic lobe (*B, open arrow*). This lesion is high signal intensity on T2 STIR and demonstrates peripheral nodular enhancement on the hepatic arterial–dominant-phase image (*B*), with centripetal progression in later phases (*D*), consistent with hemangioma type 2.

background liver tissue, whereas the lesions remain unenhanced. T1-weighted MR cholangiographic images are feasible and may represent another potential application of hepatocyte-specific contrast agents [26].

State of the art at 3T

Theoretically, the change from 1.5T to 3T magnets shows a gain in SNR that can be translated into higher spatial and temporal resolution; however, changes of relaxation kinetics [1,2] and SAR limitations [3,4] require substantial modification of abdominal sequence protocols and maturation of new technology developments. On 3T systems, T1

and T2 relaxation times of abdominal tissue are altered [1,2]. To emulate at least comparable contrast to that seen at 1.5T, a longer TR to compensate for prolonged T1 relaxation time and a shorter TE for T2-weighted sequences to compensate for the accelerated T2* decay usually are required [15]. Echo sampling time for out-of-phase and in-phase acquisition also is different at 3T. We perform two separate acquisitions for the in-phase and out-of phase images, with the first out-of-phase (1.6 milliseconds) and the first in-phase (2.2 milliseconds) echoes acquired. Because of data acquirement constraints, the first TE is not exactly out-of-phase at 3T (1.1 milliseconds). Our rationale for acquiring the first echoes for these acquisitions is to maximize

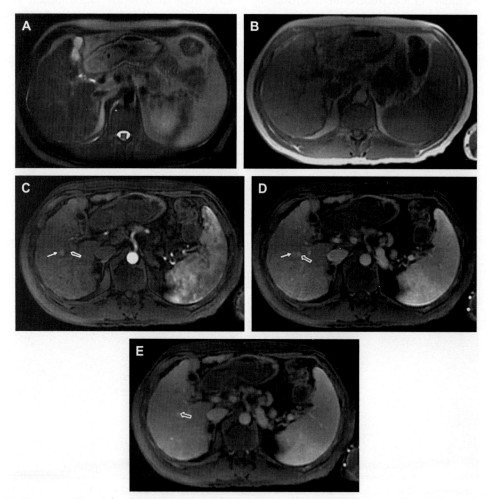

Fig. 10. Transverse T2-weighted SS-ETSE image (*A*); T1-weighted in-phase SGE image (*B*); and immediate (*C*), 45-second (*D*), and 90-second (*E*) fat-suppressed postgadolinium 3D GRE images at 3T. In this cirrhotic liver, there is one subcentimeter lesion in segment V that is not evident on T2- (*A*) or T1-weighted (*B*) images, which displays intense enhancement on the early arterial phase (*C, solid arrow*) and fades to isointensity on later phases (*C, D*). These findings are consistent with a high-grade DN. Close to the nodule, there is a signal void of the portal branch noted on the early hepatic arterial phase (*C, open arrow*) that enhances on subsequent phases (*D, E*).

T1 information. Further information on alternative sampling schemes can be found in the article on physics elsewhere in this issue.

A negative effect of the gain in SNR is increased radiofrequency (RF) energy deposition, measured as SAR, which quadruples at 3T compared with 1.5T. This limitation is particularly problematic with echo-train spin-echo sequences, which use multiple 180° RF refocusing pulses, or 2D SGE sequences with a large flip angle, resulting in high energy deposition.

To maintain SAR values below the permitted limits and avoid excess tissue heating, further sequence tradeoffs are required (eg, increased TR, decreased number of slices, decreased refocusing flip angle, decreased echo train length, or "cooling" periods). Prolonging the TR will prolong the measurement time, which helps to spread the energy over a longer time window; reducing the number of slices reduces the number of RF pulses for the same measurement time; reducing the refocusing flip angle decreases the RF field amplitude; reducing the echo train length leads to fewer RF pulses for the same TR, spreading the delivered

energy over a longer time window; and placing a pause ("cooling" periods) before or after the measurement also helps to dissipate the accumulated energy [27]. These sequence adjustments often are inevitable and may adversely affect SNR, scanning times, spatial resolution, or anatomic coverage [3,4,12,13,15].

With parallel imaging and new applicable software design, such as with "low SAR" pulses (variable-rate selective excitation; VERSE) or with variable flip angle refocusing techniques, RF exposure is decreased more efficiently.

There is substantial synergism between high-field and parallel imaging [28], with parallel imaging effectively reducing SAR. The key feature of parallel imaging is the use of different positions of surface coil elements to retrieve spatial information that otherwise would have to be obtained with additional phase-encoding steps. It decreases SAR keeping the measurement time constant [29]. Parallel imaging results in a decrease in SNR that is offset by the higher signal of 3T. In the future, increasing the number of coil elements will lead to larger anatomic coverage and higher acceleration factors, and

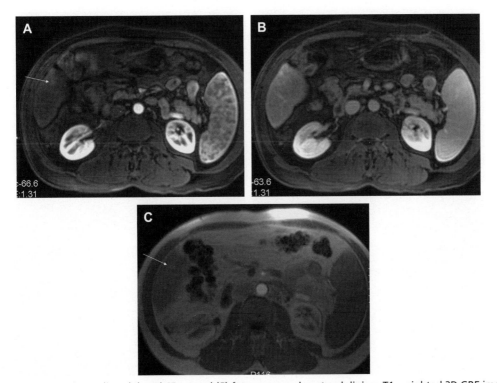

Fig. 11. Transverse immediate (*A*) and 45-second (*B*) fat-suppressed postgadolinium T1-weighted 3D GRE images at 3T. Cirrhotic liver with a subcentimeter lesion (*arrow*) in segment VI that demonstrates homogeneous enhancement on the early-phase image (*A*), but fades on the 45-second (*B*) image, consistent with a high-grade DN. Retrospectively, this lesion (*arrow*) was identified on hepatic-dominant phase (*C*) at 1.5T, but is more conspicuous at 3T.

advances in receiver technology will significantly improve the SNR [30].

Advances in pulse sequence design, such as with VERSE, can reduce peak RF power up to 40% to 60% compared with conventional techniques [30,31]. VERSE pulses use nonconstant slice select gradient amplitudes during excitation to reduce the amount of RF energy deposited [31]. This energy reduction has a particularly strong impact on long readout echo-train sequences at 3T, which previously required low flip angles for the refocusing pulses because of SAR constraints. With the VERSE pulses it is possible to use higher flip angles for the refocusing pulses—comparable to those used at 1.5T—without violating SAR constraints.

Improved adjustment procedures on echo-train sequences with application of variable flip angle–refocusing techniques (some acronyms are Hyperechoes, TRAPS, SPACE), although not so efficient, also enable reduction of RF deposition without compromising image quality. Echoes at the beginning and toward the end of the echo-train, which encode the more peripheral parts of k-space, are generated using low refocusing flip angles. Fully refocused flip angles are used only for the

important data encoding for the center part of k-space (SNR and CNR are mainly determined in the center of k-space), and, therefore, avoid signal loss resulting from the uses of low refocusing flip angles for these particular echoes [32].

Currently, 3T state-of-the-art liver imaging protocol uses the same sequence types as used at 1.5T, but they are modified to perform well at higher field strength.

Optimal sequence parameters are still evolving at 3T, and there is not much clinical experience using this field strength for abdominal evaluation at present, which is reflected by few publications on this subject. Although the quality of 3T images was reported to be equivalent to 1.5T images in a previous study [13], we believe that the quality of images varies, depending on the individual sequences and the particular machine.

Although generally able to provide diagnostic information, the quality of T1-weighted SGE images is fair. A probable explanation for fair image quality is the change in contrast at 3T [2,3]. This may reflect that the intrinsic differences in T1 relaxation times differ from one tissue to another, which affects contrast and alters the appearance compared with

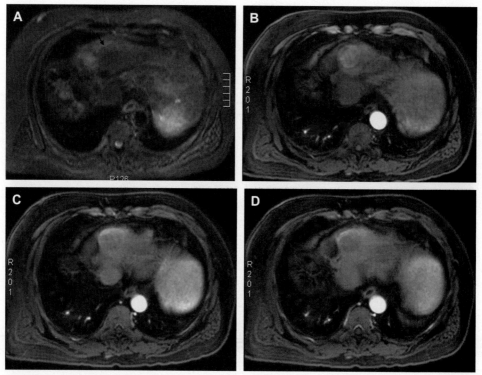

Fig. 12. Transverse STIR image (*A*) and immediate (*B*), 45-second (*C*), and 90-second (*D*) fat-suppressed postgadolinium T1-weighted 3D GRE images at 3T. There is a 3-cm mass arising from the superior aspect of the left hepatic lobe showing low signal on the STIR image (*arrow*). The lesion demonstrates heterogeneous enhancement on the immediate postcontrast image (*B*), with washout in the early hepatic venous phase (*C*) and late pseudocapsule enhancement (*D*) consistent with hypervascular HCC.

that observed and optimized at 1.5T [2,3]. For example, the detection of liver fibrosis on out-of-phase SGE sequences or the detection of fat content of the liver based on the comparison of in-phase and out-of-phase SGE sequences are more difficult at 3T compared with 1.5T. In contrast to 2D SGE sequence, 3D GRE sequences (eg, VIBE) are superior at 3T compared with 1.5T.

As illustration that sequence development and optimization is ongoing, following recent software updates on Siemens equipment that included the VERSE pulses, a significant improvement of the image quality of T2-weighted sequences was appreciated. Additionally, there was a significant decrease of the frequency and severity of artifacts for single-shot echo-train spin-echo sequences, making the image quality of T2-weighted sequences approximately equivalent to those at 1.5T.

A drawback of 3T is an increased number of types of artifacts. Certain imaging artifacts are more prominent at 3T than at 1.5T, mainly because their physical parameters are dependent on the main magnetic field strength (B0). Chemical shift artifacts of the first kind are directly proportional to the B0 and generally are twice as prominent with

3T imaging, noticeable on in-phase T1-weighted images SGE (Fig. 2). These are seen as hypointense and hyperintense bands toward the lower and higher part of the readout gradient field, observed at the fat–water interface. Susceptibility artifacts also increase with the B0 and are approximately twice as prominent at 3T as compared with 1.5T. Susceptibility artifacts appear as areas of signal loss near the interfaces of materials of substantially different magnetic susceptibility, such as metal–soft tissue or gas–soft tissue interfaces. This may be advantageous in selected cases, such as with surgical clips or pneumobilia, because they can be seen better at 3T [16]. The standard method of doubling the receiver bandwidth is effective for reducing chemical shift artifact of the first kind and susceptibility artifacts to the levels observed at 1.5T, but at the expense of SNR [16,33]. Our experience confirms previous reports that diagnostically relevant standing wave/conductivity effects are more frequent in large patients and patients who have ascites [16], and they represent an important factor in image quality deterioration. Standing wave (also called "dielectric" resonance artifacts) and conductivity effects usually occur concomitantly and become apparent

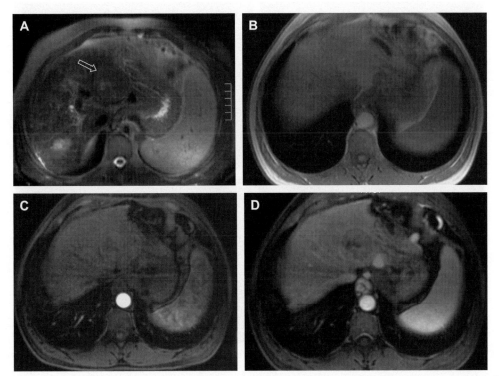

Fig. 13. Transverse STIR image (*A*); T1-weighted in-phase SGE image (*B*); and immediate (*C*) and 90-second (*D*) post-gadolinium fat-suppressed 3D GRE images at 3T. There is a 4-cm mass arising from the superior aspect of segment IV, which is slightly heterogeneous, mildly high in signal intensity on STIR (*A, arrow*), and isointense on the T1-weighted image (*B*). The lesion demonstrates negligible enhancement following gadolinium administration (*C*), with late pseudocapsule enhancement (*D*) consistent with hypovascular HCC.

in high magnetic field–strength MR systems, particularly 3T systems. This type of artifact most frequently compromises T2-weighted sequences (Fig. 3), resulting in areas of signal attenuation. Although not practical, one simple and low-cost solution to improve RF field (B1) homogeneity and reduce these artifacts is to elevate the surface coil off the individual's body using a doped aqueous pad [16,34]. This artifact is absent or insignificant in most patients on T1-weighted 3D GRE sequences. This is important because ascites is a common finding in patients who have chronic liver disease, and gadolinium-enhanced 3D GRE sequences are the most important for hepatocellular carcinoma (HCC) screening.

In vitro [35] and in vivo neuroimaging studies [36] reported better efficacy of paramagnetic contrast agents at 3T compared with 1.5T on 3D SGE sequences. We have observed that the 3T system enables acquisition of very high–quality postgadolinium T1-weighted 3D GRE sequences of the liver. Fat suppression is homogenous on 3D GRE, and thinner sections with high spatial resolution can be performed, facilitating detection and characterization of ultrasmall early enhancing lesions. These sequences are robust, relatively artifact free, and provide further reduction in slice thickness with less partial volume effects, which may render advantages for the detection of very small liver lesions.

Diffuse liver diseases

Fatty liver

Fatty liver or steatosis is defined as accumulation of lipid within hepatocytes. Nonalcoholic fatty liver disease (NAFLD) is the most common cause and often is associated with obesity and insulin resistance. NAFLD is common, present in 17% to 33% of Americans [37]. NAFLD encompasses a spectrum of hepatic histologic lesions ranging from bland hepatic steatosis to inflammatory changes with or without fibrosis, labeled nonalcoholic steatohepatitis (NASH) [38]. NASH can be present in one third of cases of NAFLD [37], and up to 28% of cases [39] may progress to cirrhosis, which carries a risk for liver failure requiring liver transplantation and HCC. No characteristic imaging findings distinguish NASH from simple steatosis.

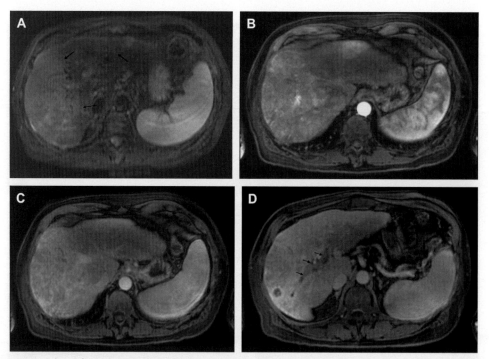

Fig. 14. T2-weighted fat-suppressed SS-ETSE image (*A*) and immediate (*B*) and 90-second (*C, D*) fat-suppressed postgadolinium 3D GRE images at 3T. The liver is diffusely heterogeneous in appearance with geographic areas of high signal intensity present throughout the right lobe and segment IV on the T2-weighted image (*A, arrows*). These areas demonstrate marked enhancement, appreciated on the immediate postgadolinium image (*B*), with diffuse mild heterogeneous washout, consistent with an infiltrating HCC. In a lower level, tumor thrombus of the main and right portal veins is appreciated (*D, arrows*), which is almost invariably present with infiltrative HCC.

Out-of-phase SGE imaging is a highly accurate technique to examine for fatty liver and to distinguish focal fat from neoplastic masses [40]. Comparing out-of-phase with in-phase SGE images, the presence of fatty metamorphosis results in signal loss because the signal from fat and water cancel out each other. MR imaging is the only imaging modality that can detect small amounts of fat (<15%), and diagnosis of steatosis can be made, even with normal laboratory evaluation. Because of the limitations of prolonged T1 relaxation at 3T with current sequence design, small amounts of lipid deposition may be harder to appreciate at 3T imaging than at 1.5T imaging (Fig. 4).

Fatty change may be uniform, patchy, focal, or spare foci of normal liver. At times, focal fatty infiltration or geographic regions of normal liver within fatty liver may mimic the appearance of mass lesions. Focal fat usually has angular, wedge-shaped boundaries and lacks mass effect.

An important ancillary observation is that uncomplicated fatty deposition within the liver enhances with gadolinium, usually indistinguishably from normal liver on in-phase images (Fig. 5).

Focal masses that contain fat generally have a rounded configuration and different enhancement. Common locations for focal fat are the central tip of segment IV and less commonly along the gallbladder. The central tip of segment IV also is a common location for focal fatty sparing. Different patterns of fatty deposition are related to variations in blood supply.

Hemochromatosis

Hemochromatosis results from abnormal iron deposition in soft tissues. Primary (hereditary) hemochromatosis is a genetic disorder of iron metabolism in which iron is absorbed excessively by the intestinal tract and accumulates in the liver, heart, joints, pancreas, and other endocrine glands. Characteristically, iron deposition is restricted to the liver in early stages. The presence of iron deposition in the pancreas correlates with irreversible changes of cirrhosis in the liver. Long-standing hemochromatosis places the patient at risk for cirrhosis and HCC.

Secondary hemochromatosis can arise in many disorders, inborn or acquired. These disorders have in common the fact that the patient is anemic.

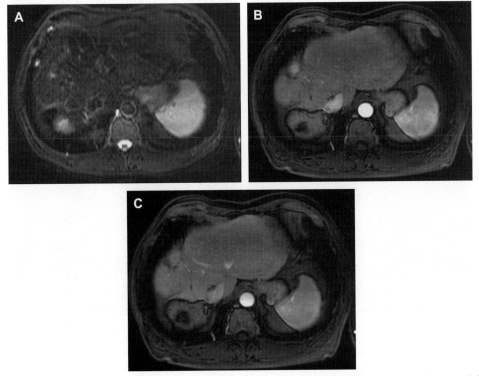

Fig. 15. Transverse STIR image (*A*) and immediate (*B*) and 45-second (*C*) fat-suppressed postgadolinium T1-weighted 3D GRE images at 3T. There is a centimeter lesion in the anterior aspect of segment VII that is not depicted clearly on T2- (*A*) and T1-weighted (not shown) images. It demonstrates intense uniform enhancement on the immediate postgadolinium image (*B*), with washout and pseudocapsule enhancement in later phases (*C*), consistent with small hypervascular HCC.

Among the hereditary forms, the most common are the thalassemias; among the acquired forms, the acquired sideroblastic anemias predominate. Blood transfusion is the most common cause of iron overload. Iron deposits in Kupffer cells and other phagocytic cells in the spleen and bone marrow and not in other organs, notably the pancreas and the heart, which distinguishes it from primary hemochromatosis. Furthermore, fibrosis usually is mild, despite even heavy iron stores, and cirrhosis is rare.

MR imaging is sensitive to hepatic iron overload because of the superparamagnetic effect of iron, leading to increased T2* decay. It can be appreciated as low signal on single-shot T2-weighted sequences comparing liver and spleen to psoas muscle because skeletal muscle is relatively spared in iron overload (Fig. 6). Calculated T2* decay values were reported to relate closely to tissue iron concentration [41]. On routine out-of-phase and in-phase acquisition, abnormal iron deposition leads to a decreased signal intensity on in-phase

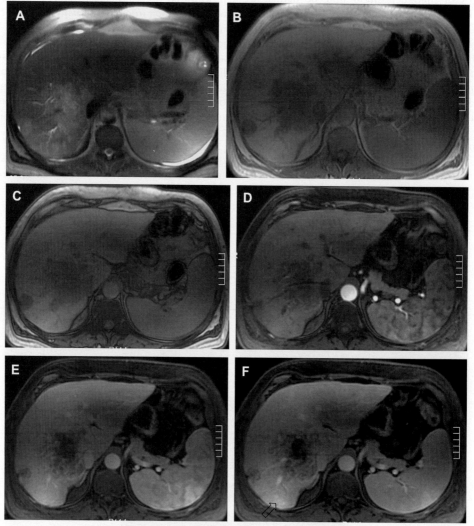

Fig. 16. Transverse T2-weighted SS-ETSE image (*A*); in-phase (*B*) and out-of-phase (*C*) SGE images; and immediate (*D*), 45-second (*E*), and 90-second (*F*) fat-suppressed postgadolinium 3D GRE images at 3T. A characteristic cauliflower-shaped colon cancer metastasis is located centrally on segment VII/VIII. A smaller subcapsular lesion and peripheral tiny nodules also are present (*arrow*). The lesions demonstrate moderately high signal intensity on the T2-weighted image (*A*) and mild low signal intensity on the in- and out-of-phase (*B, C*) images. Larger lesions show mild early enhancement, in a ring pattern, with progressive filling on venous and interstitial phases. Note that on the T1-weighted images, the small peripheral nodules are depicted only on the interstitial enhanced-phase image (*F, arrow*). Higher image quality in 3D GRE and higher T1 relaxation of gadolinium at 3T also may facilitate detection of small late-enhanced nodules.

images because of T2* decay of the longer echo time. A semiquantitative approach could be as follows: mild deposition, dark on T2, no change on T1; moderate deposition, dark on T2, gray on T1; severe deposition: dark on T2, dark on T1. Using comparable TE times at 1.5T and 3T (eg, 90 milliseconds) will result in the appearance of a lower signal in the liver at 3T, reflecting further T2* decay, which can simulate iron deposition (Fig. 7). It is critical to consider this phenomenon when interpreting studies at 3T.

Chronic hepatitis and cirrhosis

An important observation in chronic liver disease on MR images is the definition of fibrosis. At 1.5T, fibrosis is visualized best as low signal on out-of-phase (2.2 milliseconds) images, low signal on immediate postgadolinium GRE, and delayed enhancement at 2.0 minutes. The contrast on out-of-phase images (1.6 milliseconds) at 3T is not adequate to visualize subtle fibrosis, and its determination must be established on early and 2.0-minute postgadolinium images (Fig. 8).

Acute-on-chronic liver inflammation is shown as regions of transient increased enhancement on immediate postgadolinium images (Fig. 9). This pattern of enhancement must be differentiated from diffuse HCC, which tends to show heterogeneous washout and is associated invariably with portal vein tumor thrombosis [42]. Demonstration of acute-on-chronic hepatitis should be approximately equivalent for 1.5T and 3T systems.

A reticular pattern conforms to and surrounds regenerative nodules (RNs), seen as innumerable subcentimeter soft tissue nodules. RNs may accumulate iron, with low signal on all MR sequences. Nonsiderotic RNs are high in signal intensity on T1-weighted sequences and isointense on T2-weighted sequences. Because they have dominant portal vascularization, there is minimal early enhancement, comparable to or less than background liver with no washout [43]. Demonstration of RNs is comparable at 1.5T and 3T.

Dysplastic nodules (DNs) represent premalignant lesions, ranging from low- to high-grade dysplasia. HCC can develop within DNs rapidly,

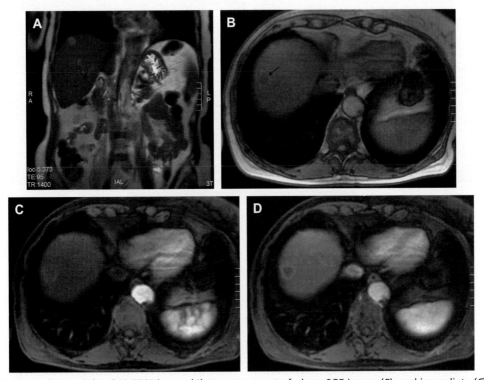

Fig. 17. Coronal T2-weighted SS-ETSE image (*A*), transverse out-of-phase SGE image (*B*), and immediate (*C*) and 90-second (*D*) fat-suppressed postgadolinium 3D GRE images at 3T in a patient with history of breast cancer. There is a fatty liver with a solitary subcapsular lesion that demonstrates high signal on T2 (*A*) and low signal on T1-weighted images (*B*), associated with a perilesional bright rim consistent with compressed liver parenchyma that is unable to deposit intracytoplasmic fat, seen on the out-of-phase image (*arrow*). On immediate postgadolinium images (*C*), the lesion exhibits a ring enhancement that persists on interstitial-phased images (*D*), consistent with hypovascular breast metastasis. This lesion was not seen on spiral CT.

within 4 months. Usually, DNs are larger than most RNs. Lesions larger than 2 cm are worrisome for HCC, especially if they exhibit early increased enhancement. Development of hepatic arterial supply may be related with higher grade of dysplasia. The imaging features include variable characteristics, depending at least partly on the degree of dysplasia and partly on variables including degree of intracellular iron and protein content. The T1 signal often is elevated, with no decrease on out-of-phase or fat-suppressed images, possibly related to high protein content. Lesions frequently show low T2 signal because of protein content or paramagnetic iron accumulation. Generally, an elevated T2 signal is observed in HCC but rarely is seen in DNs, possibly reflecting higher-grade dysplasia. DNs may show arterial enhancement but no evidence of capsule. Low-grade DNs show minimal early and late enhancement, comparable to background liver [43,44]. Because low-grade DNs may be visualized better on noncontrast T1-weighted sequences, these lesions may be shown better at 1.5T. High-grade DNs (Fig. 10) typically show intense early enhancement postgadolinium injection and fade to

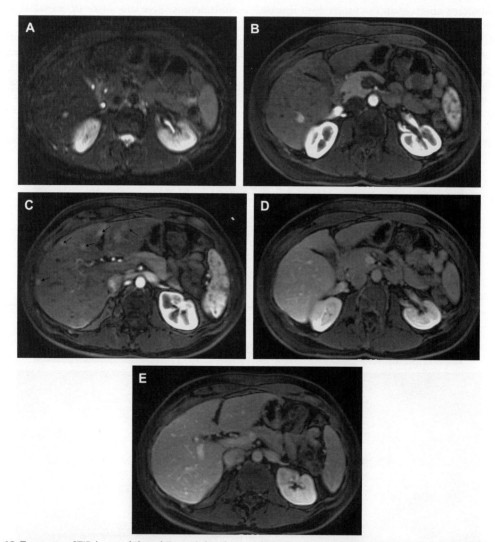

Fig. 18. Transverse STIR image (*A*) and T1-weighted immediate (*B, C*) and 45-second (*D, E*) fat-suppressed postgadolinium 3D GRE images at 3T. On the precontrast study, only one 7-mm lesion on T2-weighted sequences is visualized in segment VI with high signal intensity (*A*). This lesion is shown well as a uniform enhancing lesion on the immediate postgadolinium image (*B*); multiple other millimeter lesions get conspicuous (*C, arrows*) with the same type of enhancement. The lesions wash out rapidly and become isointense with the liver by 45 seconds (*D, E*). Small hypervascular malignant metastases commonly are shown only on the hepatic arterial–dominant phase images, and the better performance of 3D GRE postgadolinium sequences at 3T is advantageous for detection of small early-enhancing metastases.

isointensity [44]. Increased early enhancement is the critical observation to establish the diagnosis of high-grade DN. The combination of greater sensitivity for detection of small enhancing nodules and the capacity to acquire thinner slices render better conspicuity at 3T (Fig. 11).

Malignant liver lesions

Hepatocellular carcinoma

HCC is the most common primary hepatic malignancy. Although HCC may occur in the absence of any underlying liver disease [45], it generally develops in the setting of cirrhosis. In developed western countries, alcohol is the main cause of cirrhosis, although viral hepatitis is increasing steadily. Worldwide, it is related most often to viral hepatitis, with the highest frequency in East Asia. The multistep sequence carcinogenesis theory states that HCC arises from high-grade dysplastic nodules as the final stage. HCCs are solitary in 50% of cases, multifocal in 40% of cases, and diffuse in 10% of cases [46]. HCCs are predominantly hypervascular tumors, and the dominant blood supply is hepatic arterial. They have potential overlapping features with high-grade DNs because these can develop a preferential arterial supply.

HCCs possess variable T2 and T1 signal; elevated T2-weighted and low T1-weighted signal raises concern for HCC. If lesions are smaller than 1.5 cm, they frequently are isointense on T1- and T2-weighted images and are seen only on postgadolinium T1-weighted images [46]. The typical postgadolinium T1-weighted imaging findings include arterial phase intense enhancement with rapid venous and interstitial phase washout with the development of late pseudocapsule enhancement (Fig. 12). Hypovascular or isovascular HCCs are not rare, representing 10% of HCCs, and may be shown best as focal lesions that show washout on images 1 to 5 minute postgadolinium with pseudocapsule enhancement (Fig. 13).

Diffuse HCC (Fig. 14) shows irregular T2- and T1-weighted signal intensity, with irregular enhancement that has regions that washout, whereas other regions may persist [42]. Diffuse HCC is associated almost invariably with portal vein tumor thrombosis [42].

HCCs, especially small tumors, may be shown better at 3T than at 1.5T because these tumors generally are hypervascular; the higher T1 relaxation at 3T combined with thinner section acquisition and high image quality of 3D GRE render superior detection (Fig. 15).

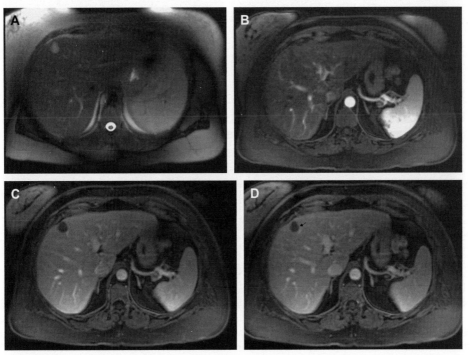

Fig. 19. Transverse T2-weighted SS-ETSE image (*A*) and transverse immediate (*B*), 45-second (*C*), and 90-second (*D*) fat-suppressed postgadolinium 3D GRE images at 3T. A 1.5-cm cystic lesion is seen superiorly in the liver, between segments VIII and IV. The lesion abuts the contour of the liver, and a thin perceptible enhancing wall is noticeable on the postgadolinium images (*D*, *arrow*), consistent with a foregut cyst. There are standing wave/conductivity effects on the T2-weighted sequence that are not perceptible on the 3D GRE sequences.

Metastases

Characterization of focal liver lesions as benign or malignant is important because patients who have known primary malignancies frequently have benign small hepatic lesions [47], which may be multiple and scattered throughout the liver.

Metastases may appear as solitary, multiple, or confluent masses and, on rare occasions, may appear infiltrative. Metastases can be classified further according to their enhancement pattern as hypo- or hypervascular.

Hypovascular metastases are the most common, and colon adenocarcinoma is the most frequent primary tumor (Fig. 16). Imaging features of hypovascular liver metastases include variable T2 signal, low signal on T1-weighted images, and mild to moderate enhancement on postgadolinium images (Fig. 17). Typically, these lesions are most conspicuous on T1-weighted GRE pre- and postgadolinium sequences, and these latter data acquisition provide maximal sensitivity and specificity for detection and diagnosis. Postgadolinium images characteristically show mild early enhancement, most often with a ring pattern, with progressive venous-interstitial phase enhancement, predominantly filling in from the outer margins. Perilesional enhancement of adjacent liver is seen frequently with adenocarcinoma metastases on immediate postgadolinium images, most commonly mucinous type from the colon, stomach, or pancreas, usually fading over time.

Hypervascular metastases show intense early enhancement. Hypervascular metastases can result from neuroendocrine tumors, including carcinoid (Fig. 18) and islet cell tumor, renal cell carcinoma, melanoma, or thyroid cancer. Breast cancer is a more common tumor to result in liver metastases, but metastases are not as consistently hypervascular. Imaging features are a variable T2 signal, but frequently moderate to moderately intense and heterogeneous signal, and a low T1 signal. Postgadolinium enhancement is most pronounced on arterial-phase images as a peripheral ring and, on delayed postgadolinium images, contrast enhancement progresses in a centripetal fashion and fades peripherally. The

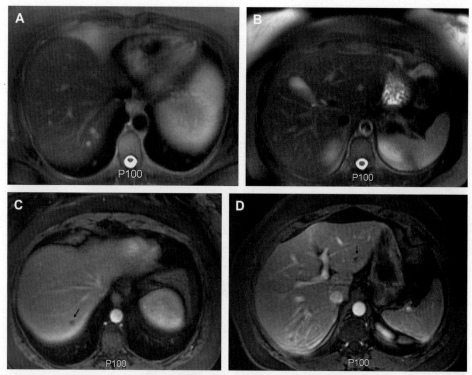

Fig. 20. Biliary hamartomas. Transverse T2-weighted SS-ETSE images (*A, B*) and transverse T1-weighted 45-second (*C, D*) fat-suppressed postgadolinium 3D GRE images. Multiple subcentimeter well-defined lesions are scattered throughout the liver. They are high signal intensity on T2-weighted images (*A, B*), and although the bigger lesions are appreciated with low signal intensity, the smaller lesions are not detected on noncontrast in- and out-of-phase T1-weighted SGE images (not shown). These lesions demonstrate thin perilesional rim enhancement on postgadolinium 3D GRE images (*C, D, arrow*), with no progressive enhancement, conferring better conspicuity at 3T, because less partial-volume effects and greater sensitivity for gadolinium are achieved consistently at this field strength compared with 1.5T.

greater sensitivity for gadolinium, thin slice acquisition, and higher image quality in 3D GRE makes 3T superior to 1.5T for the detection and characterization of hypervascular metastases.

Benign liver lesions

Cysts

Cysts are common benign liver lesions. They possess well-defined margins with homogeneous high signal intensity on T2-weighted images and low signal intensity on T1-weghted images, with no enhancement on early and late postgadolinium-enhanced images [44]. High signal intensity on T1-weighted sequences reflects the presence of protein or blood products. Other minor complications of benign cysts are lobulation of the contour and non-enhanced septations. Septal or mural nodularity enhancement should raise suspicion of biliary cystadenoma or cystadenocarcinoma. Ciliated hepatic foregut cysts (Fig. 19) are located along the convex external surface of the liver, bulge the liver contour, and usually are intersegmental. Foregut cysts usually possess a definable enhancing wall [48]. Lesions that mimic the appearance of cysts include

cystic metastases, the most common being of ovarian origin. Cysts are shown well at 1.5T and 3T. The higher SNR and thinner section acquisition permits detection and characterization of smaller cysts at 3T than at 1.5T, although this may not have clinical importance.

Bile duct hamartoma

Biliary hamartomas are small benign liver malformations, pathologically containing cystic dilated bile ducts embedded in a fibrous stroma. They occur in 3% of the population. Biliary hamartomas are seen frequently as multiple lesions 0.5 to 1 cm, usually scattered throughout both of liver lobes, especially in the subcapsular region [49]. They are high signal on T2-weighted images and low signal on T1-weighted images, indistinguishable from simple cysts. Postgadolinium imaging shows a thin peripheral enhancing rim with no progressive internal stromal enhancement [50], which aids in differentiating these lesions from cysts and hypovascular metastases. Perilesional compressed hepatic parenchyma and inflammatory cell infiltrate are believed to be responsible for the rimlike enhancement pattern [50].

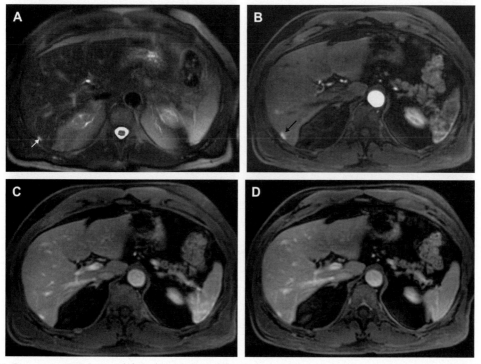

Fig. 21. Transverse STIR image (*A*) and immediate (*B*), 45-second (*C*), and 90-second (*D*) fat-suppressed 3D GRE postgadolinium images at 3T. A tiny nodule is present in segment VII that shows high signal on the T2-weighted image (*A, arrow*), low signal on the T1-weighted image (not shown), and intense uniform enhancement immediately after administration of contrast (*B, arrow*) that persists in later phases (*C, D*), consistent with small-size hemangioma, type 1 enhancement. Thin section acquisition and higher sensitivity for gadolinium at 3T confer higher confidence in diagnosing small hemangiomas.

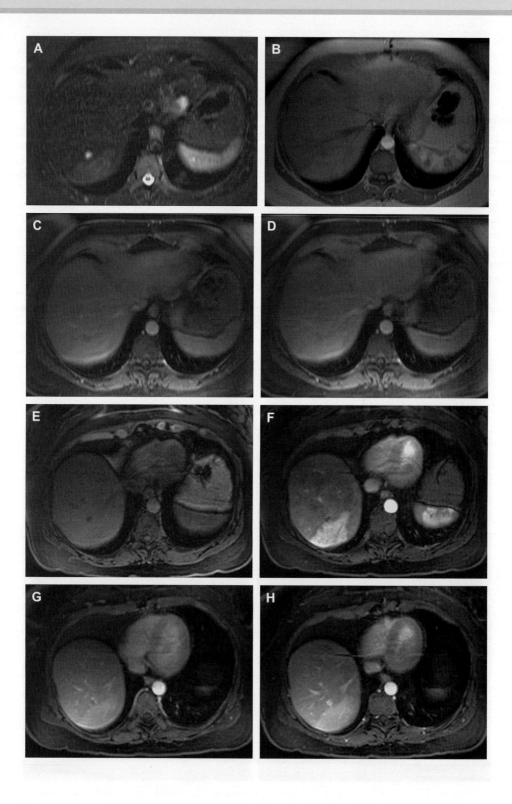

Bile duct hamartomas are shown well at 1.5T and 3T. The higher SNR and thinner section acquisition, with less partial volume at 3T, permit better detection of small lesions and clearer definition of their peripheral enhancement (Fig. 20).

Hemangiomas

Hemangiomas are the most common benign tumors in the liver, with an estimated prevalence of 0.4% to 20% in several autopsy series [51,52].

Hemangiomas range in size from subcentimeter to more than 10 cm, with most ranging from 0.5 to 5 cm. Hemangiomas are multiple in at least 50% of subjects. The imaging features include moderately high T2 signal intensity and moderately low T1 signal intensity. Postgadolinium imaging shows diagnostically specific features. The classic imaging feature is a discontinuous ring of peripheral nodules, noted on immediate postgadolinium images (see Fig. 9). Generally, smaller lesions fill more quickly, and larger lesions are more likely to show slower central filling and have thrombosis and fibrosis, seen as central persistent nonfilling. Three types of contrast enhancement patterns are described in dynamic examinations: early uniform enhancement (Fig. 21) with persistence of enhancement in the late phase (type 1); peripheral nodular enhancement with centripetal progression to uniform enhancement (type 2); and peripheral nodular enhancement with centripetal progression and persistent nonenhancing central scar tissue in the late phase (type 3). About two thirds of hemangiomas show slow progressive enhancement, whereas one third show rapid enhancement. Type 1 enhancement is present only in small tumors (<1.5 cm), whereas type 2 enhancement is the most common pattern of small- and medium (1.5–5 cm)-sized hemangiomas. Medium-sized liver lesions with type 1 enhancement represent well-differentiated tumors of hepatocellular origin or hypervascular metastasis. Giant hemangiomas usually possess a well-defined multilobular appearance, often with a central scar and invariably type 3 enhancement [53,54]. Rarely, hemangiomas can hemorrhage,

and another rare feature is transient early perilesional enhancement.

Small hemangiomas can be difficult to distinguish from hypervascular metastases. Other lesions that mimic hemangiomas include chemotherapy (antiangiogenic effect [55])-treated metastases, which may show slowly progressive central enhancement but do not show interrupted peripheral nodules that coalesce.

The thinner section acquisition and greater T1 relaxation of gadolinium at 3T renders a more confident characterization of hemangiomas. They may be particularly helpful for small lesions with slow enhancement (Fig. 22).

Focal nodular hyperplasia

FNH is a common benign liver tumor, with a reported prevalence of approximately 1%. Most often, the lesions are solitary, but can be multiple, and are most common in young adult women, probably related to hormonal stimulation. They apparently have no malignant potential, and hemorrhage is rare. Our belief is that these tumors progressively regress with age. On echo-train T2-weighted sequences, classic FNHs are isointense to very mildly hyperintense; the central core, usually described as scar (although not a true scar), may have a higher signal than the surrounding mass in approximately 50% of cases, likely related to central vessels, bile ducts, and edema in the myxomatous tissue [56]. On T1-weighted images, they are isointense to mildly hypointense; on out-of-phase images, background fatty liver is common, and, occasionally, increased fatty accumulation occurs in liver surrounding the mass (in contrast, metastases usually are associated with perilesional fatty sparing). Accumulation of intralesional fat is rare [57]. On postgadolinium images, the arterial-dominant phase shows uniform enhancement, usually very intensely. If lesions are isointense on unenhanced images, they may be visible only on arterial-phase images, which is observed often in small lesions (<1.5 cm). FNH rapidly fades in venous to interstitial phases to become isointense or slightly hyperintense to liver. No capsule is present, but

Fig. 22. Small-size hemangioma, type 2. Comparison between 1.5T and 3T. Transverse STIR image (*A*); immediate 2D SGE postgadolinium image (*B*); and 45-second (*C*) and 90-second (*D*) 3D GRE postgadolinium images at 1.5T. Transverse T1-weighted basal (*E*), immediate (*F*), 45-second (*G*), and 90-second (*H*) 3D GRE postgadolinium images at 3T. The lesion shows low signal on the T1-weighted image (*E*) and high signal on T2 STIR (*A*). At 3T, there is clear definition of the peripheral nodular enhancement on immediate (*F*) and hepatic venous–phase (*G*) images, with progression to homogeneity on the late-phase image (*H*). At 1.5T, these features are much less conspicuous, even on 45-second and 90-second images, despite almost similar thickness of the slices (3 mm on 3T and 3.5 mm on 1.5T), demonstrating greater SNR and sensitivity for gadolinium on 3D GRE sequences at 3T. There also is increased wedge-shaped arterial enhancement of the posterior aspect of the right hepatic lobe, not related to vascular thrombosis, which fades on later phases.

thin radial fibrous strands are common. The central core does not enhance on the arterial phase but becomes progressively enhanced on venous and interstitial phases in approximately 70% to 80% of cases [58]. The central core most often is not appreciated in smaller lesions (<1.5 cm).

Lesions that may mimic FNH include adenoma, HCC, hypervascular metastases, and fibrolamellar HCC. Hepatocyte-specific agents can differentiate small and atypical FNHs from adenoma accurately (Fig. 23) [25]. Gd-BOPTA and Gd-EOB-DTPA demonstrate delayed enhancement of FNH and lack of enhancement of adenomas,

which reflects accumulation in malformed bile ducts (present in FNHs and absent in adenomas). FNH should show relatively uniform enhancement and blush on hepatic arterial–dominant phase images. Irregular enhancement raises concern that the mass may represent a malignant tumor, such as HCC. Thinner section acquisition and greater T1 relaxation of gadolinium at 3T should improve the confidence of lesion characterization at 3T, particularly in older patients, because these tumors may become small; however, this difference may not be clinically necessary.

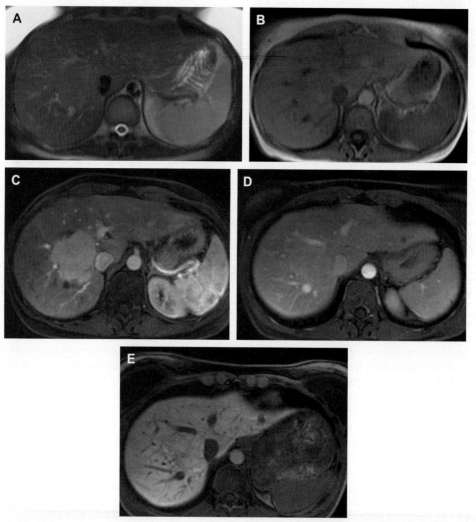

Fig. 23. Transverse T2-weighted SS-ETSE image (*A*); T1-weighted in-phase SGE image (*B*); and immediate (*C*), 90-second (*D*), and 1.5-hour (*E*) 3D GRE post–Gd-BOPTA images. Despite the large size, no lesion is appreciated clearly on the T2- (*A*) or T1-weighted (*B*) image. There is no decrease in signal intensity on the out-of-phase images (not shown) and enhances with uniform blush on hepatic arterial–dominant phase (*C*), which fades rapidly to isointensity on the late-phase image. On the 1.5-hour postcontrast image (*C*), the lesion is isointense compared to background liver, reflecting hepatocyte uptake and excretion of Gd-BOPTA. These findings are characteristic for FNH and are distinctly different from hepatic adenoma.

Adenoma

HCAs are uncommon benign liver tumors that are present mainly in women, usually of child-bearing age [59]. Their existence is associated with the use of oral contraceptives [60]. Generally, lesions will involute to a variable extent if oral contraceptives are discontinued. Because of the rarity of HCA in men and similarities in appearance with HCC, in this setting it may not be possible to confirm the diagnosis based only on MR images [61].

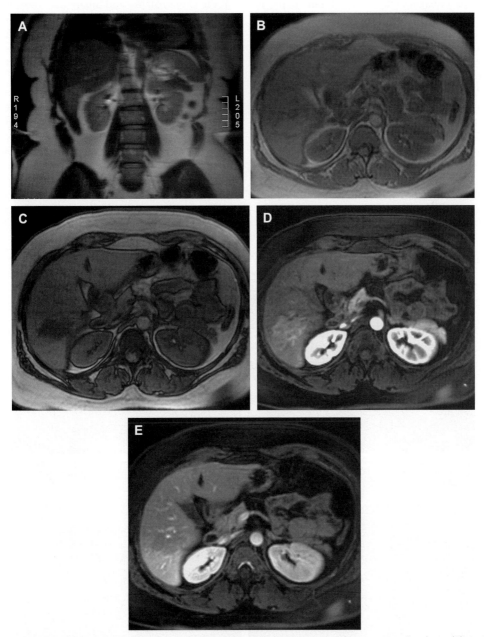

Fig. 24. Hepatic adenoma with fat. Coronal T2-weighted SS-ETSE image (*A*); transverse in-phase (*B*) and out-of-phase (*C*) SGE images; and immediate (*D*) and 45-second (*E*) fat-suppressed postgadolinium 3D GRE images. On the transverse T1-weighted SGE in-phase (*B*) and out-of-phase (*C*) images, the lesion is depicted in segment VI of the liver only on the latter one, with a decrease in signal intensity given the homogeneous intralesional fat accumulation. Its fat content renders a moderately high homogeneous signal intensity on the T2-weighted image (*A*). Diffuse blush on immediate postcontrast 3D GRE (*D*), with washout (*E*) and no pseudocapsule enhancement on late-phase images, is consistent with hepatic adenoma.

Bleeding is uncommon. The risk for bleeding is mainly dependent on tumor size and subcapsular location. Oncological indications for surgery may not be justified because malignant transformation is rare [62].

The MR imaging features (Fig. 24) include iso- to mild hyperintensity on T2-weighted images; T1-weighted imaging ranges from mildly hypo- to mildly hyperintense, depending on the presence of fat or blood products. In the presence of fat, lesions commonly are uniform and can be assessed best by in-phase and out-of-phase imaging. Fat is observed in approximately 70% of patients. If subacute blood products are present, irregular foci of high signal are apparent on T1- and T2-weighted sequences, which do not drop on out-of-phase or fat-suppressed T1-weighted sequences [63]. On postgadolinium images, an arterial-phase blush is observed most often with rapid fading, usually to hypo- or isointensity to liver. If blood products are present, enhancement may appear irregular. Fat effects on in- and out-of-phase images are shown better at 1.5T. Hence, this lesion may be evaluated

better at 1.5T; however, this may not be clinically relevant.

Infectious and inflammatory masses

Hepatic abscesses usually are caused by a bacterial infection, most often polymicrobial. Pyogenic abscess accounts for 80% of cases of hepatic abscess in the United States, and biliary tract disease is the most common predisposing factor. Fungal abscesses occur mainly in neutropenic patients, primarily as a result of *Candida albicans*. Amebic abscesses are caused by a protozoan parasite, observed mostly in developing tropical countries.

Pyogenic abscesses can be solitary or multiple. They consist of central necrotic purulent debris, with a relatively hypo or avascular core, surrounded by a fibrous rind containing inflammatory cells.

Imaging of hepatic abscesses may be comparable at 1.5T and 3T. Abscesses typically display central low T1-weighted signal and intermediate irregular T2-weighted signal. The abscess's wall enhances on the arterial phase, which persists and generally intensifies on the interstitial phase (Fig. 25). There

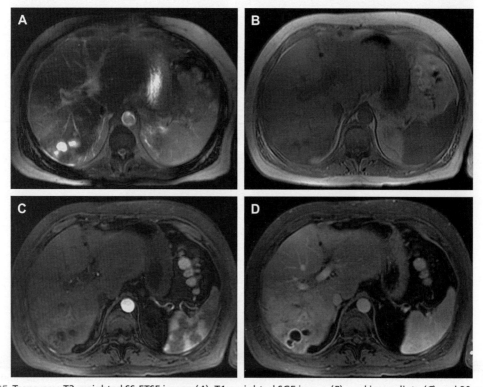

Fig. 25. Transverse T2-weighted SS-ETSE image (*A*); T1-weighted SGE image (*B*); and immediate (*C*) and 90-second (*D*) fat-suppressed postgadolinium 3D GRE images at 3T. There are multiple lesions in the right hepatic lobe that demonstrate high signal intensity on the T2-weighted image (*A*), low signal intensity on the T1-weighted image (*B*), and mild enhancement of the lesion wall immediately following administration of contrast (*C*) that persists and intensifies on the interstitial phase (*D*), with no progressive internal stromal enhancement, consistent with hepatic pyogenic abscess.

is no centripetal filling; a moderate perilesional enhancement usually is present on the arterial-dominant phase because of hyperemic inflammatory effects on adjacent liver.

Fungal abscesses generally are multiple and smaller than 1 cm. Fungal microabscesses demonstrate high T2-weighted signal (accentuated by the fact that the patient frequently has undergone blood transfusion so background liver is dark) and are signal-void on dynamic postgadolinium images, with no appreciable abscess wall enhancement.

Summary and outlook

The main advantage of liver imaging at 3T is the ability to acquire high-quality, relatively artifact-free, thin-section postgadolinium T1-weighted 3D GRE sequences. This high spatial resolution is comparable to current-generation multidetector CT, but with the advantage of unmatched intrinsic soft tissue contrast resolution. This capability gives potential advantages for the detection and characterization of small lesions. It seems that there are advantages of 3T imaging for the detection and characterization of small hypervascular malignant diseases, such as HCC and metastases. Premalignant lesions (eg, dysplastic nodules) and some enhancing small and ultrasmall benign lesions (eg, hemangiomas, FNHs, or bile duct hamartomas) may appear with better conspicuity at 3T.

Imaging at 3T is in the early phases. It requires optimization of the pulse sequence parameters normally used at 1.5T to compensate for different relaxation kinetics, and modifications need to be developed to overcome major disadvantages of higher field imaging, particularly SAR restriction. Further research and development of new sequence design are necessary to overcome the fair quality notable on in- and out-of-phase T1-weighted GRE sequences and to minimize artifacts that appear at this field strength, such as standing wave/conductivity artifact. We believe that the present limitations may reflect only the stage of development and are not intrinsic limitations of 3T in imaging the liver.

References

[1] Stanisz GJ, Odrobina EE, Pun J, et al. T1, T2 relaxation and magnetization transfer in tissue at 3.0T. Magn Reson Med 2005;54:507–12.
[2] de Bazelaire CM, Duhamel GD, Rofsky NM, et al. MR imaging relaxation times of abdominal and pelvic tissues measured in vivo at 3.0 T: preliminary results. Radiology 2004;230:652–9.
[3] Merkle EM, Dale BM. Abdominal MRI at 3.0 T: the basics revisited. AJR Am J Roentgenol 2006; 186:1524–32.
[4] Morakkabati-Spitz N, Gieseke J, Kuhl C, et al. 3.0-T high-field magnetic resonance imaging of the female pelvis: preliminary experiences. Eur J Radiol 2005;15:639–44.
[5] Gibbs GF, Huston J 3rd, Bernstein MA, et al. Improved image quality of intracranial aneurysms: 3.0-T versus 1.5-T time-of-flight MR angiography. AJNR Am J Neuroradiol 2004;25:84–7.
[6] Leiner T, de Vries M, Hoogeveen R, et al. Contrast-enhanced peripheral MR angiography at 3.0 Tesla: initial experience with a whole-body scanner in healthy volunteers. J Magn Reson Imaging 2003;17:609–14.
[7] Allkemper T, Tombach B, Schwindt W, et al. Acute and subacute intracerebral hemorrhages: comparison of MR imaging at 1.5 and 3.0 T: initial experience. Radiology 2004;232:874–81.
[8] Frayne R, Goodyear BG, Dickhoff P, et al. Magnetic resonance imaging at 3.0 Tesla: challenges and advantages in clinical neurological imaging. Invest Radiol 2003;38:385–402.
[9] Lenk S, Ludescher B, Martirosan P, et al. 3.0 T high-resolution MR imaging of carpal ligaments and TFCC. Rofo 2004;176:664–7.
[10] Eckstein F, Charles HC, Buck RJ, et al. Accuracy and precision of quantitative assessment of cartilage morphology by magnetic resonance imaging at 3.0T. Arthritis Rheum 2005;52:3132–6.
[11] Kornaat PR, Reeder SB, Koos S, et al. MR imaging of articular cartilage at 1.5T and 3.0T: comparison of SPGR and SSFP sequences. Osteoarthritis Cartilage 2005;13:338–44.
[12] Hussain SM, Wielopolski PA, Martin DR. Abdominal magnetic resonance imaging at 3.0 T: problem or a promise for the future? Top Magn Reson Imaging 2005;16:325–35.
[13] von Falkenhausen MM, Lutterbey G, Morakkabati-Spitz N, et al. High-field-strength MR imaging of the liver at 3.0 T: intraindividual comparative study with MR imaging at 1.5 T. Radiology 2006; 241:156–66.
[14] Diego R, Martin DR, Friel HT, et al. Approach to abdominal imaging at 1.5 tesla and optimization at 3 tesla. Magn Reson Imaging Clin N Am 2005;16:241–54.
[15] Schindera ST, Merkle EM, Dale BM, et al. Abdominal magnetic resonance imaging at 3.0 T: what is the ultimate gain in signal-to-noise ratio? Acad Radiol 2006;13:1236–43.
[16] Merkle E, Dale BM, Paulson EK. Abdominal MR imaging at 3.0T. Magn Reson Imaging Clin N Am 2006;14:17–26.
[17] Gaa J, Hutabu H, Jenkins RL, et al. Liver masses: replacement of conventional T2-weighted spin echo MR imaging with breath-hold MR imaging. Radiology 1996;200:459–64.
[18] De Lange EE, Mugler JP III, Bosworth JE, et al. MR imaging of the liver: breath-hold T1-weighted MP-GRE compared with conventional

T2-weighted SE imaging-lesion detection, localization, and characterization. Radiology 1994; 190:727–36.

[19] Kanematsu M, Semelka R, Matsuo M, et al. Gadolinium-enhanced MR imaging of the liver: optimizing imaging delay for hepatic arterial and portal venous phases—a prospective randomized study in patients with chronic liver damage. Radiology 2002;225:407–15.

[20] Martin DR, Semelka RC. Magnetic resonance imaging of the liver: review of techniques and approach to common diseases. Semin Ultrasound CT MR 2005;26:116–31.

[21] Rofsky NM, Lee VS, Laub G, et al. Abdominal MR imaging with a volumetric interpolated breath-hold examination. Radiology 1999;212: 876–84.

[22] Balci NC, Semelka RC. Contrast agents for MR imaging of the liver. Radiol Clin North Am 2005;43:887–98.

[23] Semelka RC, Helmberger TK. Contrast agents for MR imaging of the liver. Radiology 2001;218: 27–38.

[24] Shamsi K. Gd-EOB-DTPA, a liver-specific contrast agent for MRI: results of a placebo controlled, double blind dose ranging study in patients with focal liver lesions. Presented at the 10th Scientific Meeting and Exhibition of the International Society for Magnetic Resonance in Medicine. Honolulu, Hawaii, May 18–24, 2002.

[25] Grazioli L, Morana G, Kirchin MA, et al. Accurate differentiation of focal nodular hyperplasia from hepatic adenoma at gadobenate dimeglumine-enhanced MR imaging: prospective study. Radiology 2005;236:166–77.

[26] Lim JS, Kim M-J, Jung YY, et al. Gadobenate dimeglumine as an intrabiliary contrast agent: comparison with mangafodipir trisodium with respect to non-dilated biliary tree depiction. Korean J Radiol 2005;6:229–34.

[27] Nitz WR. SAR reduction (GRAPPA). In: Runge VM, Nitz WR, Schmeets SH, et al, editors. Clinical 3T magnetic resonance. 1st edition. New York: Thieme; 2007. p. 34–5.

[28] Pruessmann KP. Parallel imaging at high field strength: synergies and joint potential. Top Magn Reson Imaging 2004;15:237–44.

[29] Glockner JF, Hu HH, Stanley DW, et al. Parallel MR imaging: a user's guide. Radiographics 2005; 25:1279–97.

[30] Tanenbaum LN. Clinical 3T MR imaging: mastering the challenges. Magn Reson Imaging Clin N Am 2006;14:1–15.

[31] Hargreaves BA, Cunningham CH, Nishimura DG, et al. Variable-rate selective excitation for rapid MRI sequences. Magn Reson Med 2004;52:590–7.

[32] Hennig J, Weigel M, Scheffler K. Multiecho sequences with variable refocusing flip angles: optimization of signal behavior using smooth transitions between pseudo steady states (TRAPS). Magn Reson Med 2003;49:527–35.

[33] Bernstein MA, Huston J 3rd, Ward HA. Imaging artifacts at 3.0T. Magn Reson Imaging 2006;24: 735–46.

[34] Sreenivas M, Lowry M, Gibbs P, et al. A simple solution for reducing artefacts due to conductive and dielectric effects in clinical magnetic resonance imaging at 3 T. Eur J Radiol 2007;62:143–6.

[35] Sasaki M, Shibata E, Kanbara Y, et al. Enhancement effects and relaxivities of gadolinium-DTPA at 1.5 T versus 3 Tesla: a phantom study. Magn Reson Med Sci 2005;4:145–9.

[36] Nobauer-Huhmann IM, Ba-Ssalamah A, Mlynarik V, et al. Magnetic resonance imaging contrast enhancement of brain tumors at 3 tesla versus 1.5 tesla. Invest Radiol 2002;37:114–9.

[37] Farrell G, Larter C. Nonalcoholic fatty liver disease: from steatosis to cirrhosis. Hepatology 2006; 43:S99–112.

[38] Gholam PM, Flancbaum L, Machan JT, et al. Nonalcoholic fatty liver disease in severely obese subjects. Am J Gastroenterol 2007;102:399–408.

[39] Harrison SA, Neuschwander-Tetri BA. Nonalcoholic fatty liver disease and nonalcoholic steatohepatitis. Clin Liver Dis 2004;8:871–9.

[40] Mitchell DG. Focal manifestations of diffuse liver disease at MR imaging. Radiology 1992;185:1–11.

[41] Alústiza JM, Artetxe J, Castiella A, et al. MR quantification of hepatic iron concentration. Radiology 2004;230:479–84.

[42] Kanematsu M, Semelka RC, Leonardou P, et al. Hepatocellular carcinoma of diffuse type: MR imaging findings and clinical manifestations. J Magn Reson Imaging 2003;18:189–95.

[43] Krinsky GA, Lee VS. MR imaging of cirrhotic nodules. Abdom Imaging 2000;25:471–82.

[44] Martin DR, Semelka RC. Imaging of benign and malignant focal liver lesions. Magn Reson Imaging Clin N Am 2001;9(VI–VII):785–802.

[45] Winston CB, Schwartz LH, Fong Y, et al. Hepatocellular carcinoma: MR imaging findings in cirrhotic livers and noncirrhotic livers. Radiology 1999;210:75–9.

[46] Kelekis NL, Semelka RC, Woawattanakul S, et al. Hepatocellular carcinoma in North America: a multiinstitutional study of appearance on T1-weighted, T2 weighted, and serial gadolinium-enhanced gradient-echo images. AJR Am J Roentgenol 1998;170:1005–13.

[47] Bruneton JN, Raffaelli C, Maestro C, et al. Benign liver lesions: implications of detection in cancer patients. Eur Radiol 1995;5:387–90.

[48] Shoenut JP, Semelka RC, Levi C, et al. Ciliated hepatic foregut cysts: US, CT, and contrast-enhanced MR imaging. Abdom Imaging 1994; 19:150–2.

[49] Chung EB. Multiple bile-duct hamartomas. Cancer 1970;26:287–96.

[50] Semelka RC, Hussain SM, Marcos HB, et al. Biliary hamartomas: solitary and multiple lesions shown on current MR techniques including gadolinium enhancement. J Magn Reson Imaging 1999;10:196–201.

[51] Craig J, Peters R, Edmonson H. Tumors of the liver and intrahepatic bile ducts. In: Hartman H, Sobin L, editors. Atlas of tumor pathology. 2nd edition. Washington, DC: Armed Forces Institute of Pathology.

[52] Karhunen PJ. Benign hepatic tumours and tumour like conditions in men. J Clin Pathol 1986;39:183–8.

[53] Semelka RC, Brown ED, Ascher SM, et al. Hepatic hemangiomas: a multi-institutional study of appearance on T2-weighted and serial gadolinium-enhanced gradient-echo MR images. Radiology 1994;192:401–6.

[54] Danet IM, Semelka RC, Braga L, et al. Giant cavernous hemangioma of the liver: MR imaging characteristics in 24 patients. Magn Reson Imaging 2003;21:95–101.

[55] Semelka RC, Worawattenakul S, Noone K, et al. Chemotherapy-treated liver metastases mimicking hemangiomas on MR images. Abdom Imaging 1999;24:378–82.

[56] Vilgrain Valérie. Focal nodular hyperplasia. Eur J Radiol 2006;58:236–45.

[57] Stanley G, Jeffrey RB, Feliz B. CT findings and histopathology of intratumoral steatosis in focal nodular hyperplasia: case report and review of the literature. J Comput Assist Tomogr 2002;26: 815–7.

[58] Mortele KJ, Praet M, van Vlierberghe H, et al. CT and MR imaging findings in focal nodular hyperplasia of the liver: radiologic-pathologic correlation. AJR Am J Roentgenol 2000;175: 687–92.

[59] Wiener Y, Dushnitzky T, Slutzki S, et al. Synchronous bleeding of liver adenomatosis and possible relation to acoustic trauma. HPB Surg 2001; 3:267–9.

[60] Chiche L, Dao T, Salame E, et al. Liver adenomatosis: reappraisal, diagnosis, and surgical management: eight new cases and review of the literature. Ann Surg 2000;231:74–81.

[61] Evlampia A, Psatha EA, Semelka RC, et al. Hepatocellular adenomas in men: MRI findings in four patients. J Magn Reson Imaging 2005; 22:258–64.

[62] Foster JH, Berman MM. The malignant transformation of liver cell adenomas. Arch Surg 1994; 129:712–7.

[63] Paulson EK, McClellan JS, Washington K, et al. Hepatic adenoma: MR characteristics and correlation with pathologic findings. AJR Am J Roentgenol 1994;163:113–6.

MAGNETIC RESONANCE IMAGING CLINICS

Magn Reson Imaging Clin N Am 15 (2007) 349–353

MR Imaging of the Pancreas: 1.5T versus 3T

Robert R. Edelman, MD[a,b],*

- References

Pancreatic cancer is the ninth or tenth most commonly diagnosed cancer, but the third leading cause of cancer death in men and the fourth in women [1]. Of the approximately 30,000 individuals diagnosed with this highly lethal cancer each year in the United States, most cases are unresectable and approximately 97% of patients die as a result of the disease [2,3]. Early detection promises a better prognosis, however. For instance, one study of pancreatic cancers smaller than 2 cm found that all lesions were resectable [4]. Survival is reported to approach 100% for tumors smaller than 1 cm and limited to the intraductal epithelium without parenchymal, vascular, perineural, or lymphatic invasion [5]. Several imaging tests are currently available for diagnosis and staging, including CT, endoscopic ultrasound (EUS), MR imaging, and positron emission tomography. Each imaging test offers advantages and limitations [6].

CT is moderately sensitive for pancreatic cancer. A retrospective study reported a sensitivity of 72% and specificity of 100% to detect pancreatic cancers 2 cm or smaller with helical CT [7]. Interestingly, one retrospective study found that CT findings diagnostic or suspicious for pancreatic cancer were present in as many as 50% of patients up to 18 months before the clinical diagnosis of pancreatic cancer [8]. The most reliable early finding in these cases was pancreatic duct dilatation. Extremely small tumors (<1 cm) often show ductal dilatation without an associated mass [9].

EUS is the most sensitive test (approaching 100%), but the invasive nature of the test limits its potential as a screening test for early-stage tumors [10]. Use of EUS for screening may be justifiable in certain high-risk individuals, however [11,12].

The pancreas is a technically challenging organ for evaluation by MR imaging [13]. It moves with respiration. Positioned within the retroperitoneum, it is adjacent to air-containing motile small bowel loops that can produce blurring and ghost artifacts. The central location within the abdomen and distant positioning from the elements of a phased-array coil reduce the available signal-to-noise ratio (SNR). Moreover, various disease processes affect the pancreas and may have similar presentations. For instance, pancreatic cancer may cause inflammatory changes that are indistinguishable from pancreatitis caused by a stone in the ampulla. In comparing MR imaging with CT, several studies suggest that MR imaging is comparable or superior for detection and staging of pancreatic cancer [14,15]. Moreover, MR imaging is generally superior to CT for evaluation of the hepatobiliary ducts.

Compared with imaging at 1.5T, 3T offers the potential of a twofold improvement in the SNR. A twofold improvement in the SNR equates to

[a] Department of Radiology, Evanston Northwestern Healthcare, Walgreen Building, Room G534, 2650 Ridge Avenue, Evanston, IL 60201, USA
[b] Feinberg School of Medicine, Northwestern University, Evanston, Illinois, USA
* Department of Radiology, Evanston Northwestern Healthcare, Walgreen Building, Room G534, 2650 Ridge Avenue, Evanston, IL 60201.
E-mail address: redelman@enh.org

1064-9689/07/$ – see front matter © 2007 Elsevier Inc. All rights reserved.
mri.theclinics.com
doi:10.1016/j.mric.2007.06.005

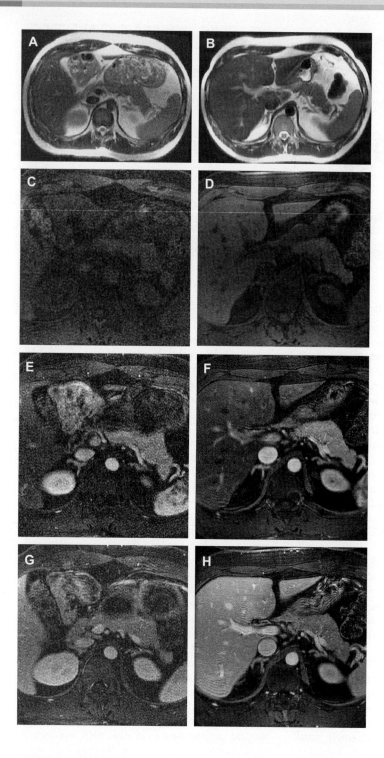

Fig. 1. Comparison of images acquired at 1.5T and 3T in a normal subject. The improved SNR at 3T is manifested as a markedly reduced level of image graininess. The differences in image quality between 3T and 1.5T are made obvious by the small fields of view used. Examples of a 1.5T single-shot fast spin-echo acquisition (*A*), a 3T single-shot fast spin-echo acquisition (*B*), a 1.5T precontrast fat-suppressed three-dimensional (3D) acquisition (*C*), a 3T precontrast fat-suppressed 3D acquisition (*D*), a 1.5T arterial phase fat-suppressed 3D acquisition (*E*), a 3T arterial phase fat-suppressed 3D acquisition (*F*), a 1.5T delayed postcontrast fat-suppressed 3D acquisition (*G*), and a 3T delayed postcontrast fat-suppressed 3D acquisition (*H*). (*From* Edelman RR, Salanitri G, Brand R, et al. Magnetic resonance imaging of the pancreas at 3.0 tesla: qualitative and quantitative comparison with 1.5 tesla. Invest Radiol 2006;41:177; with permission.)

a fourfold reduction in scan time, which would improve patient tolerance, reduce the likelihood of respiratory motion artifact, and improve the temporal resolution of multiphase contrast-enhanced studies. Alternatively, one could reduce the slice thickness in half or decrease the field of view by approximately 40%. Moreover, parallel imaging techniques generally work better at the higher field strength, providing additional flexibility in the choice of imaging protocol.

There are several reasons why the theoretic twofold improvement in SNR may not be achievable in practice, however [16]. The T1 relaxation times of the abdominal organs are on the order of 20%

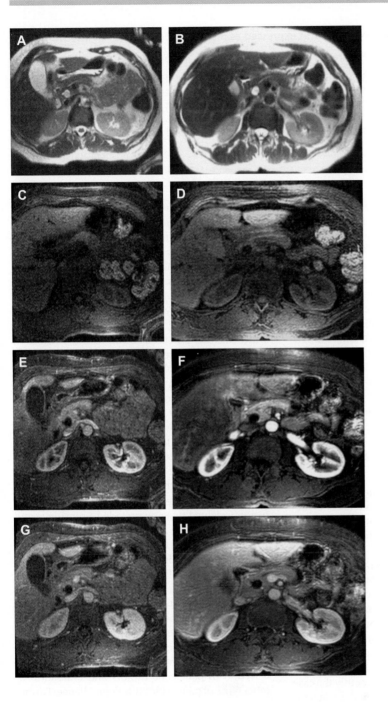

Fig. 2. Patient with cyst in the head of the pancreas. Examples of a 1.5T single-shot fast spin-echo acquisition (*A*) and a 3T single-shot fast spin-echo acquisition (*B*). Although the SNR is obviously better in *B*, there is also greater signal nonuniformity across the image compared with *A*. Examples of a 1.5T precontrast fat-suppressed three-dimensional (3D) acquisition (*C*), a 3T precontrast fat-suppressed 3D acquisition (*D*), a 1.5T arterial phase fat-suppressed 3D acquisition (*E*), a 3T arterial phase fat-suppressed 3D acquisition (*F*), a 1.5T delayed postcontrast fat-suppressed 3D acquisition (*G*), and a 3T delayed postcontrast fat-suppressed 3D acquisition (*H*). (*From* Edelman RR, Salanitri G, Brand R, et al. Magnetic resonance imaging of the pancreas at 3.0 tesla: qualitative and quantitative comparison with 1.5 tesla. Invest Radiol 2006;41:177; with permission.)

to 30% higher at 3T than at 1.5T [17]. Chemical shift artifact is twice as large at 3T. Although a concern for low bandwidth acquisitions, this has not proven to be a significant limitation using typical acquisition parameters. Moreover, it becomes irrelevant for commonly used fat-suppressed acquisitions, such as volumetric interpolated breath hold examination (VIBE) or liver acquisition volume acceleration (LAVA).

The fourfold higher rate of power deposition at 3T is also a concern. The VIBE and LAVA sequences use small excitation flip angles, however. Because the power deposition quadratically depends on flip angle, power deposition is not a significant limitation. Of greater concern is the impact on single-shot turbo spin-echo sequences that use trains of refocusing pulses. The specific absorption rate (SAR) limitations are readily overcome using

Table 1:   **SNR ratios at 3T compared with 1.5T expressed as mean (SD)**

	Pancreas	Liver	Spleen	Muscle
SSFSE	1.63 (0.39)	1.82 (0.39)	1.45 (0.18)	2.01 (0.16)
Precontrast 3D	1.28 (0.29)	1.26 (0.30)	1.16 (0.27)	1.76 (0.45)
Postcontrast 3D (arterial phase)	2.02 (0.28)	1.60 (0.42)	1.47 (0.26)	1.94 (0.32)
Postcontrast 3D (delayed phase)	1.63 (0.51)	2.01 (0.25)	1.66 (0.06)	2.31 (0.47)

Abbreviations: 3D, breath-hold fat-suppressed 3D gradient-echo sequence; SSFSE, single-shot fast spin-echo sequence.

refocusing pulses with flip angles less than 180°, variable rate selective excitation (VERSE) techniques, hyperechoes, or parallel imaging.

The author and his colleagues performed a study comparing 1.5T and 3T for imaging of the pancreas (Figs. 1 and 2) [18]. Imaging parameters were nearly identical, as were the configurations of the phased-array coils. The SNR benefit of 3T was significantly greater on contrast-enhanced as compared with noncontrast T1-weighted three-dimensional (3D) gradient-echo images (Table 1). With qualitative comparison of images obtained at the two magnetic field strengths, the fat-suppressed 3D gradient-echo images obtained at 3T were preferred, whereas the single-shot turbo spin-echo images obtained at 1.5T were preferred because of better signal homogeneity.

Allowing for the small size of this study, the findings can be summarized as follows:

1. There is a substantial improvement in the SNR for precontrast imaging of the pancreas. As predicted from the longer T1 relaxation times, this improvement is less than the potential factor of 2.
2. After the administration of contrast agent, a full twofold improvement in the SNR is obtained. This is a promising result, particularly because the use of contrast enhancement is the norm for detection and characterization of pancreatic lesions. Note that the T1 relaxivities of the standard extracellular paramagnetic contrast agents used by Rohrer and colleagues [19] are comparable at 3T and 1.5T. This is not necessarily the case for newer contrast agents that bind to macromolecules for the purpose of relaxivity enhancement. Such agents tend to demonstrate lower T1 relaxivity at the higher field strength.

Image artifacts did not seem worse over the pancreatic region at 3T than at 1.5T. Susceptibility artifact is acceptable so long as a short echo time (eg, <2 milliseconds) and reasonably high sampling bandwidth are used for gradient-echo acquisitions. Turbo spin-echo acquisitions are naturally resistant to such artifacts. Dielectric artifacts, which can be significant over the left lobe of the liver, did not prove to be particularly noticeable over the pancreatic bed. Such artifacts are much more severe in patients with gross ascites, however, particularly with turbo spin-echo pulse sequences; thus, imaging of such patients is better done at 1.5T.

These results would suggest that one can reasonably reduce the slice thickness by a factor of 2 for pancreatic imaging at 3T compared with 1.5T, which has the potential to improve the detection rate of small pancreatic tumors substantially. Another potential application of the improved SNR at 3T is for diffusion imaging of the pancreas. Diffusion imaging monitors the random motion of water molecules, which can be more or less restricted because of local variations in tissue structure. Although the technique is primarily used on a clinical basis for early detection of stroke, there is growing interest in its use for detection of abdominal malignancies. In one study of diffusion imaging used to detect pancreatic adenocarcinoma, high b-value diffusion-weighted imaging provided a sensitivity and specificity of 96.2% and 98.6%, respectively [20].

Pancreas imaging typically includes evaluation of the hepatobiliary ducts using MR cholangiopancreatography (MRCP). Although there are few publications comparing MRCP at 3T with that at 1.5T, early results suggest that image quality is as good or better at the higher field strength [21].

In summary, given the intrinsic SNR improvement from the higher static magnetic field strength, 3T holds considerable promise as a means for early detection of pancreatic tumors and evaluation of other types of pancreatic pathologic change. Further improvements are expected as phased-array coil designs evolve, higher relaxivity or tissue-specific contrast agents become available, and methods like transmit sensitivity encoding (SENSE) are implemented to improve image uniformity.

References

[1] Available at: www.pancreatica.org. Accessed June 15, 2007.

[2] Jemal A, Murray T, Samuels A, et al. Cancer statistics, 2003. CA Cancer J Clin 2003;53:5–26.

[3] Poston GJ, Williamson RC. Causes, diagnosis, and management of exocrine pancreatic cancer. Compr Ther 1990;16:36–42.

[4] Tsuchiya R, Noda T, Harada N, et al. Collective review of small carcinomas of the pancreas. Ann Surg 1986;203:77–81.

[5] Ariyama J, Suyama M, Satoh K, et al. Imaging of small pancreatic ductal adenocarcinoma. Pancreas 1998;16:396–401.

[6] Santo E. Pancreatic cancer imaging: which method? JOP 2004;5(4):253–7.

[7] Bronstein YL, Evelyne M, Loyer EM, et al. Detection of small pancreatic tumors with multiphasic helical CT. AJR Am J Roentgenol 2004;182: 619–23.

[8] Gangi S, Fletcher JG, Nathan MA, et al. Time interval between abnormalities seen on CT and the clinical diagnosis of pancreatic cancer: retrospective review of CT scans obtained before diagnosis. AJR Am J Roentgenol 2004;182:897–903.

[9] Ishikawa O, Ohigashi H, Imaoka S, et al. Minute carcinoma of the pancreas measuring 1 cm or less in diameter: collective review of Japanese case reports. Hepatogastroenterology 1999;46:8–15.

[10] Hunt GC, Faigel DO. Assessment of EUS for diagnosing, staging, and determining resectability of pancreatic cancer: a review. Gastrointest Endosc 2002;55:232–7.

[11] Canto M, Wroblewski L, Goggins M, et al. Screening for pancreatic neoplasia in high-risk individuals: the Johns Hopkins experience [abstract]. Gastroenterology 2002;122(Suppl 1):A17.

[12] Goggins M, Canto M, Hruban R. Can we screen high-risk individuals to detect early pancreatic carcinoma? J Surg Oncol 2000;74:243–8.

[13] Keogan M, Edelman R. Technologic advances in abdominal MR imaging. Radiology 2001;220: 310–20.

[14] Sheridan MB, Ward J, Guthrie JA, et al. Dynamic contrast enhanced MR imaging and dual-phase helical CT in the preoperative assessment of suspected pancreatic cancer: a comparative study with receiver operating characteristic analysis. AJR Am J Roentgenol 1999;173:583–90.

[15] Schima W, Fugger R, Schober E, et al. Diagnosis and staging of pancreatic cancer: comparison of mangafodipir trisodium-enhanced MR imaging and contrast enhanced helical hydro-CT. AJR Am J Roentgenol 2002;179:717–24.

[16] Merkle EM, Dale BM. Abdominal MRI at 3.0 T: the basics revisited. AJR Am J Roentgenol 2006; 186:1524–32.

[17] de Bazelaire CMJ, Duhamel GD, Rofsky NM, et al. MR imaging relaxation times of abdominal and pelvic tissues measured in vivo at 3.0 T: preliminary results. Radiology 2004;230:652–9.

[18] Edelman RR, Salanitri G, Brand R, et al. Magnetic resonance imaging of the pancreas at 3.0 tesla qualitative and quantitative comparison with 1.5 tesla. Invest Radiol 2006;41:175–80.

[19] Rohrer M, Bauer H, Mintorovitch J, et al. Comparison of magnetic properties of MRI contrast media solutions at different magnetic field strengths. Invest Radiol 2005;40(11):715–24.

[20] Ichikawa1 T, Erturk SM, Motosugi U, et al. High-b value diffusion-weighted MRI for detecting pancreatic adenocarcinoma: preliminary results. AJR Am J Roentgenol 2007;188:409–14.

[21] Merkle EM, Haugan PA, Thomas J, et al. 3.0-versus 1.5-T MR cholangiography, 2006 cholangiography: a pilot study. AJR Am J Roentgenol 2006;186:516–21.

MAGNETIC
RESONANCE
IMAGING CLINICS

Magn Reson Imaging Clin N Am 15 (2007) 355–364

MR Cholangiopancreatography: 1.5T versus 3T

Sebastian T. Schindera, MD[a], Elmar M. Merkle, MD[b],*

- MR imaging of the biliary tract system
  Quantitative comparison of 3T with 1.5T
  Qualitative comparison of 3T with 1.5T
  Comparison of MR
    cholangiopancreatography sequences
    within 3T
  Contrast-enhanced MR cholangiography
- MR imaging of the pancreatic ductal
  system

- *Impact of susceptibility artifacts on*
  MR cholangiopancreatography images
  at 3T
- *Impact of B1-inhomogeneity artifacts on*
  MR cholangiopancreatography images
  at 3T
- Summary
- Acknowledgment
- References

Evaluation of the biliary tract system with MR imaging using heavily T2-weighted sequences was first described in 1991 [1]. Since then, MR imaging of the pancreaticobiliary tree, referred to as MR cholangiopancreatography (MRCP), has achieved widespread success as a diagnostic tool among radiologists, gastroenterologists, and hepatobiliary surgeons for two reasons: because the technique relies on the inherent contrast-related properties of fluid-filled compartments, no administration of exogenous contrast agents is required for MRCP examinations, and MRCP does not require radiation. The main competitor of MRCP in the assessment of the pancreaticobiliary tree is endoscopic retrograde cholangiopancreatography (ERCP), owing to its higher spatial resolution and potential for image-guided therapy; however, ERCP is an invasive technique that has a reported complication rate (eg, duodenal perforation, pancreatitis, bleeding and sepsis) of up to 5.0% [2,3]. ERCP also is more expensive and operator dependent than MRCP. Furthermore, MRCP has a high sensitivity

and specificity for the evaluation of various pancreaticobiliary pathologies [4–13]. For all of these reasons, MRCP has replaced diagnostic ERCP in the last few years, unless an intervention or tissue sampling is required.

In recent years, high-field whole-body MR imaging at 3T has gained substantial clinical interest as dedicated torso array receive-only coils for 3T MR systems became available. The main reason for the increased clinical use of 3T units is the desire for an increased signal-to-noise ratio (SNR) at the higher magnetic field strength compared with standard 1.5T. Substantial benefits of 3T units have been demonstrated for imaging the brain and the musculoskeletal system but not for body MR imaging [14]. Regarding MRCP, it is unclear whether the higher magnetic field strength is clearly superior to the standard field strength of 1.5T. This article summarizes the peer-reviewed literature available on 3T MRCP and discusses the advantages and disadvantages of the higher magnetic field strength for MRCP in comparison with 1.5T.

[a] Interventional and Pediatric Radiology, University Hospital of Bern, Institute for Diagnostic, Inselspital Bern, Freiburgstrasse 10, CH-3010 Bern, Switzerland
[b] Department of Radiology, Duke University Medical Center, DUMC Box 3808, Durham, NC 27710, USA
* Corresponding author.
E-mail address: elmar.merkle@duke.edu (E.M. Merkle).

1064-9689/07/$ – see front matter © 2007 Elsevier Inc. All rights reserved.
mri.theclinics.com

doi:10.1016/j.mric.2007.06.009

MR imaging of the biliary tract system

In the past decade, MRCP at the standard field strength of 1.5T has proven highly accurate for the evaluation of the extrahepatic biliary system [4,5,8,9,13]. For the evaluation of the intrahepatic biliary system, however, particularly in the absence of obstructive biliary disease, MRCP has several diagnostic limitations caused by the limited spatial resolution and poor SNR of 1.5T [15]. These limitations may be overcome by using high-field whole-body 3T MR systems, which increase the SNR substantially. The greater SNR can be maintained to improve image quality or be traded in for increased spatial or temporal resolution [14,16]. Figs. 1–4, acquired on 3T MR systems and demonstrating several cases of biliary pathologies, exemplify the excellent image quality offered by these high-field MR systems.

In the past few years, several studies of healthy volunteers or patients who did or did not have biliary dilatation quantitatively and qualitatively compared MRCP examinations at 3T with those at 1.5T [17–20]. Overall, the quantitative image analysis revealed superior results at 3T, whereas no distinct preference in terms of image quality was found for either of the two field strengths [17–20].

Quantitative comparison of 3T with 1.5T

In a pilot study of 15 healthy volunteers, our group compared three MRCP sequences: a breath-hold, multi-slice, T2-weighted half-Fourier single-shot turbo-spin echo (HASTE) sequence; a breath-hold, single-slice, T2-weighted rapid acquisition with relaxation enhancement (RARE) sequence; and a respiratory-triggered, multi-slice, three-dimensional (3D) T2-weighted turbo-spin echo (TSE). All

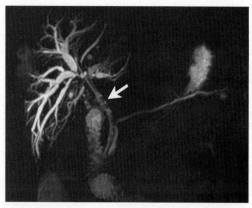

Fig. 1. Coronal maximum-intensity projection of a respiratory-triggered, 3D fast spin echo MRCP dataset acquired at 3T demonstrating a dilated intrahepatic biliary system due to hilar cholangiocarcinoma. Filling defects (*arrow*) in the common bile duct represent blood clots next to the biliary stent.

sequences were acquired on a 3T and a 1.5T MR system [17]. Contrast-to-noise ratios (CNRs) between the intra- and extrahepatic biliary ductal system and the periductal tissue were higher at 3T than at 1.5T. These differences were statistically significant for the respiratory-triggered TSE sequence in three different locations (common bile duct, left hepatic duct, and right posterior segmental branch), for the RARE sequence in two locations (common bile duct and right posterior segmental branch), and for the HASTE sequence in one location (left hepatic duct).

In a subsequent investigation, our group quantitatively assessed the MR image datasets of 100 patients who did or did not have biliary dilatation undergoing MRCP on a 3T or a 1.5T unit [20]. The MR sequence protocol consisted of a breath-hold, single-slice RARE and a respiratory-triggered, 3D TSE sequence. The CNR at 3T increased, on average up to 38.1%, thus confirming our preliminary data gathered in healthy volunteers.

A study by O'Regan and colleagues [18] yielded diverse quantitative data in 10 patients undergoing an MRCP on a 3T and a 1.5T MR system. A significantly higher CNR was seen at 3T between the common bile duct and the liver on a HASTE sequence, whereas a thick-slab TSE sequence did not demonstrate an improvement in CNR at the higher field strength. This lack of increased CNR was attributed to the use of different receiver coils, namely a built-in whole-body coil at 3T and a dedicated torso array coil at 1.5T. In a study by Isoda and colleagues [19], consisting of 14 healthy volunteers, the CNR ratio between the intrahepatic bile ducts and the liver increased, on average, by 62% at 3T on heavily T2-weighted images obtained with a breath-hold, multi-slice HASTE sequence.

CNR increases at 3T are expected because twice the number of free water protons per voxel contributes to the MR signal at 3T compared with the lower field strength; however, the measured increase in CNR in all studies mentioned above was less than twofold [17–20]. One major reason is that increasing the magnetic field strength results in an increase of the T1 relaxation time and perhaps a slight decrease of the T2 relaxation time; both of these factors combine to reduce the net increase in MR signal to less than twofold [21]. Minor reasons for the diminished increase in CNR at 3T include the immature hardware and software, B1-inhomogeneity artifacts, and increased susceptibility artifacts.

Qualitative comparison of 3T with 1.5T

In both of our studies, qualitative image analysis of the visualization of the extrahepatic biliary ductal structures did not reveal any significant preference for either field strength [17,20]. In the study on

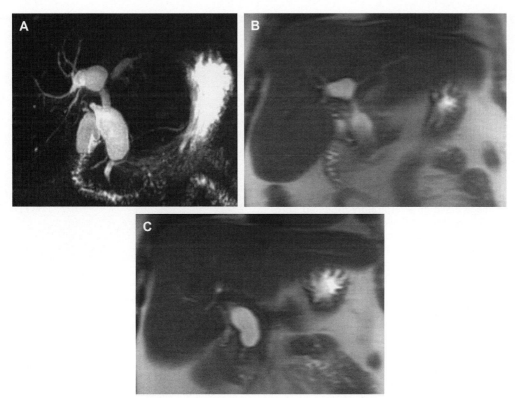

Fig. 2. (*A*) Coronal maximum-intensity projection of a respiratory-triggered, 3D fast spin echo MRCP dataset acquired at 3T showing a Todani-type IVa choledochal cyst in the intrahepatic biliary system and the common bile duct. Note a pancreas divisum. (*B*, *C*) Coronal, single-shot fast spin echo images again show the cystic dilations of the extrahepatic and intrahepatic biliary ductal system.

15 volunteers, the depiction of the common bile duct and the delineation of cystic duct insertion were graded subjectively by three readers as similar on both MR systems. In our study on 100 patients, three independent readers scored the overall diagnostic quality of the MRCP examinations acquired at both field strengths as moderate [20]. In contrast, O'Regan and colleagues [18] demonstrated a significantly better visualization of the pancreaticobiliary tree at 3T compared with 1.5T on HASTE and thick-slab TSE sequences. Isoda and colleagues [19] also reported a trend toward superior visualization of the cystic duct and the common bile duct with 3T using HASTE and 3D TSE sequences.

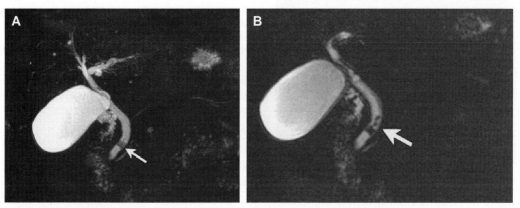

Fig. 3. Coronal maximum-intensity projection 3T MRCP image based on a respiratory-triggered, coronal, 3D T2-weighted TSE sequence (*A*) and coronal source MR image (*B*) show a filling defect in the distal common bile duct (*arrow*) that represents a gallstone.

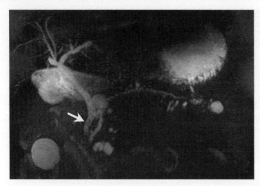

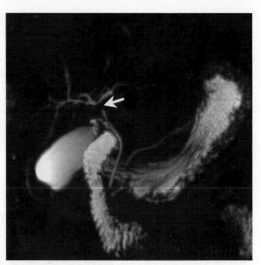

Fig. 4. Coronal maximum-intensity projection 3T MRCP image based on a respiratory-triggered, coronal, 3D T2-weighted TSE sequence shows a filling defect in the distal common bile duct (*arrow*) and a prominent, irregular pancreatic duct in a patient who has choledocholithiasis and chronic pancreatitis. Note the pseudocysts and the cystic dilations of the pancreatic side branches.

Fig. 6. Coronal maximum-intensity projection of a respiratory-triggered, 3D fast spin echo MRCP dataset acquired at 3T demonstrating the intrahepatic biliary system without pathologic finding. The right posterior segmental branch fuses with the right anterior segmental branch to form the right hepatic duct. The right hepatic duct fuses with the left hepatic duct to form the common hepatic duct. This is the most common normal biliary anatomy (seen in ∼60% of individuals) [22]. Note the band-like artifact in the common hepatic duct mimicking a biliary obstruction (*arrow*). This artifact is caused by the crossing right hepatic artery.

Besides the assessment of the extrahepatic biliary ductal system, we analyzed the presence of intrahepatic biliary ductal variants in our volunteer study [17]. The 3T magnet offered better sensitivity and specificity in the detection of intrahepatic biliary variants (Figs. 5 and 6) [22]. The biggest change was seen in the sensitivity in the detection of intrahepatic biliary variants when using the 3D-TSE sequence (53% at 1.5T versus 87% at 3T). This result may reflect the advantage of 3T MR units in which MR signal gain is particularly helpful in sequences with thin slices in the range of 1 mm. Furthermore, the confidence levels for the detection of biliary ductal variants were significantly higher for all three readers for the 3T magnet than for the 1.5T magnet. Thus, the higher magnetic field strength helped to improve the radiologist's confidence in diagnosing biliary ductal variants. This improved confidence is particularly valuable in the preoperative radiological assessment of living liver lobe donor candidates. In the future, 3T MR imaging might completely replace invasive preoperative planning in these patients, who usually are healthy subjects. Our preliminary findings are supported by Isoda and colleagues [19], who also saw a significant improvement in the visualization of intrahepatic bile ducts with 3T MR imaging.

Comparison of MR cholangiopancreatography sequences within 3T

Within 3T, maximum-intensity projections reconstructed from the source data of respiratory-triggered, 3D TSE sequences offered significantly higher CNR values in subjects who did not have biliary dilatation compared with other MRCP

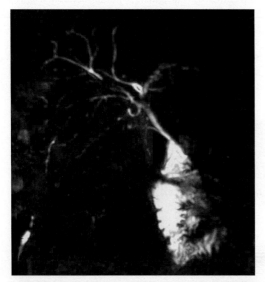

Fig. 5. Coronal maximum-intensity projection of a respiratory-triggered, 3D fast spin echo MRCP dataset acquired at 3T demonstrating normal depiction of the intrahepatic biliary ductal system and the biliary–enteric anastomosis in a patient with status post Whipple procedure.

sequences, such as the HASTE and RARE sequences [17,20]. In patients with a dilated common bile duct, however, there was no significant difference in CNR between the 3D TSE and the RARE sequences [20]. The superior CNR values on the 3D TSE sequence are in accordance with various other reports of 1T and 1.5T MR systems [23,24]. This increased CNR is not necessarily obvious, because the smaller voxel size of any 3D TSE sequence should generally decrease CNR. In this case, CNR increased because of respiratory triggering, which permits a dramatic increase in acquisition time.

In our study of 15 volunteers, we also saw a clear trend for superior visualization of the nondilated biliary tree at 3T with 3D TSE compared with the RARE and HASTE images [17]. Using a 1.5T MR system, Asbach and colleagues [24] found that the respiratory-triggered TSE sequence also demonstrated significantly better results regarding the depiction of the biliary tree compared with a breath-hold single-shot technique. This trend was not seen in our study of 100 patients [20]. Nevertheless, we continue to recommend, along with Asbach and colleagues [24], incorporation of respiratory-triggered TSE sequences, in addition to standard breath-hold MRCP sequences, into routine MR cholangiography sequence protocols.

Contrast-enhanced MR cholangiography

Although T2-weighted MRCP relies on the inherent contrast-enhanced properties of the fluid-filled pancreaticobiliary system, it lacks a functional component (eg, it cannot assess bile excretion dynamics). To overcome this limitation, T1-weighted MR cholangiography after the intravenous administration of hepatobiliary MR contrast agents, such as mangafodipir trisodium, has been introduced. Mangafodipir trisodium is a manganese-based contrast agent that is approved in Europe and other non-European countries for MR imaging of the hepatobiliary system, but is no longer available in the United States. Mangafodipir trisodium shortens T1 and is primarily excreted by way of bile. Contrast-enhanced MR cholangiography with mangafodipir trisodium has shown promising results for the assessment of bile duct leaks, intrahepatic anatomy, and biliary–enteric anastomoses [25–28]. To the best of our knowledge, no published reports are available on contrast-enhanced MR cholangiography with mangafodipir trisodium acquired at 3T.

Other potential contrast agents for contrast-enhanced MR cholangiography examinations are gadobenate dimeglumine and gadoxetic acid; both are gadolinium-based contrast agents. Gadobenate dimeglumine is approved in the United States for MR imaging of the central nervous system, and it is approved in Europe and non-European countries for MR imaging of the central nervous system and the liver. Up to 5% of the injected dose of gadobenate dimeglumine is eliminated from the body through the hepatobiliary pathway, resulting in hepatobiliary enhancement on T1-weighted images acquired between 1 and 3 hours after its administration [29]. Gadoxetic acid, a liver-specific contrast agent was approved recently in Europe and other non-European countries, but it has not been approved in the United States [30]. Up to 50% of gadoxetic acid is excreted unmetabolized by way of the hepatobiliary pathway [31–33]. The efficiency of gadobenate dimeglumine–enhanced and gadoxetic acid–enhanced MR cholangiography still has to be evaluated on 3T MR systems.

MR imaging of the pancreatic ductal system

It is well known from studies on 1.5T MR systems that MR imaging of the pancreatic ductal system is a challenge owing to the central location of the pancreas in the abdomen, which can diminish the MR signal substantially [34]. Furthermore, gas-filled bowel loops adjacent to the pancreas can cause susceptibility artifacts. Because these artifacts increase with the magnetic field strength, they are slightly larger at 3T than at 1.5T. In theory, it is possible that these enlarged susceptibility artifacts at 3T may obscure important findings within the ductal pancreatic system that may have been visualized at standard 1.5T MRCP. Isoda and colleagues [19] recently reported a clear trend toward improved visualization of the pancreatic duct in volunteers at 3T with a HASTE and a 3D TSE sequence. To the best of our knowledge, the impact of 3T MRCP on the image quality of the pancreas and its ductal system has not been reported in patients who have pancreatic disorders. Additional research is needed to assess the clinical usefulness of 3T MR imaging for the pancreas.

Impact of susceptibility artifacts on MR cholangiopancreatography images at 3T

Increased susceptibility artifacts at higher magnetic field strengths can cause impaired image quality of MRCP examinations at 3T [35]. These artifacts usually are caused by gas, metal implants, surgical debris, or physiologic or pathologic conditions accompanied by iron deposition, such as hemosiderosis and hemochromatosis [36,37]. Because susceptibility artifacts appear as areas of central signal void surrounded by a small, hyperintense rim, they may obscure the visualization of relevant anatomic structures, such as the pancreaticobiliary system, and prevent adequate image analysis [38].

To assess the extent of susceptibility artifacts from surgical clips from prior cholecystectomy at 3T, our group conducted an in vitro and in vivo study [35]. In the in vitro portion of the study, susceptibility artifacts were larger at 3T compared with 1.5T for two-dimensional, dual-echo, in- and opposed-phase T1- and T2-weighted MRCP sequences, with the differences being statistically significant. Susceptibility artifacts were most pronounced on the gradient echo sequence with the longer echo time and on multi-slice, 3D T2-weighted TSE images. The smallest susceptibility artifacts were noted on multi-slice T2-weighted HASTE imaging. In vivo MRCP image quality was impaired by susceptibility artifacts in 3 of 21 cases at 3T and in 2 of 21 cases at 1.5T. These artifacts were most pronounced on the gradient echo image with the longer echo time, with the differences being statistically significant within 1.5T and 3T (Fig. 7). Biliary pseudo-obstructions due to susceptibility artifacts from cholecystectomy surgical clips were not substantially more common on 3T MRCP. Based on this study, patients with a history of cholecystectomy should not be excluded from 3T MRCP.

Susceptibility artifacts also occur next to gas-filled structures. The enlarged susceptibility artifacts at 3T due to a gas and soft tissue interface can be helpful in the detection of intrahepatic pneumobilia (Fig. 8); however, intrahepatic pneumobilia in patients with a biliary–enteric anastomosis can make the evaluation of the biliary ductal system challenging at 3T.

Impact of B1-inhomogeneity artifacts on MR cholangiopancreatography images at 3T

In addition to the exacerbation of artifacts occurring at a field strength of 1.5T, specific 3T artifacts (eg, B1-inhomogeneity artifacts) can substantially impair the image quality of the pancreatic ductal system. These artifacts particularly affect the MR appearance of the pancreas and its ductal system at 3T because they occur mainly in the center of the MR

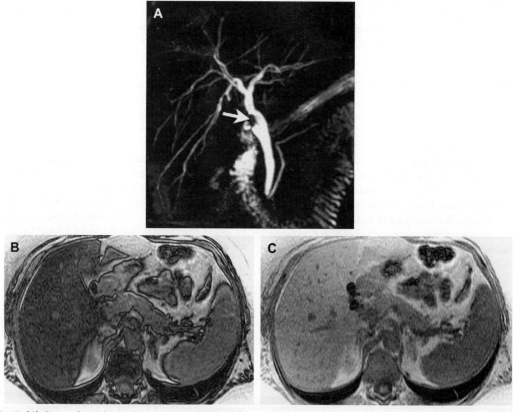

Fig. 7. (A) Coronal maximum-intensity projection of a respiratory-triggered, 3D turbo-spin echo MRCP dataset acquired at 3T shows a metal-induced susceptibility artifact (*arrow*) adjacent to the cystic duct remnant in a patient postcholecystectomy. The metal-induced susceptibility artifact causes a pseudo-obstruction of the common bile duct. (B) Axial gradient echo opposed-phase image showing a subtle hypointense area in the gallbladder fossa representing a metal-induced susceptibility artifact. (C) Axial gradient echo in-phase image shows a markedly larger susceptibility artifact in the gallbladder fossa compared with the artifact in (B), the gradient echo opposed-phase image. This is due to the longer echo time used to collect the in-phase echo.

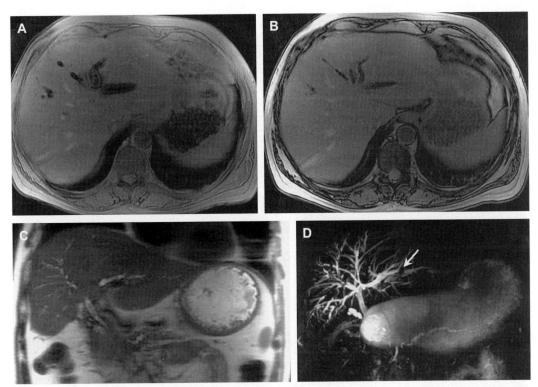

Fig. 8. Susceptibility artifacts due to pneumobilia shown on gradient echo in-phase (*A*) and opposed-phase images (*B*), coronal T2-weighted HASTE image (*C*), and coronal maximum-intensity projection image (*D*). All images were acquired on a 3T system. The axial gradient echo in-phase image acquired with an echo time of 4.4 milliseconds (*A*) shows markedly larger susceptibility artifacts due to pneumobilia compared with (*B*), the gradient echo opposed-phase image acquired with an echo time of 1.3 milliseconds. The gas-induced susceptibility artifacts in the biliary system also are seen as filling defects in the coronal HASTE image (*C*) and on the coronal maximum-intensity projection MRCP image (*arrow; D*).

image, distant from the receiver coil on TSE T2-weighted sequences. These artifacts can be substantial and, in selected cases, can obscure the entire pancreas. The origin of B1-inhomogeneity artifacts is described in detail elsewhere in this issue (see the article by Soher and colleagues on 3T MR physics). Although T1-weighted gradient echo imaging usually is not compromised by these artifacts, they often are problematic in T2-weighted TSE sequences, such as MRCP sequences [37,39]. Strong signal variations can be seen across an image, especially brightening or dark "holes," in regions away from the receiver coil, which are caused by constructive or destructive interference from the standing waves. These artifacts become more pronounced the larger the region of interest is relative to the wavelength (ie, they are seen more in obese patients with a distended abdomen than in thin patients).

In the last few years, different vendors have introduced radiofrequency (RF) cushions (also known as dielectric pads) to improve the homogeneity of the B1-field during abdominal MR imaging at 3T

[39]. They consist of ultrasound gel encapsulated in synthetic material. To eliminate the MR signal from the gel itself, the gel is mixed with a highly concentrated gadolinium- or manganese-based MR contrast agent. RF cushions can be used in conjunction with a body coil or a dedicated receive-only torso array coil. The dielectric cushion has a high dielectric constant and low conductivity that are designed to passively alter the geometry of the imaged object and change the phase of the radiofrequency standing waves in the abdomen. In many cases, the result is sufficient to reduce, eliminate, or move the B1-inhomogenity signal voids.

At our institution, we recently investigated in 20 volunteers the qualitative impact of an RF cushion on abdominal MR imaging at 3T [40]. Our data demonstrated a statistically significant benefit of the RF cushion on the image quality during TSE-based, T2-weighted imaging of the abdomen. This positive effect was achieved by decreasing the B1-inhomogeneity artifacts that commonly appear in the center of the abdomen—left hepatic lobe, epigastric region, and pancreas—when imaging without the

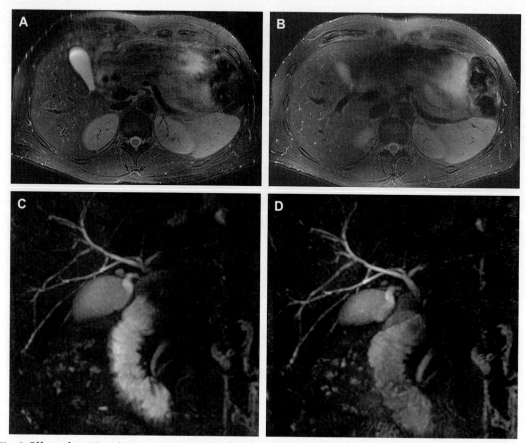

Fig. 9. Effect of an RF cushion on image quality of axial T2-weighted fast spin echo images (*A, B*), and coronal maximum-intensity projections (*C, D*) based on respiratory-triggered, 3D turbo-spin echo MRCP datasets acquired on a 3T system. The image acquired with the RF cushion in place (*A*) shows slightly less image degradation in the left hepatic lobe. The image acquired without the RF cushion (*B*) shows more B1-inhomogeneity artifacts that obscure parts of the left hepatic lobe. During MRCP imaging, no substantial difference in B1-inhomogeneity artifacts is seen between the image with the RF cushion (*C*) and the image without the RF cushion (*D*).

RF cushion, thus improving visualization of the liver parenchyma and pancreas. The decrease in B1-inhomogeneity artifacts was independent of the body habitus (eg, body mass index or fraction of body fat), as indicated by no or only poor correlation between these two parameters and the appearance of artifacts. These RF cushions do not solve the problem of B1-inhomogeneity artifacts in all patients; thus, they are considered an interim solution at best until better and more sophisticated solutions become available (Fig. 9).

Summary

The published data on MRCP at 3T indicate that the technique is feasible and ready for routine clinical use [17–20]. Studies of MRCP at 3T compared with 1.5T showed a trend toward increased CNR and improved visualization of the pancreaticobiliary system; however, expectations for MRCP at 3T should remain reserved. Because the sequences, the RF transmitter, and the receiver technology at 3T are considered immature, the maximum image quality possible at 3T has not been achieved. In addition, several underlying physical principles, susceptibility artifacts, and the limitations in specific absorption rate make MRCP at 3T challenging [14]. In the last 2 years, VERSE (VariablE-Rate Selective Excitation) and SPACE (Sampling Perfection with Application optimized Contrasts using different flip angle Evolutions) have been introduced for MRCP at 3T [41]. These sequences, coupled with the implementation of parallel-imaging techniques, may shorten acquisition time substantially while maintaining excellent spatial resolution and sufficient SNR. The use of variable flip angles can decrease acquisition time further while decreasing the specific absorption rate [41–43].

MRCP at 3T has to be considered equal, not superior, to 1.5T; however, with the progressive development of 3T hardware and software, MRCP at 3T holds great promise to improve the diagnosis of pancreaticobiliary diseases.

Acknowledgment

The authors are grateful to Richard Youngblood, MA, for reviewing the manuscript.

References

[1] Wallner BK, Schumacher KA, Weidenmaier W, et al. Dilated biliary tract: evaluation with MR cholangiography with a T2-weighted contrast-enhanced fast sequence. Radiology 1991;181(3): 805–8.

[2] Masci E, Toti G, Mariani A, et al. Complications of diagnostic and therapeutic ERCP: a prospective multicenter study. Am J Gastroenterol 2001; 96(2):417–23.

[3] Loperfido S, Angelini G, Benedetti G, et al. Major early complications from diagnostic and therapeutic ERCP: a prospective multicenter study. Gastrointest Endosc 1998;48(1):1–10.

[4] Romagnuolo J, Bardou M, Rahme E, et al. Magnetic resonance cholangiopancreatography: a meta-analysis of test performance in suspected biliary disease. Ann Intern Med 2003;139(7): 547–57.

[5] Aube C, Delorme B, Yzet T, et al. MR cholangiopancreatography versus endoscopic sonography in suspected common bile duct lithiasis: a prospective, comparative study. AJR Am J Roentgenol 2005;184(1):55–62.

[6] Valls C, Alba E, Cruz M, et al. Biliary complications after liver transplantation: diagnosis with MR cholangiopancreatography. AJR Am J Roentgenol 2005;184(3):812–20.

[7] Vitellas KM, El-Dieb A, Vaswani KK, et al. MR cholangiopancreatography in patients with primary sclerosing cholangitis: interobserver variability and comparison with endoscopic retrograde cholangiopancreatography. AJR Am J Roentgenol 2002;179(2):399–407.

[8] Ragozzino A, De Ritis R, Mosca A, et al. Value of MR cholangiography in patients with iatrogenic bile duct injury after cholecystectomy. AJR Am J Roentgenol 2004;183(6):1567–72.

[9] Ward J, Sheridan MB, Guthrie JA, et al. Bile duct strictures after hepatobiliary surgery: assessment with MR cholangiography. Radiology 2004; 231(1):101–8.

[10] Sahani DV, Kadavigere R, Blake M, et al. Intraductal papillary mucinous neoplasm of pancreas: multi-detector row CT with 2D curved reformations–correlation with MRCP. Radiology 2006;238(2):560–9.

[11] Tamura R, Ishibashi T, Takahashi S. Chronic pancreatitis: MRCP versus ERCP for quantitative caliber measurement and qualitative evaluation. Radiology 2006;238(3):920–8.

[12] Gillams AR, Kurzawinski T, Lees WR. Diagnosis of duct disruption and assessment of pancreatic leak with dynamic secretin-stimulated MR cholangiopancreatography. AJR Am J Roentgenol 2006;186(2):499–506.

[13] Soto JA, Barish MA, Alvarez O, et al. Detection of choledocholithiasis with MR cholangiography: comparison of three-dimensional fast spin-echo and single- and multisection half-Fourier rapid acquisition with relaxation enhancement sequences. Radiology 2000;215(3):737–45.

[14] Merkle EM, Dale BM, Paulson EK. Abdominal MR imaging at 3T. Magn Reson Imaging Clin N Am 2006;14(1):17–26.

[15] Goldman J, Florman S, Varotti G, et al. Noninvasive preoperative evaluation of biliary anatomy in right-lobe living donors with mangafodipir trisodium-enhanced MR cholangiography. Transplant Proc 2003;35(4):1421–2.

[16] Frayne R, Goodyear BG, Dickhoff P, et al. Magnetic resonance imaging at 3.0 Tesla: challenges and advantages in clinical neurological imaging. Invest Radiol 2003;38(7):385–402.

[17] Merkle EM, Haugan PA, Thomas J, et al. 3.0- versus 1.5-T MR cholangiography: a pilot study. AJR Am J Roentgenol 2006;186(2):516–21.

[18] O'Regan DP, Fitzgerald J, Allsop J, et al. A comparison of MR cholangiopancreatography at 1.5 and 3.0 Tesla. Br J Radiol 2005;78(934): 894–8.

[19] Isoda H, Kataoka M, Maetani Y, et al. MRCP imaging at 3.0 T vs. 1.5 T: preliminary experience in healthy volunteers. J Magn Reson Imaging 2007;25(5):1000–6.

[20] Schindera ST, Miller CM, Ho LM, et al. Magnetic resonance (MR) cholangiography: quantitative and qualitative comparison of 3.0 Tesla with 1.5 Tesla. Invest Radiol 2007;42(6):399–405.

[21] de Bazelaire CM, Duhamel GD, Rofsky NM, et al. MR imaging relaxation times of abdominal and pelvic tissues measured in vivo at 3.0 T: preliminary results. Radiology 2004;230(3):652–9.

[22] Mortele KJ, Rocha TC, Streeter JL, et al. Multimodality imaging of pancreatic and biliary congenital anomalies. Radiographics 2006;26(3): 715–31.

[23] Papanikolaou N, Karantanas AH, Heracleous E, et al. Magnetic resonance cholangiopancreatography: comparison between respiratory-triggered turbo spin echo and breath hold single-shot turbo spin echo sequences. Magn Reson Imaging 1999;17(9):1255–60.

[24] Asbach P, Klessen C, Kroencke TJ, et al. Magnetic resonance cholangiopancreatography using a free-breathing T2-weighted turbo spin-echo sequence with navigator-triggered prospective acquisition correction. Magn Reson Imaging 2005;23(9):939–45.

[25] Kapoor V, Peterson MS, Baron RL, et al. Intrahepatic biliary anatomy of living adult liver donors: correlation of mangafodipir trisodium-enhanced MR cholangiography and intraoperative

cholangiography. AJR Am J Roentgenol 2002; 179(5):1281–6.

[26] Vitellas KM, El-Dieb A, Vaswani KK, et al. Using contrast-enhanced MR cholangiography with IV mangafodipir trisodium (Teslascan) to evaluate bile duct leaks after cholecystectomy: a prospective study of 11 patients. AJR Am J Roentgenol 2002;179(2):409–16.

[27] Lee VS, Rofsky NM, Morgan GR, et al. Volumetric mangafodipir trisodium-enhanced cholangiography to define intrahepatic biliary anatomy. AJR Am J Roentgenol 2001;176(4): 906–8.

[28] Hottat N, Winant C, Metens T, et al. MR cholangiography with manganese dipyridoxyl diphosphate in the evaluation of biliary-enteric anastomoses: preliminary experience. AJR Am J Roentgenol 2005;184(5):1556–62.

[29] Grazioli L, Morana G, Kirchin MA, et al. Accurate differentiation of focal nodular hyperplasia from hepatic adenoma at gadobenate dimeglumine-enhanced MR imaging: prospective study. Radiology 2005;236(1):166–77.

[30] Dahlstrom N, Persson A, Albiin N, et al. Contrast-enhanced magnetic resonance cholangiography with Gd-BOPTA and Gd-EOB-DTPA in healthy subjects. Acta Radiol 2007;48(4):362–8.

[31] Carlos RC, Hussain HK, Song JH, et al. Gadolinium-ethoxybenzyl-diethylenetriamine pentaacetic acid as an intrabiliary contrast agent: preliminary assessment. AJR Am J Roentgenol 2002;179(1):87–92.

[32] Carlos RC, Branam JD, Dong Q, et al. Biliary imaging with Gd-EOB-DTPA: is a 20-minute delay sufficient? Acad Radiol 2002;9(11):1322–5.

[33] Bluemke DA, Sahani D, Amendola M, et al. Efficacy and safety of MR imaging with liver-specific contrast agent: U.S. multicenter phase III study. Radiology 2005;237(1):89–98.

[34] Edelman RR, Salanitri G, Brand R, et al. Magnetic resonance imaging of the pancreas at 3.0 Tesla: qualitative and quantitative comparison with 1.5 Tesla. Invest Radiol 2006;41(2): 175–80.

[35] Merkle EM, Dale BM, Thomas J, et al. MR liver imaging and cholangiography in the presence of surgical metallic clips at 1.5 and 3 Tesla. Eur Radiol 2006;16(10):2309–16.

[36] Merkle EM, Nelson RC. Dual gradient-echo in-phase and opposed-phase hepatic MR imaging: a useful tool for evaluating more than fatty infiltration or fatty sparing. Radiographics 2006;26(5):1409–18.

[37] Schick F. Whole-body MRI at high field: technical limits and clinical potential. Eur Radiol 2005;15(5):946–59.

[38] Allkemper T, Schwindt W, Maintz D, et al. Sensitivity of T2-weighted FSE sequences towards physiological iron depositions in normal brains at 1.5 and 3.0 T. Eur Radiol 2004;14(6):1000–4.

[39] Merkle EM, Dale BM. Abdominal MRI at 3.0 T: the basics revisited. AJR Am J Roentgenol 2006; 186(6):1524–32.

[40] Franklin KM, Dale BM, Merkle EM. Improvement in B1-inhomogeneity artifacts in the abdomen at 3 tesla MR imaging using a radiofrequency cushion. J Magn Reson Imaging 2007, in press.

[41] Haystead C, Merkle E, Dale B. MRC at 3 Tesla with SPACE. Presented at the Annual Meeting of International Society for Magnetic Resonance in Medicine, Seattle, WA, May 6–12, 2006.

[42] Hargreaves BA, Cunningham CH, Nishimura DG, et al. Variable-rate selective excitation for rapid MRI sequences. Magn Reson Med 2004;52(3): 590–7.

[43] Hennig J, Scheffler K. Hyperechoes. Magn Reson Med 2001;46(1):6–12.

MAGNETIC RESONANCE IMAGING CLINICS

Magn Reson Imaging Clin N Am 15 (2007) 365–372

MR Imaging of the Adrenal Glands: 1.5T versus 3T

Elmar M. Merkle, MD[a],*, Sebastian T. Schindera, MD[b]

- Chemical shift imaging
- Sequence protocol for adrenal MR imaging at 1.5T
- Adrenal MR imaging at 3T
- Common adrenal lesions: comparison of 1.5T and 3T

- Adrenal adenoma
- Adrenocortical carcinoma
- Pheochromocytoma
- Metastasis
- Summary
- References

Over the past 15 years, MR imaging has become the prime imaging modality for characterization of adrenal lesions. Many of those lesions are discovered incidentally on cross-sectional imaging, thus called "incidentalomas" [1–3]. Adrenal masses of at least 1 cm in size are discovered in up to 1.5% of the population during abdominal CT [3]. Although most of these lesions are benign adenomas, even in patients who have extra-adrenal malignancy, the adrenal gland also is a common site for metastasis, most commonly from lung cancer [4,5]. Therefore, it is of utmost importance to characterize all adrenal tumors precisely to plan an appropriate clinical approach.

Chemical shift imaging

Soon after its introduction to clinical MR imaging in the late 1980s, a gradient echo in-phase and opposed-phase (IP/OP) sequence has become a routine part of every adrenal MR imaging protocol. This sequence is used primarily to characterize focal adrenal lesions using the chemical shift cancellation artifact (also known as fat/water cancellation artifact, black lining artifact, or India ink artifact). OP images demonstrate a sharply defined black rim around organs with a fat/water interface, such as the adrenal glands. Because this is a phase-cancellation effect, it is not limited to the frequency encoding direction, such as the classic chemical shift artifact, but may be seen in all pixels along the fat/water interface. In the past, the IP and the OP images were acquired within separate breath-holds, which caused suboptimal registration between the corresponding IP and OP images. This problem has been solved, allowing acquisition of the IP and OP images within the same breath-hold and resulting in perfect registration between corresponding images [6–8].

The diagnostic efficiency of IP/OP MR imaging for characterization of adrenal lesions originates from its high sensitivity for distinguishing tissues with different intracytoplasmic lipid content, using the interference of fat and water signals caused by the change in chemical frequency shift [9]. In contrast to nonadenomas, adrenal adenomas generally

[a] Department of Radiology, Duke University Medical Center, DUMC Box 3808, Durham, NC 27710, USA
[b] Interventional and Pediatric Radiology, University Hospital of Bern, Institute for Diagnostic, Inselspital Bern, Freiburgstrasse 10, CH-3010 Bern, Switzerland
* Corresponding author.
E-mail address: elmar.merkle@duke.edu (E.M. Merkle).

1064-9689/07/$ – see front matter © 2007 Elsevier Inc. All rights reserved.

doi:10.1016/j.mric.2007.06.008

contain variable amounts of intracytoplasmic lipid, such as cholesterol, fatty acids, and neutral fat [1,10,11]. This lipid content causes a decrease in MR signal on OP imaging, thus allowing the characterization of these lesions as adrenal adenomas [12]. Unfortunately, some of the adrenal adenomas are lipid poor, whereas other nonadenomas, such as adrenocortical carcinoma, hepatocellular carcinoma metastases, and metastases from clear cell carcinoma of the kidney, and liposarcoma may contain small amounts of fat.

Over the past 15 years, a wealth of literature has become available demonstrating the high diagnostic efficiency of IP/OP MR imaging for characterizing adrenal lesions at magnetic field strengths ranging from 0.5T to 1.5T. An excellent review was provided by Hussain and Korobkin [1] summarizing these data in a clearly arranged form.

Analysis of signal loss in an adrenal mass often is performed by comparing the signal intensity of the lesion on OP imaging to that on IP imaging and to the signal of a reference tissue, such as the liver, paraspinal muscle, or spleen. This comparison can be performed qualitatively by simple visual analysis or quantitatively by using region-of-interest measurements. Various equations to calculate the relative change in signal have been published in the past; the two most reliable formulas are the signal intensity (SI) index and the adrenal-to-spleen ratio (ASR) [1,10,13,14].

$$SI \text{ index} = \left[\left(SI_{\text{in-phase}} - SI_{\text{opposed-phase}} \right) / \left(SI_{\text{in-phase}} \right) \right] \times 100\%$$

$$ASR = \left[\left(SI(\text{addrenal})_{\text{opposed-phase}} / SI(\text{spleen})_{\text{opposed-phase}} \right) / \left(SI(\text{addrenal})_{\text{in-phase}} / SI(\text{spleen})_{\text{in-phase}} \right) - 1 \right]$$

Various thresholds, ranging from -25 to 0.8 for the ASR [11,15,16] and from 1% to 16.5% for the SI index [10,13,17,18], have been used at 1.5T for the differentiation of adenomas from nonadenomas, indicating that no optimal threshold has been elucidated. The main reason for the wide variability of these thresholds likely is related to differences in data collection. At 1.5T, the frequency shift between water and fat signals is approximately 225 Hz, resulting in IP signals at echo times (TE) of 0.0, 4.4, 8.8 milliseconds, and so on, and OP signals at TEs of 2.2, 6.6, 11.0 milliseconds, and so on. Although data acquisition during the most recent studies has been performed

at 2.2 and 4.4 milliseconds—corresponding to the first OP and first IP echo—earlier studies used longer echo times of up to 13 milliseconds.

Sequence protocol for adrenal MR imaging at 1.5T

Whenever possible, a dedicated torso array coil should be used for signal reception to optimize the signal-to-noise ratio. Following a dual-plane localizer, the dedicated adrenal MR sequence protocol in our institution consists of:

- Axial T1-weighted (T1w) breath-hold dual-echo spoiled gradient recalled echo (repetition time [TR] 100–200 milliseconds, TE 2.2 and 4.4 milliseconds, flip angle 70°, slice thickness <5 mm). Both echoes are acquired within the same breath-hold, allowing reliable coregistration of the corresponding IP and OP images. This sequence is used for the differentiation of adrenal adenomas from nonadenomas.
- Axial breath-hold T2-weighted (T2w) single-shot fast-spin echo (TR 1000 milliseconds, TE 100 milliseconds, flip angle 90°, slice thickness<5 mm). This sequence is used mainly for the characterization of pheochromocytomas.
- Data analysis: If the adrenal lesion is smaller than 3 cm in size and demonstrates an SI index greater than 16.5% or an ASR ratio of less than 0.71, the adrenal mass is characterized as an adrenal adenoma, and the data acquisition is considered complete.
- In all other cases, an axial breath-hold three-dimensional (3D) T1w gradient echo recalled sequence (TR 5.1 milliseconds, TE 2.5 milliseconds, flip angle 10°) with chemical shift fat saturation before and after the administration of a gadolinium-containing contrast agent is added. This sequence is used primarily for the evaluation of malignant lesions (organ origin and vascular invasion).

Adrenal MR imaging at 3T

To the best of our knowledge, no scientific manuscript has been published on IP/OP MR imaging for characterization of adrenal tumors using a 3T MR system. On these MR systems, the TE pairs for IP/OP MR imaging need to be adjusted because the frequency difference is double that of standard 1.5T MR systems [19]. Using a 3T MR system, fat and water protons are OP at 1.1, 3.3, 5.5 milliseconds, and so on, and IP at 2.2, 4.4, 6.6 milliseconds, and so on. The acquisition of the first OP echo at 1.1 milliseconds and the first IP echo at 2.2 milliseconds within the same breath-hold would require unacceptably high receiver bandwidths at 3T. The most obvious solution is to acquire the first OP echo and first IP echo in different breath-holds; however, this approach can make the quantitative analysis of particularly smaller adrenal lesions less reliable because of differences in slice selection. Therefore, all three major MR vendors (GE Healthcare, Philips Medical Systems, and Siemens Medical Solutions) recommend the collection of the first IP signal and the third OP signal or the first OP signal and the second IP signal [20,21]. This difference in data collection significantly influences the characterization of adrenal lesions, as presented recently during the 2007 annual meeting of the International Society of Magnetic Resonance in Medicine [22]. When obtaining the first OP echo before the second IP echo, there was no overlap of SI index values between 14 adenomas and four nonadenomas [22]. In contrast, acquisition of the first IP image before the third OP image demonstrated a substantial overlap of SI index values between the adenomas and nonadenomas. Two studies using a shorter TE for the IP echo than for the OP echo described similar overlap margins of SI index values between adenomas and nonadenomas at field strengths less than 3T [18,23]. In these studies, several malignant tumors presented a misleading signal loss on the OP images.

If the OP echo is collected after the IP echo, two factors influence signal loss on OP images: chemical shift effects due to intracytoplasmic fat and T2* decay. The latter provides the most plausible explanation for the misleading signal loss of nonadenomas with little or no lipid content on OP images when the IP echo is acquired before the OP echo. This scenario would yield a positive SI index value, whereas reverse TE selection most likely would yield a negative SI index value. Radiologists selecting a shorter TE for the IP echo than for the OP echo are confronted with a diagnostic dilemma when detecting a signal loss in an adrenal lesion on the OP images, because they are unable to distinguish whether signal loss is due to chemical shift effect in a fat-containing adenoma or T2* decay in a malignant lesion with little or no fat. In 1995, Tsushima and Dean [24] already noted the impact of the selection of TEs on the SI index for IP/OP MR imaging when characterizing adrenal tumors. In these cases, the use of an internal reference tissue has been suggested to reduce the impact of T2* decay [11,13,15,25]. Reference tissues used have included the spleen, liver, and paraspinal muscle. Several recent investigations have considered the spleen as the most suitable reference tissue, because fatty infiltration of the liver or paraspinal muscle may influence the quantitative evaluation

substantially [11,13,15]; however, the SI of the spleen also may be subject to alteration, namely in the case of hemosiderosis. In the recent study presented during the 2007 annual meeting of the International Society of Magnetic Resonance in Medicine, the adrenal-to-liver ratio and the ASR represented excellent discriminators between adrenal adenomas and nonadenomas when the IP echo was collected first [22]; however, radiologists acquiring the IP before the OP echo and using the liver or spleen as an internal reference tissue must be attentive to hepatic steatosis and splenic or hepatic iron deposition. Our current adrenal MR sequence protocol performed on a 3.0-T platform using a torso array coil for signal reception is as follows:

Axial T1w breath-hold dual-echo spoiled gradient recalled echo (TR 100–200 milliseconds, TE 1.6 and 4.9 milliseconds, flip angle 90°, slice thickness<5 mm). Both echoes are acquired within the same breath-hold, allowing reliable coregistration of the corresponding IP and OP images.

Axial breath-hold T2w single-shot fast-spin echo (TR 1000 milliseconds, TE 80 milliseconds, flip angle 90°, slice thickness<5 mm).

Data analysis: If the adrenal lesion is smaller than 3 cm in size and demonstrates an SI index greater than 1.7%, the adrenal mass will be characterized as an adrenal adenoma, and the data acquisition is considered complete. The threshold of 1.7% is based on a small sample size of 21 patients [22]. Thus, this threshold qualifies as "preliminary" at best, and larger studies are needed to better define this SI index threshold for differentiation of adenomas from nonadenomas at 3T.

In cases with a lesion size of more than 3 cm or an SI index of less than 1.7%, an axial breath-hold 3D T1w gradient echo recalled sequence (TR 3.4 milliseconds, TE 1.4 milliseconds, flip angle 13°) with chemical shift fat saturation before and after the administration of a gadolinium-containing contrast agent is added.

The latest efforts in chemical shift imaging at 3T focus on the development of 3D dual-echo techniques that allow the acquisition of the first OP and the first IP echo within the same breath-hold [26–28]. These sequences offer good image quality and probably will become available commercially in 2008. Besides offering an IP and an OP image, these sequences allow the automated reconstruction of "water-only" and "fat-only" images based on a two-point Dixon technique.

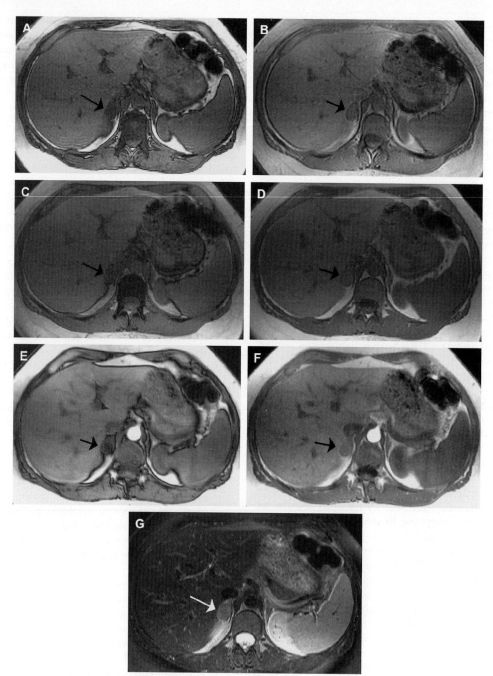

Fig. 1. 3-T MR imaging in a 39-year-old woman with a right-sided adrenal adenoma (*arrow*) measuring 2.6 cm × 1.8 cm. Image pairs A and B, C and D, and E and F were acquired within the same breath-hold. This figure illustrates how the selection of the echo pair impacts the quantitative analysis of adrenal lesions. (*A*) Axial two-dimensional (2D) gradient echo image, first OP echo acquired with an echo time of 1.6 milliseconds: the SI of the adrenal lesion measures 132. (*B*) Axial 2D gradient echo image, second IP echo acquired with an echo time of 4.9 milliseconds: the SI of the adrenal lesion measures 191. Based on the image pair A and B, the SI index of 30.9% is indicative of an adrenal adenoma. (*C*) Axial 2D gradient echo image, third OP echo acquired with an echo time of 5.7 milliseconds: the SI of the adrenal lesion measures 152. (*D*) Axial 2D gradient echo image, first IP echo acquired with an echo time of 2.2 milliseconds: the SI of the adrenal lesion measures 329. Based on the image pair C and D, the SI index of 53.8% is indicative of an adrenal adenoma. (*E*) Axial 3D gradient echo image, first OP echo acquired with an echo time of 1.1 milliseconds: the SI of the adrenal lesion measures 16. (*F*) Axial 3D gradient echo image, first IP echo acquired with an echo time of 2.2 milliseconds: the SI of the adrenal lesion measures 71. Based on the image pair E and F, the SI index of 77.5% is indicative of an adrenal adenoma. (*G*) Axial T2w turbo spin echo image with fat saturation.

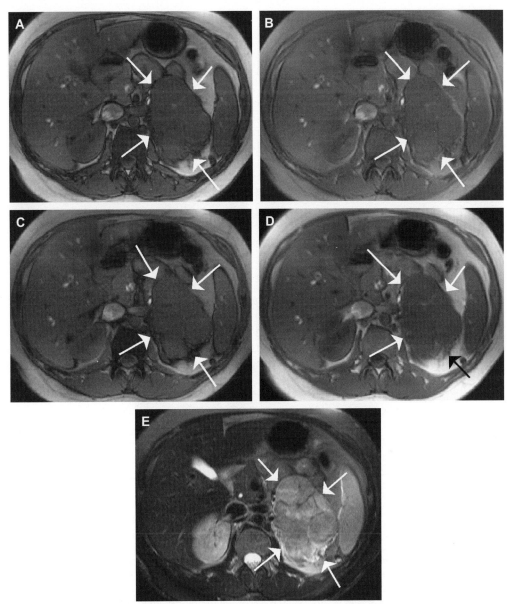

Fig. 2. 3T MR imaging in a 26-year-old woman with a left-sided adrenocortical carcinoma (*arrows*) measuring 9.6 cm × 7.5 cm. Image pairs A and B and C and D were acquired within the same breath-hold. This figure again illustrates how the selection of the echo pair impacts the quantitative analysis of adrenal lesions. (*A*) Axial 2D gradient echo image, first OP echo acquired with an echo time of 1.6 milliseconds: the SI of the adrenal lesion measures 290. (*B*) Axial 2D gradient echo image, second IP echo acquired with an echo time of 4.9 milliseconds: the SI of the adrenal lesion measures 274. Based on the image pair A and B, the SI index of −5.8% is indicative of a nonadenoma. (*C*) Axial 2D gradient echo image, third OP echo acquired with an echo time of 5.7 milliseconds: the SI of the adrenal lesion measures 266. (*D*) Axial 2D gradient echo image, first IP echo acquired with an echo time of 2.2 milliseconds: the SI of the adrenal lesion measures 307. Based on the image pair C and D, the SI index of 13.4% is suggestive of an adenoma. (E) Axial T2w turbo spin-echo image with fat saturation.

Common adrenal lesions: comparison of 1.5T and 3T

Adrenal adenoma

Nonfunctioning adrenal adenomas are the most common adrenal masses, with a prevalence of approximately 3% [29]. Most of these lesions contain various amounts of intracytoplasmic fat, do not exceed 3 cm in size, and are round or oval with smooth and well-defined margins. These lesions are homogeneous on T2w and T1w imaging (Fig. 1). Chemical shift imaging is the single most

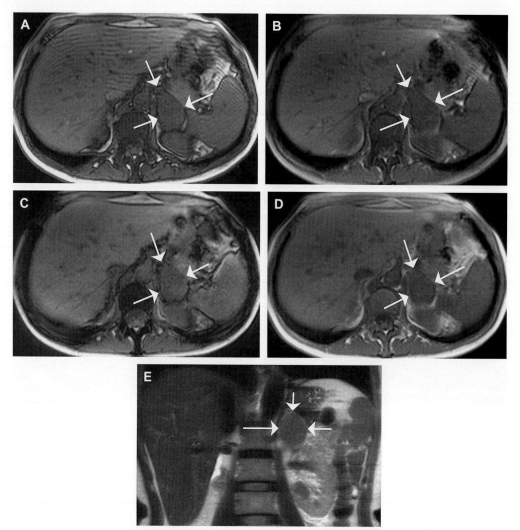

Fig. 3. 3T MR imaging in a 51-year-old woman with a left-sided adrenal metastasis (*arrows*) from cervical squamous cell cancer measuring 3.9 cm × 2.9 cm. Image pairs A and B and C and D were acquired within the same breath-hold. This figure again illustrates how the selection of the echo pair impacts the quantitative analysis of adrenal lesions. (*A*) Axial 2D gradient echo image, first OP echo acquired with an echo time of 1.6 milliseconds: the SI of the adrenal lesion measures 388. (*B*) Axial 2D gradient echo image, second IP echo acquired with an echo time of 4.9 milliseconds: the SI of the adrenal lesion measures 340. Based on the image pair A and B, the SI index of −14.1% is indicative of a nonadenoma. (*C*) Axial 2D gradient echo image, third OP echo acquired with an echo time of 5.7 milliseconds: the SI of the adrenal lesion measures 361. (*D*) Axial 2D gradient echo image, first IP echo acquired with an echo time of 2.2 milliseconds: the SI of the adrenal lesion measures 430. Based on the image pair C and D, the SI index of 16.1% is suggestive of an adenoma. (*E*) Coronal T2w turbo spin-echo image without fat saturation.

important MR technique for the precise characterization of these lesions because most adenomas (except lipid poor) demonstrate a substantial decrease in MR signal on OP imaging. Although a wealth of data exists at 1.5T with reasonably well-defined thresholds, limited data are available at 3T. Based on the laws of MR physics, the SI index thresholds for the differentiation of adenomas from nonadenomas at 1.5T and 3T are likely different.

1.5T MR imaging is considered the standard of reference. Whether 3T MR imaging will substantially improve the differentiation of adenoma from nonadenoma remains uncertain.

Adrenocortical carcinoma

Patients who have adrenocortical carcinoma often present with abdominal pain or a mass because these tumors usually are larger than 6 cm in size at the time of presentation (Fig. 2). Most are functional, producing hormones or precursors. Adrenocortical carcinomas may contain areas of hemorrhage, fat, and central necrosis, which explains the heterogeneous appearance on T2w, T1w, and gadolinium-enhanced imaging. Diagnosis of an adrenocortical carcinoma usually is not a problem with 1.5T MR imaging because these tumors often are large, and the imaging appearance is fairly characteristic. It is doubtful whether 3T MR imaging will improve the diagnosis of this entity.

Pheochromocytoma

These tumors originate from the adrenal medulla and have been called "10% tumors" because approximately 10% are bilateral, extra-adrenal, familial, malignant, or occur in children [30,31]. Pheochromocytomas also are larger than 3 cm, in general, and may contain necrosis, hemorrhage, and cystic areas with fluid–fluid levels [30]. The classic MR appearance of pheochromocytomas is homogeneous hypointensity on T1w; lack of signal loss on OP imaging; and marked uniform hyperintensity on T2w imaging, occasionally referred to as "light bulb bright." Rarely, pheochromocytomas are purely cystic and need to be considered as a differential diagnosis in the presence of cystic adrenal tumors [32]. Following gadolinium administration, these tumors usually demonstrate marked enhancement. Diagnosis of pheochromocytomas usually is not a problem with 1.5T MR imaging because these tumors are large, the imaging appearance is fairly characteristic, and the clinical setting is appropriate. It is doubtful whether 3T MR imaging will improve the diagnostic capabilities in this clinical scenario.

Metastasis

The adrenal gland is the fourth most common site of metastatic disease following lung, liver, and bone, which is remarkable considering the small organ size. The primary tumors most often involved originate from the lung, breast, thyroid, and colon [33,34]. On MR imaging, metastases to the adrenal gland usually are hypointense on T1w imaging and mildly hyperintense on T2w imaging relative to the liver (Fig. 3) [29]. Of utmost importance is the fact that metastases do not demonstrate a loss of signal on OP imaging unless the primary cancer already contains intracytoplasmic fat (eg, liposarcoma, clear cell cancer from the kidney, and, occasionally, hepatocellular cancer). Therefore, an adrenal metastasis must be considered as a differential diagnosis for each lesion without a substantial decrease in signal on OP imaging. MR imaging at 1.5T remains the standard of reference in the workup of adrenal metastases, given the aforementioned problems related to chemical shift imaging at 3T.

Summary

MR imaging at 1.5T must be considered the standard of reference for the characterization of adrenal lesions. At 3T, the collection of the first OP echo and the first IP echo, although desirable, is technically not feasible on current commercially available pulse sequences. Therefore, the first IP echo and the third OP echo or the first OP echo and the second IP echo are collected. This selection of the echo time pair for IP/OP MR imaging greatly affects the quantitative analysis of adrenal tumors at 3T. To avoid misclassification of adrenal tumors on IP/OP MR images, the SI index should be applied when the TE of the IP echo is longer than the TE of the OP echo. If the IP echo is collected before the OP echo, the use of an internal reference tissue, such as the spleen or liver, to correct for $T2^*$ decay effects is recommended. These problems will be overcome soon as 3D dual-echo sequences are developed. This new type of pulse sequence will allow the collection of the first OP and first IP echo at a field strength of 3T; however, quantitative analysis thresholds for the differentiation of adenomas from nonadenomas may be different at 1.5T and 3T, and more data need to be gathered to establish these thresholds for 3T MR platforms.

References

[1] Hussain HK, Korobkin M. MR imaging of the adrenal glands. Magn Reson Imaging Clin N Am 2004;12:515–44.

[2] Korobkin M, Francis IR, Kloos RT, et al. The incidental adrenal mass. Radiol Clin North Am 1996;34:1037–54.

[3] Glazer HS, Weyman PJ, Sagel SS, et al. Nonfunctioning adrenal masses: incidental discovery on computed tomography. AJR Am J Roentgenol 1982;139(1):81–5.

[4] Burt M, Heelan RT, Coit D, et al. Prospective evaluation of unilateral adrenal masses in patients with operable non-small-cell lung cancer. Impact of magnetic resonance imaging. J Thorac Cardiovasc Surg 1994;107:584–9.

[5] Oliver TW Jr, Bernardino ME, Miller JI, et al. Isolated adrenal masses in non small-cell bronchogenic carcinoma. Radiology 1984;153(1):217–8.

[6] Martin J, Puig J, Falco J, et al. Hyperechoic liver nodules: characterization with proton fat-water chemical shift MR imaging. Radiology 1998;207:325–30.

[7] Wang Y, Li D, Haacke EM, et al. A three-point Dixon method for water and fat separation using 2D and 3D gradient-echo techniques. J Magn Reson Imaging 1998;8:703–10.

[8] Zhang W, Goldhaber DM, Kramer DM. Separation of water and fat MR images in a single scan at .35 T using "sandwich" echoes. J Magn Reson Imaging 1996;6:909–17.

[9] Mitchell DG, Kim I, Chang TS, et al. Fatty liver. Chemical shift phase-difference and suppression magnetic resonance imaging techniques in animals, phantoms, and humans. Invest Radiol 1991;26:1041–52.

[10] Tsushima Y, Ishizaka H, Matsumoto M. Adrenal masses: differentiation with chemical shift, fast low-angle shot MR imaging. Radiology 1993;186:705–9.

[11] Mayo-Smith WW, Lee MJ, McNicholas MM, et al. Characterization of adrenal masses (<5 cm) by use of chemical shift MR imaging: observer performance versus quantitative measures. AJR Am J Roentgenol 1995;165:91–5.

[12] Korobkin M, Giordano TJ, Brodeur FJ, et al. Adrenal adenomas: relationship between histologic lipid and CT and MR findings. Radiology 1996;200:743–7.

[13] Fujiyoshi F, Nakajo M, Fukukura Y, et al. Characterization of adrenal tumors by chemical shift fast low-angle shot MR imaging: comparison of four methods of quantitative evaluation. AJR Am J Roentgenol 2003;180:1649–57.

[14] Israel GM, Korobkin M, Wang C, et al. Comparison of unenhanced CT and chemical shift MRI in evaluating lipid-rich adrenal adenomas. AJR Am J Roentgenol 2004;183:215–9.

[15] Bilbey JH, McLoughlin RF, Kurkjian PS, et al. MR imaging of adrenal masses: value of chemical-shift imaging for distinguishing adenomas from other tumors. AJR Am J Roentgenol 1995;164:637–42.

[16] Outwater EK, Siegelman ES, Huang AB, et al. Adrenal masses: correlation between CT attenuation values and chemical shift ratio at MR imaging with in-phase and opposed-phase sequences. Radiology 1996;200:749–52.

[17] Namimoto T, Yamashita Y, Mitsuzaki K, et al. Adrenal masses: quantification of fat content with double echo chemical shift in-phase and opposed-phase FLASH MR images for differentiation of adrenal adenomas. Radiology 2001;218:642–6.

[18] Slapa RZ, Jakubowski W, Dabrowska E, et al. Magnetic resonance imaging differentiation of adrenal masses at 1.5T: T2-weighted images, chemical shift imaging, and Gd-DTPA dynamic studies. MAGMA 1996;4:163–79.

[19] Merkle EM, Dale BM. Abdominal MRI at 3T: the basics revisited. AJR Am J Roentgenol 2006;186:1524–32.

[20] Merkle EM, Nelson RC. Dual gradient-echo in-phase and opposed-phase hepatic MR imaging: a useful tool for evaluating more than fatty infiltration or fatty sparing. Radiographics 2006;26:1409–18.

[21] von Falkenhausen MM, Lutterbey G, Morakkabati-Spitz N, et al. High-field-strength MR imaging of the liver at 3T: intraindividual comparative study with MR imaging at 1.5T. Radiology 2006;241:156–66.

[22] Merkle EM, Soher BJ, Dale BM, et al. Characterization of adrenal tumors with single breath-hold in-phase/opposed-phase MR imaging at 3.0 Tesla: comparison of different echo time pairs. Presented at the joint annual meeting ISMRM-ESMRMB 2007, Berlin, Germany, No. 2737.

[23] Reinig JW, Stutley JE, Leonhardt CM, et al. Differentiation of adrenal masses with MR imaging: comparison of techniques. Radiology 1994;192:41–6.

[24] Tsushima Y, Dean PB. Characterization of adrenal masses with chemical shift MR imaging: how to select echo times. Radiology 1995;195:285–6.

[25] Schwartz LH, Panicek DM, Koutcher JA, et al. Adrenal masses in patients with malignancy: prospective comparison of echo-planar, fast spin-echo, and chemical shift MR imaging. Radiology 1995;197:421–5.

[26] Dale BM, Merkle EM. A new 3D approach for clinical in- and opposed-phase MRI at 3 T. Abstract, presented an the joint annual meeting ISMRM-ESMRMB 2007, Berlin, Germany, No. 2723.

[27] Low RN, Knowles A, Vu AT, et al. LAVA dual echo with water reconstruction: preliminary experience with a novel pulse sequence for gadolinium-enhanced abdominal MR imaging. Abstract, presented an the joint annual meeting ISMRM-ESMRMB 2007, Berlin, Germany, No. 726.

[28] Ma J. Breath-hold water and fat imaging using a dual-echo two-point Dixon technique with an efficient and robust phase-correction algorithm. Magn Reson Med 2004;52:415–9.

[29] Peppercorn PD, Reznek RH. State-of-the-art CT and MRI of the adrenal gland. Eur Radiol 1997;7:822–36.

[30] Rha SE, Byun JY, Jung SE, et al. Neurogenic tumors in the abdomen: tumor types and imaging characteristics. Radiographics 2003;23(1):29–43.

[31] Francis IR, Korobkin M. Pheochromocytoma. Radiol Clin North Am 1996;34:1101–12.

[32] Belden CJ, Powers C, Ros PR. MR demonstration of a cystic pheochromocytoma. J Magn Reson Imaging 1995;5(6):778–80.

[33] Abrams HL, Spiro R, Goldsein N. Metastases in carcinoma. Analysis of 1000 autopsied cases. Cancer 1950;3:74–85.

[34] Korobkin M. Overview of adrenal imaging/adrenal CT. Urol Radiol 1989;11(4):221–6.

MAGNETIC
RESONANCE
IMAGING CLINICS

Magn Reson Imaging Clin N Am 15 (2007) 373–382

Kidneys and MR Urography

John R. Leyendecker, MD*, David D. Childs, MD

- Potential benefits of 3T imaging of the urinary tract: signal-to-noise ratio
- Potential benefits of 3T imaging of the urinary tract: contrast enhancement
- Reality check: potential disadvantages of urinary tract imaging at 3T
- Future directions: nonanatomic (functional) evaluation of the urinary tract with 3T MR imaging
- Summary
- References

MR imaging of the urinary tract presents several challenges not relevant to high field strength imaging of the brain or joints. The kidneys, ureters, and bladder span nearly the entire length of the abdomen and pelvis, requiring the capacity to image large fields-of-view efficiently for a comprehensive examination of the urinary tract. Respiratory motion requires that sequences be exceptionally time efficient, motion resistant, or have the capacity for respiratory triggering. Temporal resolution is likewise important for gadolinium-enhanced imaging to assess the renal vasculature or evaluate the enhancement characteristics of a renal mass or the bladder wall. When diuretic-enhanced imaging is performed, overall examination time must be minimized to avoid patient discomfort or involuntary voiding related to a full urinary bladder. Coincident with these requirements is the need for sufficient contrast resolution to reliably detect small lesions of the renal parenchyma and sufficient spatial resolution to facilitate detection of small urothelial tumors.

At a given field strength, improvements in temporal and spatial resolution often are obtained at the expense of the signal-to-noise ratio (SNR). An increase in field strength from 1.5T to 3T provides a potential improvement in SNR that can be applied toward these improvements in temporal and spatial resolution, while maintaining SNR at acceptable levels. Although this potential would seem to make urinary tract imaging at 3T extremely compelling, there has been surprisingly little published literature addressing MR imaging of the urinary tract at 3T.

Potential benefits of 3T imaging of the urinary tract: signal-to-noise ratio

The increase in SNR experienced at 3T compared with 1.5T is visually apparent in images obtained of the kidneys using a variety of clinically relevant sequences (Figs. 1 and 2). Schindera and colleagues [1] reported a significant in vivo gain in measured SNR of the renal cortex for a vendor-optimized half-Fourier acquisition single-shot turbo spin-echo (HASTE) sequence performed at 3T compared with a similar sequence performed on a 1.5T scanner. Definite, although less impressive, gains also were seen with in-and-out of phase T1-weighted imaging in this study. To maximize gains in SNR while maintaining the clinical usefulness of sequences, adjustments must be made for increases in tissue T1-relaxation times, specific absorption rate (SAR), and artifacts encountered at 3T.

Department of Radiology, Wake Forest University School of Medicine, Medical Center Boulevard, Winston-Salem, NC 27157, USA
* Corresponding author.
E-mail address: jleyende@wfubmc.edu (J.R. Leyendecker).

1064-9689/07/$ – see front matter © 2007 Elsevier Inc. All rights reserved.
mri.theclinics.com

doi:10.1016/j.mric.2007.06.007

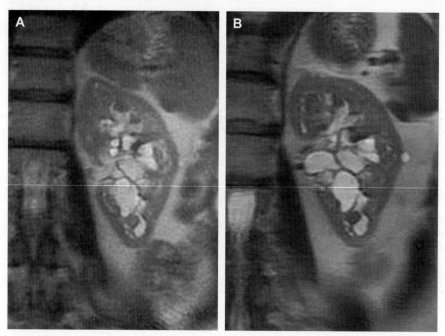

Fig. 1. Coronal single-shot fast spin-echo MR images through the left kidney in patient who has renal sinus cysts performed with an eight-channel body array coil using parallel imaging at 1.5T (*A*) and 3T (*B*). Slice thickness was 8 mm in each case. An increase in SNR is readily visible at 3T.

Improvements in SNR potentially can improve anatomic detail and aid in the detection and characterization of small renal lesions. This potential benefit remains theoretic; no study has been published specifically comparing the evaluation of renal lesions at 3T versus other field strengths. Because the urine-filled ureters have intrinsically high SNR on unenhanced T2-weighted and enhanced T1-weighted excretory phase images, the MR evaluation of the ureters is not signal limited. In this case, the additional signal available at 3T can be compromised in the interest of spatial or temporal resolution while maintaining SNR equivalent to or better than that obtainable with 1.5T. The increased signal available at 3T also permits high-resolution imaging of the entire urinary tract in the coronal plane during a single breath hold (Fig. 3). Despite the large area of coverage required of MR urography, excellent detail and uniformity of SNR can be maintained at 3T. With our current 1.5T scanners, similar SNR and resolution only can be obtained by imaging the upper and lower portions of the urinary tract with separate acquisitions. Therefore, we have found that our 3T MR urograms are more time efficient than those performed on our clinical 1.5T scanners. The higher spatial resolution potentially achievable at 3T does not eliminate the need for ureteral distention when performing MR urography. Therefore, diuretic administration or hydration usually is necessary for adequate ureteral distention at 3T as for 1.5T [2–4].

Because the effects of increasing field strength from 1.5T to 3T on T2 relaxation times of tissues are minimal, and urine has intrinsically high signal intensity at both field strengths, static MR urography requires few adaptations at 3T (Fig. 4). Theoretically, higher resolution images may contribute to better detection of small urinary calculi or urothelial tumors, although this has not been validated in a comparison study to date (Fig. 5). Despite the potential for improved resolution at 3T, it is likely that the diagnosis of ureteral calculi will still rely heavily upon indirect signs, to include persistent ureteral dilatation above the calculus (Fig. 6). For this reason, we continue to perform multiple sequential heavily T2-weighted thick-slab acquisitions to assess for fixed areas of narrowing or obstruction in the ureters [5]. When performing multiple sequential thick-slab heavily T2-weighted acquisitions at 3T, as with 1.5T, it is important to allow sufficient time between acquisitions to avoid saturation effects that result in progressive signal loss.

Although caution is warranted in extrapolating magnetic resonance cholangiopancreatography (MRCP) data to the application of MR urography, one can assume the same physical principles apply to the urine-filled collecting systems as apply to the bile-filled biliary tree. Initial pilot data comparing 3T MRCP images to those obtained at 1.5T were encouraging, suggesting that at least some sequences used for MRCP were qualitatively and

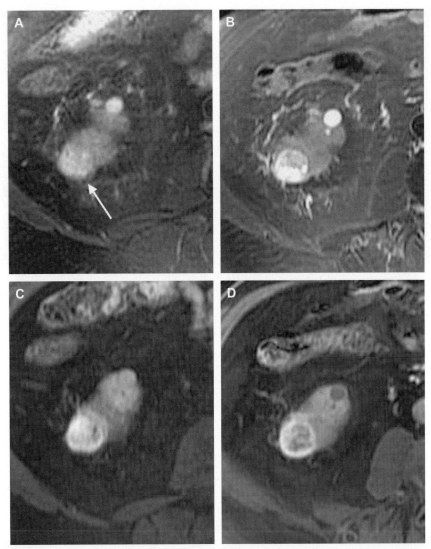

Fig. 2. Axial respiratory-triggered fast spin-echo T2-weighted MR images (*A, B*) and gadolinium-enhanced fat-suppressed 3D gradient-echo images (*C, D*) through the right kidney of patient who has renal cell carcinoma (*arrow*). All images were obtained using an eight-channel body array coil and parallel imaging. (*A, C*) 1.5T. (*B, D*) 3T.

quantitatively (in terms of contrast-to-noise ratio [CNR]) significantly better when obtained at 3T [6,7]. More recently, Schindera and colleagues [8] compared quantitative and qualitative image quality of MR cholangiography at 1.5T and 3T. CNRs between the biliary ductal system and the periductal tissues generally were higher at 3T compared with 1.5T, although this difference failed to reach statistical significance. Qualitative assessment of the images obtained also failed to show a statistically significant benefit of 3T. Extrapolation of these results to the urinary-collecting systems suggests that T2-weighted (static fluid) MR urography may benefit from higher field strength, although that benefit alone is probably not sufficient to warrant the preferential use of 3T for MR urography.

Potential benefits of 3T imaging of the urinary tract: contrast enhancement

The relaxivity of gadolinium decreases with increasing field strength, although this effect is small relative to the increase in the T1 prolongation of water [9]. Studies of the effectiveness of gadolinium chelates used for neurologic applications suggest that, despite decreases in gadolinium chelate relaxivity, the conspicuity of gadolinium enhancement increases as field strength increases from 1.5T to 3T [10–12]. This has potential benefit for the detection of subtle areas of enhancement within renal lesions and the detection of small urothelial neoplasms. With recent reports linking nephrogenic systemic fibrosis, a systemic disease with severely debilitating

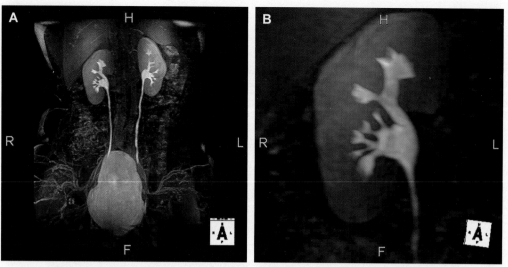

Fig. 3. Coronal maximum-intensity projection images from excretory MR urogram performed on a 3T scanner with eight-channel body array coil using parallel imaging during a single breath hold. 0.05 mmol/kg Gd-BOPTA and 5 mg intravenous furosemide were administered. Through-plane resolution is 2 mm. Note the excellent detail (*B*) despite the large field of view (*A*).

skin manifestations, to gadolinium administration in the setting of severe renal insufficiency, there is likely to be renewed interest in gadolinium dose-reduction strategies in MR imaging [13–18]. Although the use of gadolinium doses less than 0.1 mmol/kg has never been examined systematically for urologic applications at 3T, Krautmacher and colleagues [12] showed that using half the standard dose of gadolinium diethylenetriaminepentaacetic acid (Gd-DTPA) for brain imaging at 3T produced tumor-to-brain contrast similar to that obtained with a standard

0.1 mmol/kg dose at 1.5T. At our institution, we perform MR urography at 3T using a 0.05 mmol/kg dose of gadolinium benzyloxypropionictetraacetate (Gd-BOPTA), because Gd-BOPTA maintains superior relaxivity in human blood plasma in vitro compared with other agents at 3T (Figs. 7 and 8) [19] Urinary tract imaging with Gd-BOPTA represents an off-label use of this agent in the United States, however, and there are no data available comparing the use of a reduced dose of Gd-BOPTA with a standard dose of an alternative gadolinium-based contrast

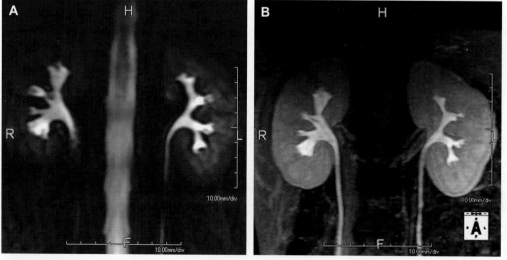

Fig. 4. Coronal thick-slab T2-weighted static fluid MR urogram (*A*) and maximum-intensity projection excretory MR urogram (*B*) of a normal patient performed on a 3T scanner using an eight-channel body array coil and parallel imaging. 0.05 mmol/kg Gd-BOPTA and 5 mg furosemide were administered for the excretory MR urogram.

One additional benefit of 3T MR imaging may improve the conspicuity of enhancement after administration of paramagnetic contrast agents. The improved spectral resolution available at 3T results in improved fat suppression compared with 1.5T MR imaging. Because the kidneys, ureters, and bladder are surrounded by fat, improved fat suppression can indirectly improve the conspicuity of enhancement of these structures and their abnormalities. The improvement in the conspicuity of enhancement as a result of better fat suppression at 3T was reported for magnetic resonance angiography (MRA) of the abdomen by Fukatsu [20], who observed that similar MRA image quality could be obtained using a half-standard dose of gadolinium at 3T compared with a standard dose of gadolinium at 1.5T.

Reality check: potential disadvantages of urinary tract imaging at 3T

Although it is clear that 3T MR imaging offers some potential benefits over 1.5T imaging of the urinary tract, there are considerable challenges to be overcome at 3T [21–23]. The T1 relaxation times of tissues increase with increasing field strength, and this alteration in T1 relaxation times is not uniform across all tissue types [24,25]. The difference in T1 relaxation times of various tissues between 1.5T and 3T potentially translates into visibly altered T1-weighted image contrast. The extent to which this impedes diagnosis is unknown, although the effect is likely to be minimal for most clinically

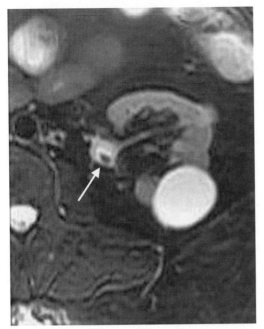

Fig. 5. Respiratory-triggered fast spin-echo MR image performed on a 3T scanner using an eight-channel body array coil through the left kidney in patient who has small urinary calculus within the left renal pelvis (*arrow*).

agent for urinary tract imaging at 3T. Gadolinium-enhanced excretory MR urography using any available contrast agent is unlikely to succeed in patients who have severely compromised renal function and should be avoided.

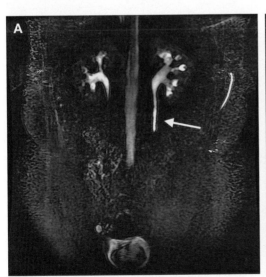

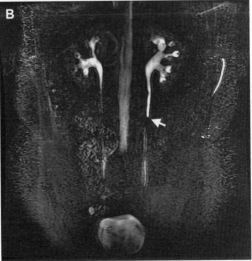

Fig. 6. Two successive images from series of sequential thick-slab T2-weighted MR urograms performed at 3T in patient who has a small ureteral calculus resulting in a standing column of urine (*arrow, A*). Note that urine is seen distending the ureter below the level of the calculus (*arrowhead*) on the subsequent image (*B*), confirming that calculus is only partially obstructing.

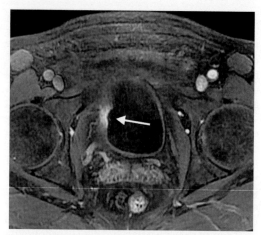

Fig. 7. Axial gadolinium-enhanced fat-suppressed 3D gradient-echo image obtained through the bladder as part of 3T MR urogram in patient who has transitional cell carcinoma of the right bladder wall. Note that enhancement is clearly visible at site of tumor using 0.05 mmol/kg Gd-BOPTA. Shallow ulceration is present centrally at site of prior biopsy (*arrow*).

relevant questions. The effects of higher field strength on T1-weighted image contrast can be compensated for at the expense of acquisition time through increases in repetition time (TR). Inversion prepulses also can be used to produce images with acceptable T1-weighted image contrast in a time-efficient manner.

The noticeable increase in chemical shift artifact (of the first kind) encountered at 3T could result in obscuration of subtle findings at the interface between the renal or bladder surface and surrounding fat (eg, small subcapsular renal hematoma or subtle transmural bladder tumor extension) (Fig. 9). A potential advantage of increased chemical shift artifact can be found in the identification of small foci of fat in renal angiomyolipomas. If chemical shift artifact becomes clinically detrimental for a given case, it can be reduced by increasing the receiver bandwidth (with a resulting loss of SNR).

Chemical shift imaging using in-phase and opposed-phase echo times is important for the diagnosis of some renal angiomyolipomas and clear cell carcinomas of the kidney. In- and opposed-phase imaging performed at a field strength of 3T differs slightly from chemical shift imaging at 1.5T. Most available MR scanners are capable of performing a dual echo in- and opposed-phase gradient echo acquisition. At 1.5T, the opposed-phase echo is acquired first, followed by the in-phase echo at approximately 4.4 milliseconds. As discussed in the article on physics elsewhere in this issue, the in- and opposed-phase echo times change at 3T, with the first opposed-phase echo potentially obtainable at 1.1 milliseconds. Rather than acquire opposed-phase and in-phase echoes at 1.1 and 2.2 milliseconds, respectively, many available MR scanners obtain the opposed-phase echo at approximately 6 milliseconds. This reversal of the in- and

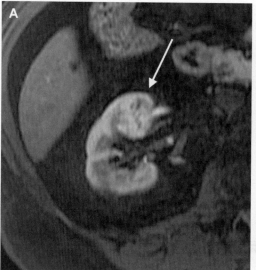
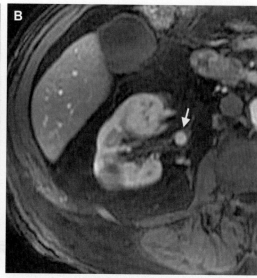

Fig. 8. Axial gadolinium-enhanced fat-suppressed gradient echo images performed through the right kidney in patient who has multiple renal cell carcinomas (*arrow*) and metastasis to the renal pelvis (*arrowhead*). (*A*) Image obtained at 1.5T after 0.1 mmol/kg Gd-DTPA. (*B*) Image obtained at 3T after 0.05 mmol/kg Gd-BOPTA. Both images performed using same sequence using eight-channel coil and parallel imaging. Note that metastatic focus (*arrowhead*) has grown during the interval between studies.

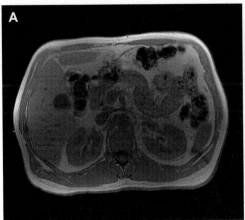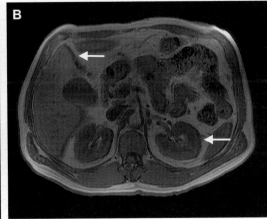

Fig. 9. Axial T1-weighted in-phase gradient echo images obtained at 1.5T (*A*) and 3T (*B*). Note the improved SNR and increased chemical shift artifact (*arrows*) in (*B*).

opposed-phase echo times results in greater susceptibility artifact on the opposed-phase images. The clinical effects of this difference between dual-echo chemical shift imaging at 1.5T and 3T are likely to be small; however, one should exercise caution so as not to interpret signal loss due to the presence of hemosiderin on long echo time (TE) opposed-phase images as evidence of intracellular lipid. Of course, this problem can be avoided by acquiring in- and opposed-phase images as separate acquisitions, using a shorter TE for the opposed-phase image.

The increased susceptibility artifact present at 3T becomes particularly important in the abdomen, because of the large volume of air within the gastrointestinal tract at any given time. This becomes problematic in parts of the genitourinary tract in close proximity to air-filled bowel (Fig. 10). Having the patient fast before imaging may help to alleviate this problem. Susceptibility artifact related to surgical clips, hip prostheses, or other orthopedic hardware also is magnified at higher field strengths and can interfere significantly with evaluation of the urinary tract. Susceptibility artifact can be minimized by using as short a TE as possible and increasing receiver bandwidth (at the expense of SNR).

Standing wave and conductivity effects are particularly problematic for abdominal imaging at 3T [21]. These effects usually translate into poor signal homogeneity (Fig. 11). This loss of signal can be alleviated—but not eliminated entirely—through the use of a pad, specifically designed for this purpose, placed over the abdomen (see Fig. 11) [26,27].

A final disadvantage encountered, when increasing field strength from 1.5T to 3T, with urinary tract implications is the significant increase in SAR. This is a significant problem for long echo-train spin-echo sequences that use series of closely spaced

refocusing pulses. Such sequences constitute a significant component of most urinary tract imaging protocols. Many of the solutions to this problem, such as shortening the echo train length, result in unacceptable trade-offs (eg, increased acquisition times). Adjustments in flip angle, the use of parallel imaging technologies, or the application of "hyperechoes" can be beneficial [28–30].

Future directions: nonanatomic (functional) evaluation of the urinary tract with 3T MR imaging

Despite the lack of comparative data objectively evaluating 3T MR applications for anatomic urinary

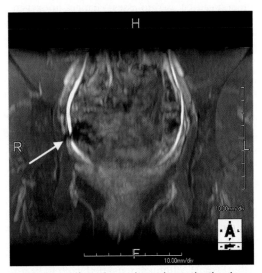

Fig. 10. Coronal maximum-intensity projection image of excretory MR urogram created from axial data set demonstrates signal loss in region of right distal ureter (*arrow*) as a result of susceptibility artifact from adjacent gas-filled bowel.

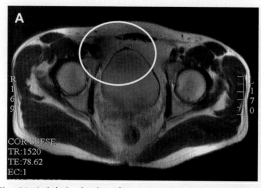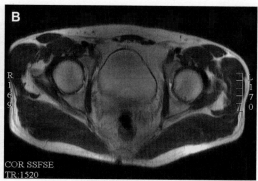

Fig. 11. Axial single-shot fast spin-echo images performed through the pelvis on a 3T MR scanner without (*A*) and with (*B*) the use of a "dielectric" pad designed to improve signal homogeneity. Note area of signal loss in (*A*) (*circle*). Signal intensity of urine within the bladder is more uniform in (*B*).

tract imaging, there has been some interesting research conducted evaluating novel nonanatomic or functional applications of renal imaging at 3T. Noninvasive measurements of renal physiology could have important applications for the evaluation of renal parenchymal disease, and the increased SNR, susceptibility effect, and spectral resolution at higher field strengths make functional renal imaging at 3T an enticing prospect [31]. Although these techniques may be considered investigational, they have the potential to become part of routine urinary tract imaging protocols.

Blood oxygen level–dependent (BOLD) contrast MR imaging is a method of measuring blood oxygenation that stands to benefit from increasing scanner field strength. The parameter R_2^* (= $1/T_2^*$) is related to the level of tissue deoxyhemoglobin and can be used to assess changes in oxygenation. BOLD imaging at 3T has been used to study renal medullary oxygenation levels during water loading without and with naproxen [32].

Maril and colleagues [33] used Na-23 MR imaging at 3T to perform functional imaging of the kidney. The investigators were able to image and map the sodium distribution within the kidney, including a quantitative measurement of the corticomedullary sodium gradient. Because in vivo Na-23 MR images exhibit an SNR four orders of magnitude lower than that of in vivo H-1 MR images, the gain in signal-to-noise with 3T was crucial.

Michaely and colleagues [34] investigated first-pass renal perfusion using gadolinium chelates with high temporal resolution turbo fast low-angle shot (TurboFLASH) at 1.5T and 3T, as well as time-resolved echo-shared angiographic technique (TREAT) at 3T. Although renal perfusion indicators of time to peak signal intensity and mean transit time were similar at 1.5T and 3T with TurboFLASH, use of the TREAT sequence at 3T also provided additional vascular anatomic information. Boss and

colleagues [35] also used the gain in SNR at 3T to perform perfusion quantification and perfusion mapping of the kidneys without intravenously administered contrast using the flow-sensitive alternating inversion recovery-true fast imaging in steady precision method with arterial spin labeling. In healthy volunteers, they were able to achieve highly resolved perfusion images of one single slice, as well as whole-kidney perfusion mapping. The advantage of such a technique is the lack of need for gadolinium-based contrast agents in patients who have severely compromised renal function.

The greater resonant frequency difference between fat and water at 3T compared with 1.5T allows for better spectral resolution in MR spectroscopy (MRS). Katz-Brull and colleagues [36] showed the feasibility of abdominal proton MRS using 3T MR imaging. The three most important factors enabling successful abdominal MRS were high magnetic field strength, use of a torso multicoil array, and breath holding. The same group of investigators used multiple breath hold averaged hydrogen MRS at 3T to aid in the characterization of renal masses [37]. Ten healthy volunteers and 14 patients who had renal cell carcinoma underwent frame-by-frame single voxel point resolved spectroscopy. In comparison with the normal subjects, the renal cell carcinomas tended to show a metabolic shift consisting of a decrease in free cholesterol and the degree of unsaturation of fatty acids.

Summary

3T MR imaging of the kidneys and urinary-collecting system is feasible and capable of producing high-quality images, although data comparing the results of urinary tract imaging at 3T with those obtained at 1.5T are lacking. The primary potential advantages of 3T imaging of the urinary tract over 1.5T imaging are similar to those of other parts of the body and include an increase in SNR and greater conspicuity of gadolinium-based contrast enhancement. As in other areas of the body, the increased SNR available at 3T often is sacrificed partially in the interest of improved spatial or temporal resolution, whereas the improved conspicuity of gadolinium-based contrast agents creates the potential for contrast dose-reduction strategies. Although all of the sequences used to evaluate the urinary tract at 1.5T can be used at 3T, adjustments in scan parameters and strategies to manage SAR and increased artifact conspicuity are necessary. Although anatomic MR imaging of the urinary tract may derive only limited benefit from increases in field strength from 1.5T to 3T, functional MR imaging of the kidneys potentially has much to gain. As a result, functional renal MR imaging likely will represent an area of rapid growth in the 3T MR imaging arena.

References

[1] Schindera S, Merkle E, Dale B, et al. Abdominal magnetic resonance imaging at 3.0T: what is the ultimate gain in signal-to-noise ratio? Acad Radiol 2006;13:1236–43.

[2] Nolte-Ernsting C, Adam G, Bücker A. Contrast-enhanced magnetic resonance urography: first experimental results with a polymeric gadolinium bloodpool agent. Invest Radiol 1997;32:418–23.

[3] El-Diasty T, Mansour O, Farouk A. Diuretic contrast-enhanced magnetic resonance urography versus intravenous urography for depiction of nondilated urinary tracts. Abdom Imaging 2003;28:135–45.

[4] Ergen FB, Hussain HK, Carlos RC, et al. 3D excretory MR urography: improved image quality with intravenous saline and diuretic administration. J Magn Reson Imaging 2007;25:783–9.

[5] Tsubota M, Takahara T, Nitatori T, et al. Utility of cine MR urography of the urinary tract and comparison with static MR urography. Radiat Med 2004;22:212–7.

[6] Merkle EM, Haugan PA, Thomas J, et al. 3.0T versus 1.5T MR cholangiography: a pilot study. AJR Am J Roentgenol 2006;186:516–21.

[7] O'Regan DP, Fitzgerald J, Allsop J, et al. A comparison of MR cholangiopancreatography at 1.5 and 3.0 Tesla. Br J Radiol 2005;78:894–8.

[8] Schindera ST, Miller CM, Ho LM, et al. Magnetic resonance (MR) cholangiography: quantitative and qualitative comparison of 3.0 Tesla with 1.5Tesla. Invest Radiol 2007;42:399–405.

[9] Sasaki M, Shibata E, Kanbara Y, et al. Enhancement effects and relaxivities of gadolinium-DTPA at 1.5 versus 3 Tesla: a phantom study. Magn Reson Med Sci 2005;4:145–9.

[10] Trattnig S, Pinker K, Ba-Ssalamah A, et al. The optimal use of contrast agents at high field MRI. Eur Radiol 2006;16:1280–7.

[11] Nöbauer-Huhmann IM, Ba-Ssalamah A, Mlynarik V, et al. Magnetic resonance imaging contrast enhancement of brain tumors at 3 Tesla versus 1.5 Tesla. Invest Radiol 2002;37:114–9.

[12] Krautmacher C, Willinek WA, Tschampa H, et al. Brain tumors: full- and half-dose contrast-enhanced MR imaging at 3.0T compared with 1.5T—initial experience. Radiology 2005;237:1014–9.

[13] Grobner T. Gadolinium: a specific trigger for the development of nephrogenic fibrosing dermopathy and nephrogenic systemic fibrosis? Nephrol Dial Transplant 2006;21:1104–8.

[14] Marckmann P, Skov L, Rossen K, et al. Nephrogenic systemic fibrosis: suspected causative role of gadodiamide used for contrast-enhanced magnetic resonance imaging. J Am Soc Nephrol 2006;17:2359–62.

[15] Khurana A, Runge VM, Narayanan M, et al. Nephrogenic systemic fibrosis: a review of 6 cases temporally related to gadodiamide injection (Omniscan). Invest Radiol 2007;42:139–45.

[16] Broome DR, Girguis MS, Baron PW, et al. Gadodiamide-associated nephrogenic systemic fibrosis: why radiologists should be concerned. AJR Am J Roentgenol 2007;188:586–92.

[17] Sadowski EA, Bennett LK, Chan MR, et al. Nephrogenic systemic fibrosis: risk factors and incidence estimation. Radiology 2007;242:148–57.

[18] Kanal E, Barkovich AJ, Bell C, et al. ACR guidance document for safe MR practices: 2007. AJR Am J Roentgenol 2007;188:1447–74.

[19] Pintaske J, Martirosian P, Graf H, et al. Relaxivity of Gadopentetate Dimeglumine (Magnevist), Gadobutrol (Gadovist), and Gadobenate Dimeglumine (MultiHance) in human blood plasma at 0.2, 1.5, and 3 Tesla. Invest Radiol 2006;41:213–21.

[20] Fukatsu H. 3T MR for clinical use: update. Magn Reson Med Sci 2003;2:37–45.

[21] Merkle E, Dale B, Paulson E. Abdominal MR imaging at 3T. Magn Reson Imaging Clin N Am 2006;14:17–26.

[22] Bernstein M, Huston J III, Ward H. Imaging artifacts at 3.0T. J Magn Reson Imaging 2006;24:735–46.

[23] Tanenbaum L. Clinical 3T MR imaging: mastering the challenges. Magn Reson Imaging Clin N Am 2006;14:1–15.

[24] Bottomley P, Foster T, Argersinger R, et al. A review of normal tissue hydrogen NMR relaxation times and relaxation mechanisms from 1-100 MHz: dependence on tissue type, NMR frequency, temperature, species, excision, and age. Med Phys 1984;11:425–48.

[25] Staniz G, Odrobina EE, Pun J, et al. T1, T2 relaxation and magnetization transfer in tissue at 3T. Magn Reson Med 2005;54:507–12.

[26] Schmitt M, Feiweier T, Horger W, et al. Improved uniformity of RF-distribution in clinical whole

body imaging at 3T by means of dielectric pads. Presented at the 12th Annual Meeting of ISMRM. Kyoto, Japan, May 15–21, 2004.

[27] Sreenivas M, Lowry M, Gibbs P, et al. A simple solution for reducing artefacts due to conductive and dielectric effects in clinical magnetic resonance imaging at 3 T. Eur J Radiol 2007;62:143–6.

[28] Pruessmann KP. Parallel imaging at high field strength: synergies and potential. Top Magn Reson Imaging 2004;15:237–44.

[29] Busse R. Reduced RF power without blurring: correcting for modulation of refocusing flip angle in FSE sequences. Magn Reson Med 2004; 51:1031–7.

[30] Hennig J, Scheffler K. Hyperechoes. Magn Reson Med 2001;46:6–12.

[31] Michaely HJ, Herrmann KA, Nael K, et al. Functional renal imaging: nonvascular renal disease. Abdom Imaging 2007;32:1–16.

[32] Tumkur SM, Vu AT, Li LP, et al. Evaluation of intra-renal oxygenation during water diuresis: a time-resolved study using BOLD MRI. Kidney Int 2006;70:139–43.

[33] Maril N, Rosen Y, Reynolds G, et al. Sodium MRI of the human kidney at 3 Tesla. Magn Reson Med 2006;56:1229–34.

[34] Michaely H, Nael K, Schoenberg SO, et al. Renal perfusion: comparison of saturation-recovery TurboFLASH measurements at 1.5 T with saturation-recovery TurboFLASH and time-resolved echo-shared angiographic technique (TREAT) at 3.0T. J Magn Reson Imaging 2006; 24:1413–9.

[35] Boss A, Martirosian P, Graf H, et al. High resolution MR perfusion imaging of the kidneys at 3 Tesla without administration of contrast media. Rofo 2005;177:1625–30.

[36] Katz-Brull R, Rofsky NM, Lenkinski RE. Breath-hold abdominal and thoracic proton MR spectroscopy at 3T. Magn Reson Med 2003;50:461–7.

[37] Katz-Brull R, Rofsky NM, Morrin MM, et al. Decreases in free cholesterol and fatty acid unsaturation in renal cell carcinoma demonstrated by breath-hold magnetic resonance spectroscopy. Am J Physiol Renal Physiol 2005; 288:F637–41.

MAGNETIC
RESONANCE
IMAGING CLINICS

Magn Reson Imaging Clin N Am 15 (2007) 383–393

Small Bowel MR Imaging: 1.5T versus 3T

Michael A. Patak, MD[a],*, Constantin von Weymarn, PhD[b],
Johannes M. Froehlich, PhD[b]

- Patient preparation
- MR imaging
- Pulse sequences for 1.5T and 3T imaging of the small bowel
  - Half-Fourier acquisition single-shot turbo spin echo/single-shot fast spin echo imaging
  - Steady-state free-precession/balanced fast-field echo/fast imaging employing steady state acquisition
  - Dynamic three-dimensional T1-weighted volumetric interpolated breath-hold

examination/liver acquisition with volume acceleration/3D T1-high resolution isotropic volume examination
  - Two-dimensional T1-weighted fast low-angle shot
- Inflammatory bowel disease
- Summary
  - 3T imaging of the small bowel: what's hot, what's not
- References

Direct visual assessment of the small bowel is possible in a limited way only. Capsule endoscopy is on the edge of becoming clinical routine, and thin long endoscopes are being used only occasionally [1,2]. Both techniques are able to visualize the surface of the small bowel but not the deeper layers. Most of the diseases of the small bowel, however, affect the entire bowel wall, the adjacent fat, or the mesentery, making the need for an imaging modality to visualize all layers obvious [3].

For a long time, x-ray enteroclysis was the sole technique for imaging the small bowel using naso-duodenal intubation for contrast administration and distension (Fig. 1). With the catheter tip in the proximal jejunum just beyond the ligament of Treitz, a contrast agent is pumped into the lumen to visualize and distend the bowel. Homogeneous opacification, surface coating, and adequate

distension are key to allow for a correct diagnosis. Placement of the catheter can be cumbersome, and is perceived as invasive and traumatizing by patients [4], particularly if they have to undergo this procedure repeatedly (eg, patients who have Crohn's disease [CD]).

Although new techniques like CT enteroclysis (Fig. 2) [5] and magnetic resonance (MR) enteroclysis [6] are on the edge of becoming clinical routine, these methods still use nasoduodenal intubation to achieve optimal distension of the intestinal loops.

CT enterography using oral administration of mannitol (Fig. 3) [7] or Volumen (EZ-EM; Lake Success, New York) is being used more frequently as the technique of choice for evaluation of the small bowel [8]. In addition to the burden of radiation, however, CT enterography still offers inferior

[a] Institute of Diagnostic, Interventional and Pediatric Radiology, Inselspital, University Hospital, 3010 Bern, Switzerland
[b] MR Research Group, Cantonal Hospital, Brauerstrasse 15, 8400 Winterthur, Switzerland
* Corresponding author.
E-mail address: michael.patak@insel.ch (M.A. Patak).

1064-9689/07/$ – see front matter © 2007 Elsevier Inc. All rights reserved.   doi:10.1016/j.mric.2007.07.002
mri.theclinics.com

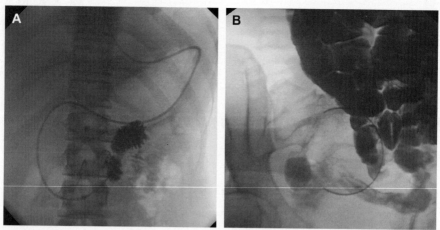

Fig. 1. Conventional enteroclysis has been the standard of reference for small bowel imaging. Conventional radiography has the highest image resolution but needs intubation for the procedure. (*A*) This tube has to be placed beyond the ligament of Treitz, which is perceived by patients as being traumatizing. Afterward, contrast is applied under continuous flow. (*B*) This patient has the typical presentation of ileitis terminalis, presenting with narrowing of the lumen and ulceration. This imaging technique is purely projectional and provides only information about the bowel wall.

soft tissue contrast when compared with MR imaging.

Another advantage of MR imaging is its ability to monitor small bowel wall changes dynamically in a fashion equivalent to fluoroscopy. The recent introduction of whole-body 3T MR imaging scanners brings the potential benefits of the higher field

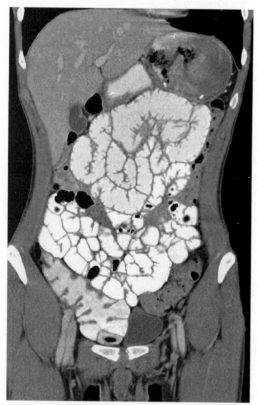

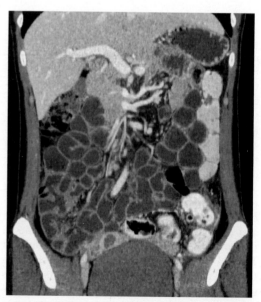

Fig. 2. CT enteroclysis. With the same techniques as for the conventional enteroclysis, a nasojejunal tube is placed and contrast is applied over the tube. Afterward, a CT scan is acquired with high intraluminal attenuation and high contrast to the bowel wall. (*Courtesy of* S. Wildermuth, MD, St. Gallen, Switzerland.)

Fig. 3. CT enterography. After oral administration of 3% mannitol solution at a dose of 1000 mL over the period of 1 hour, the multidetector CT scan is acquired. There is constant and high distension throughout the whole small bowel. Also, the contrast between the lumen and the bowel wall is high after administration of intravenous contrast.

strength to clinical applications, such as small bowel imaging.

This article is intended to provide practical information regarding patient preparation schemes for small bowel MR imaging and about a dedicated pulse sequence protocol for 1.5T and 3T MR imaging scanners, with specific emphasis on the advantages and remaining limitations of the higher field strength.

Patient preparation

Two important prerequisites must be considered to achieve optimal imaging results of the small bowel: adequate intraluminal distension and sufficient contrast. It is almost impossible to diagnose subtle changes in the collapsed bowel [5,9,10]. Therefore, distension is needed to unfold the bowel loops and to keep the bowel wall apart during the MR imaging examination. Intraluminal contrast, conversely, is needed to delineate the bowel wall and separate it from the content of the bowel lumen and the surrounding mesenteric fat. Ideally, for the preparation of the small bowel, a substance is chosen that addresses both of these prerequisites.

There are two fundamentally different approaches to achieve contrast and distension: by oral uptake or by administration of a distending agent by means of a tube placed in the duodenum or proximal jejunum. The term *MR enterography* is generally used for the noninvasive peroral use of contrast, whereas the term *MR enteroclysis* is used for the placement of the tube. Both techniques are widely used in clinical practice at 1.5 T [11]. The most common oral contrast for delineating the bowel lumen is tap water [12]. It is a bimodal contrast agent providing a bright signal on T2-weighted images and a low signal on T1-weighted images, which is particularly desired in combination with intravenous contrast. Other oral contrast agents with similar imaging characteristics have been described [12], with most of them not being used in daily routine. Water alone is not able to provide adequate distension because of its hyposmolarity, leading to rapid absorption after oral uptake [13]. To prevent this absorption from the gastrointestinal tract, osmotic active ingredients, such as sorbitol [14], mannitol [15], or other not absorbable saccharides have to be added. A second group of additives are high-molecular gelifiers or fiber-rich soluble polymers, such as methylcellulose, agar, and psyllium (Metamucil, Procter&Gamble, Ohio) (Fig. 4) [16]. Locust bean gum [17], polyethilenglycol (PEG) [18], and barium sulfate are also used to keep the water inside the bowel tube without significantly changing the MR signal characteristics.

In their institutions, the authors prefer MR enterography (ie, noninvasive administration of

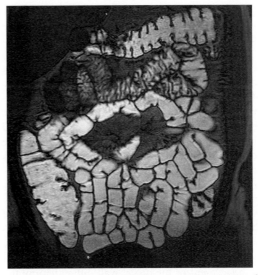

Fig. 4. MR enterography with oral administration of Metamucil and Gd-DOTA (Dotarem, Guerbet, Roissy, France). Without intravenous contrast, there is high contrast of the bowel lumen, which allows imaging in high resolution. Even without intubation, the distension of the small bowel is good and allows good delineation of the bowel wall.

contrast) with the poorly absorbed sugar monomer mannitol as an oral contrast. Mannitol is a ready-to-use white powder that can be dissolved easily in water, yielding a slightly sweet-tasting solution that is well accepted by the authors' patients. Mannitol at a dose of 30 g is dissolved in water (1000 mL), achieving a 3% solution, which is slightly hyposmolar compared with blood plasma. The patient is encouraged to drink the mannitol/water mixture (approximately 1–1.5 L) at regular intervals over a period of 1 hour before the examination. Shortly before the MR imaging examination, the patient is again asked to drink another 200 mL to achieve adequate distension of the stomach and duodenum.

Some mild adverse events have been reported, ranging from bloating to diarrhea. These adverse events are rare, usually mild, and self-limiting. They occur mainly after the termination of the MR imaging examination. Because of the high osmotic capacity of mannitol, water is kept inside the bowel lumen, and thus limits the filling of the bladder, which is advantageous in case of longer examination times but, conversely, might cause diarrhea in susceptible patients.

Whenever possible, the patient should be placed prone in the scanner. This limits the displacement of bowel segments during the examination (acquired at end-inspiration), because the spine is lifted from the MR imaging table and not from the areas in which most of the small bowel segments are located. The patient's arms should be extended over the head to avoid aliasing artifacts. Dedicated torso array receive-only coils should be used whenever possible to optimize signal reception.

Ideally, the oral distending agent should be combined with intravenous contrast and an inhibitor of bowel motion (ie, spasmolytic agent). Dynamic T1-weighted sequences with water-rich intraluminal solutions lead to a good contrast between the bowel wall and the lumen [19]. In particular, solid lesions and inflammatory bowel diseases can be optimally assessed with the use of intravenous contrast [20,21]. The authors generally use a dynamic scan protocol after the administration of a gadolinium-containing contrast agent at a body weight of 0.1 mmol/kg with an injection rate of 4 mL/s, followed by a flush of 20 mL saline (0.9% sodium chloride [NaCl]) at a rate of approximately 4 mL/s. Recent studies have shown that ideal enhancement of the bowel wall differs temporally from the peak enhancement of the liver [19]. Therefore, in the authors' imaging protocol, an additional enteric imaging phase at 60 seconds after the initiation of contrast has been implemented. Three-dimensional (3D), contrast-enhanced, T1-weighted, gradient-recalled echo (GRE) scanning is usually started after a fixed delay of 15 seconds, acquiring the arterial phase, followed by a second acquisition after 60 seconds for an ideal display of the bowel wall and, finally, a 90-second delay for the assessment of extraluminal pathologic findings and delayed contrast enhancement.

T1-weighted imaging is sensitive to motion and must be improved by using spasmolytic agents that reduce the peristaltic movement of the bowel loops. Depending on their availability, agents like glucagon or the antimuscarinic hyoscine butyl bromide (Buscopan; Boehringer Ingelheim, Ingelheim, Germany) are routinely administered. Because of the short efficiency window of these agents, the intravenous application cannot take place before the examination, and the agent has to be applied within the scanner. The best timing is shortly before the high-resolution, contrast-enhanced, 3D imaging starts. The authors use glucagon at a dose of 1 mg or hyoscine butyl bromide at a dose of 40 mg administered intravenously, followed by a saline flush of approximately 20 mL. There are several other administration techniques with glucagon, such as splitting the dosage in two, with half applied intramuscularly and the other applied intravenously shortly before dynamic scanning.

MR imaging

The MR imaging examination is usually started with a half-Fourier acquisition single-shot turbo spin echo (HASTE) sequence, followed by steady-state free-precession (TrueFisp, balanced fast-field echo [FFE], fast imaging employing steady state acquisition [FIESTA]) sequences. After the administration of an antiperistaltic agent, the first phase of the contrast-enhanced dynamic imaging with 3D T1-weighted sequences is performed. The contrast medium is administered as described previously, followed by dynamic 3D GRE scans acquired after 15, 60, and 90 seconds. Finally, 2D T1-weighted images are obtained. Postprocessing is often performed using the 3D T1-weighted data sets for the reconstruction of maximum-intensity projections (MIPs) or multiplanar reconstructions or, sometimes, to render dynamic images in other imaging planes (Fig. 5).

The inherent higher signal-to-noise ratio (SNR) at 3T with approximately 1.7 times the SNR allows the use of parallel imaging and to scan up to two to four times faster at 3T compared with 1.5T without losing the SNR [22]. Various kinds of artifacts have been described for abdominal 3T studies (eg, chemical shift, peripheral image distortion, dielectric effects), causing partial darkening. In the authors' experience, dielectric effects occur more frequently in thinner patients with variable severity and can usually be resolved by changing the acquisition plane. In the following section, the various sequences are discussed in greater detail for 1.5T and 3T (Table 1).

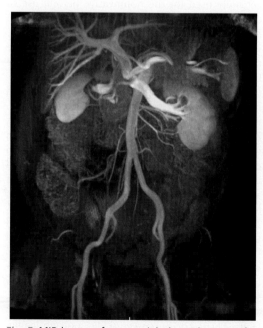

Fig. 5. MIP image of an arterial phase data set after intravenous contrast administration during a small bowel imaging protocol acquired on a 3T scanner. The 3D T1-weighted images are acquired without and 15 seconds, 60 seconds, and 90 seconds after administration of intravenous contrast.

Table 1:   **Overview of sequence parameters at 1.5T and 3T for small bowel imaging**

Field strength	Vendor	Sequence acronym	Parameters						
			TR	TE	Flip	Matrix	Slice thickness	Parallel imaging factor
1.5T	Philips[a]	3D bFFE ax and cor	4.4	1.3	20	512 × 512	1.5	2
		3D T1 THRIVE cor	4.8	1.3	20	512 × 512	1.5	2
		2D T1 trans	170	Min	80	512 × 512	7	
	Siemens[b]	HASTE ax and cor	1010	80	90	512 × 512	6	
		TruFisp ax and cor	3.8	1.9	57	512 × 384	6	
		3D VIBE cor	2.5	1	20	288 × 320	1.3	
		2D FLASH ax and cor	111	4.8	70	512 × 512	6	
	GE[c]	SSFSE	Min	140	90	384 × 128	10	
		FIESTA	X	Min-full	75	288 × 200	10	
		3D LAVA cor	3.3	X	12	288 × 192	4.4	2
3T	Philips[a]	SSFSE ax and cor	1485.5	80	90	512 × 512	5	2
		3D T1 THRIVE cor	6.8	3.5	22	512 × 512	3	2
		2D T1	450	2.8	75	512 × 512	5	2
	Siemens[b]	HASTE cor	2000	92	90	320 × 320	5	
		TruFisp ax	4.4	2.2	70	320 × 320	5	
		3D T1 VIBE	2.7	1.1	20	512 × 512	1	2
		2D T1 FLASH	128	3.7	70	384 × 288	3	2
	GE[c]	SSFSE	Min	120	90	512 × 224	8	
		FIESTA	X	Min-full	30	288 × 224	8	
		LAVA	4.1	X	12	288 × 192	4.4	2

Abbreviations: ax, axial; cor, coronal; FIESTA, fast imaging employing steady state acquisition; FLASH, fast low-angle shot; LAVA, liver acquisition with volume acceleration; Min, minimum possible; SSFSE, single-shot fast spin echo; THRIVE, 3D T1-high resolution isotropic volume examination; trans, transverse; VIBE, volumetric interpolated breath-hold examination; X.
[a] Philips Medical Systems, Best, The Netherlands.
[b] Siemens Medical Systems, Erlangen, Germany.
[c] GE Healthcare, Diagnostic Imaging, Milwaukee, Wisconsin.

Pulse sequences for 1.5T and 3T imaging of the small bowel

Half-Fourier acquisition single-shot turbo spin echo/single-shot fast spin echo imaging

This T2-weighted pulse sequence is ideal to begin the examination. It provides a rapid general overview of the whole abdomen. As a single-shot technique, this sequence is robust and almost insensitive to motion artifacts. Therefore, it is most helpful in cases of noncooperative patients who are unable to hold their breath [23]. The normal bowel wall usually has a low signal on these sequences, whereas fat and water present with a high signal. This excellent contrast allows visualization of the bowel wall separate from the luminal content and surrounding mesenteric tissue. The detailed structures of the bowel wall can be seen on these fast sequences even without the use of spasmolytic agents. In bowel segments with a normal structure, the valvulae conniventes are easily seen on these images (Fig. 6). Bowel wall edema, extraintestinal fluid accumulations, and mesenteric edema are clearly seen. Also, lymph nodes can easily be depicted, particularly in the coronal imaging plane.

Unfortunately, at 3T, higher specific absorption rate (SAR) levels are often a limiting factor within this sequence (Fig. 7). It takes approximately

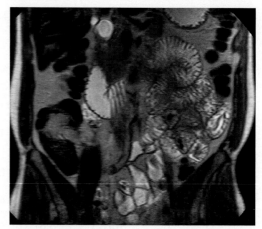

Fig. 7. Single-shot fast spin echo (SSFSE) images acquired on a 3T system. These images are stable and insensitive to motion and are ideal to achieve a fast overview, especially in patients who are not able to hold their breath. In addition to the detailed structures of the bowel wall, this pulse sequence is good for the display of wall edema or for the presence of extraintestinal fluid or mesenteric edema.

10 minutes to cover the entire abdomen in a transverse imaging plane, because one has to split the data acquisition into approximately five stacks in a normal-sized patient. Parallel imaging techniques may help in reducing the data acquisition time by decreasing SAR, and thereby allowing greater coverage, but this is at the expense of the SNR. The authors recently modified their small bowel sequence protocol and now skip the acquisition in the axial plane, using single-shot fast spin echo imaging because it simply takes too long even with parallel imaging.

Steady-state free-precession/balanced fast-field echo/fast imaging employing steady state acquisition

This 2D TrueFisp sequence offers T2-weighted over T1-weighted image contrast and is the preferred pulse sequence to evaluate the mesentery and the bowel wall. The vascular structures in the mesentery are clearly visible and easy to assess, because all structures with flow are signal intense, and are thus highlighted on these images. All structures with a fat/water interface are nicely outlined by a small dark rim because of a chemical shift artifact of the second kind (ie, India ink artifact). Thus, the lymph nodes are also easily depicted. In the authors' experience, the assessment of the bowel wall itself is also easy with this sequence, because wall edema and layering within the wall can be displayed [24]. Broader chemical shift artifacts might hamper the image quality. To overcome this

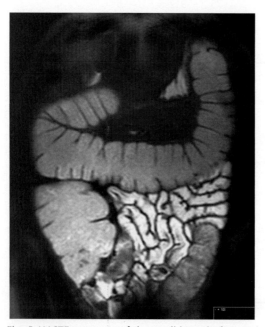

Fig. 6. HASTE sequence of the small bowel after oral preparation with mannitol. These images allow imaging of detailed bowel wall structures even without the use of spasmolytic agents. The valvulae convenientes are easily seen on these images in normal segments.

problem, there could be a benefit with the use of fat saturation [25].

For 3T MR imaging, chemical shift artifacts may even be increased and may seriously hamper the image quality. TrueFisp sequences are not always applicable at 3T because of distortion artifacts. The authors currently use a 2D sequence that takes longer to acquire but is stable enough with a good SNR of the bowel wall (Fig. 8).

Dynamic three-dimensional T1-weighted volumetric interpolated breath-hold examination/liver acquisition with volume acceleration/3D T1-high resolution isotropic volume examination

These dynamic T1-weighted sequences are excellent for the assessment of the enhancement pattern of the bowel wall. This is of utmost clinical importance, especially for the evaluation of inflammatory small bowel disease. These data sets have to be acquired during breath hold and in short intervals between the different contrast phases. This can be challenging for the patient. In the authors' experience, it is helpful to communicate to the patient the importance of apnea. The authors normally inform the patient and simulate or train the course of the dynamic examination before the data acquisition, because these images are usually rendered nondiagnostic without the patient's cooperation.

Partially because of the excellent through-plane spatial resolution, the unenhanced 3D data sets

often present with low signal. These images are only useful for subtraction purposes and when there is a T1-weighted hyperintense lesion on the unenhanced images. During the course of the administration of the contrast agent, a strong gain in the SNR and contrast-to-noise ratio (CNR) is observed. It is important to look at the small changes of contrast in the bowel wall or mucosa to detect subtle lesions. Because the sequence is a 3D acquisition, various image reconstructions can be performed. The authors routinely reconstruct an MIP image of the arterial and portal-venous phases to obtain a general overview of the mesenteric vessels.

Dynamic scanning on 3T MR imaging systems is feasible and provides a twofold higher SNR, and perhaps an even further improved CNR. The in-plane spatial resolution is as high as with 1.5T imaging; however, because of the higher SNR, the through-plane resolution can be improved. Usually, the fat suppression is more pronounced on 3T images and helps to display the vessels and the small bowel wall even better (Fig. 9).

Two-dimensional T1-weighted fast low-angle shot

This gradient-echo sequence is usually performed when the contrast is evenly distributed within the vascular and interstitial spaces corresponding to the late phase. It is acquired approximately 3 to 5 minutes after the administration of intravenous contrast. The highly vascularized bowel wall demonstrates strong uptake of contrast, and therefore a good CNR. Actively inflamed tissue may be differentiated from normal or chronically ill tissue to a certain extent. Because it is usually performed late, the effect of spasmolytic agents starts to fade and motion artifacts may hamper the image quality. Nevertheless, this is a clinically important sequence. Because of the excellent SNR, these images allow for the detection of subtle lesions of the small bowel wall. Reassessment of these areas on the dynamic scans allows further lesion characterization. It is also the preferred sequence for extraintestinal contrast-enhanced findings, such as lymph node imaging.

At 3T imaging, these gradient-echo sequences can easily be implemented. They are robust and show good and strong contrast of the bowel wall and the surrounding tissues. Because of the excellent SNR and CNR, these images can be acquired in a higher spatial resolution compared with 1.5T (Fig. 10).

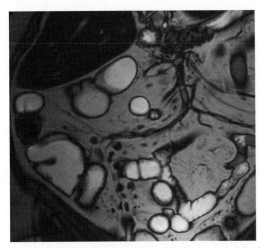

Fig. 8. TrueFisp sequence. This pulse sequence is ideal for the display of the vascular structures and the display of the mesentery. Lymph nodes are also clearly visible on these images. This patient has CD, and the terminal ileum is affected by the disease. There are several enlarged lymph nodes about the terminal ileum that can be easily identified on these TrueFisp images.

Inflammatory bowel disease

CD is a chronic inflammatory transmural disease of any part of the gastrointestinal tract [3,26]. The

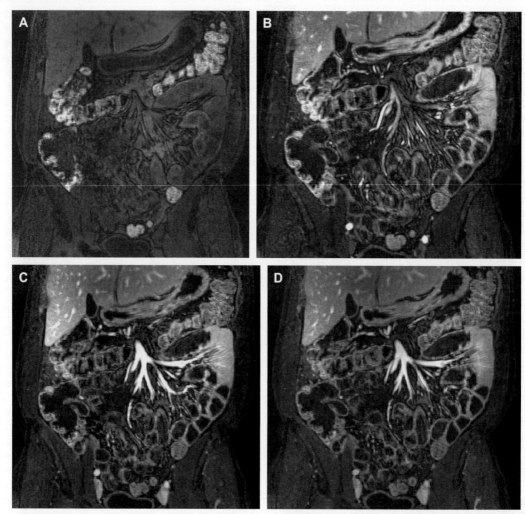

Fig. 9. Dynamic imaging of the small bowel. The dynamic acquisition after intravenous administration of contrast is crucial for the clinical assessment of the small bowel wall. A 3D T1-weighted sequence is acquired before (*A*), 15 seconds after (*B*), 60 seconds after (*C*), and 90 seconds after (*D*) contrast administration. The images were acquired on a 3T system. The contrast uptake of the bowel wall and its segmental assessment has high sensitivity and specificity for different pathologic findings of the small bowel.

disease is of unknown etiology, ill-defined, and unpredictable and shows a variable response to medical or surgical therapy [27,28]. The course of the disease is prolonged and unpredictable with alternating exacerbations and remissions. As a consequence of the chronic recurrent course, repeated diagnostic controls are necessary.

MR imaging has proven to be a good tool to evaluate the extent and activity of the disease and the presence of extraluminal complications [11]. MR imaging is also able to identify the type of the disease: the active/inflammatory, fistulizing/perforating, fibrostenosing, or reparative/regenerative type [29].

Because this entity is one of the main indications for small bowel imaging, it is further discussed in

this section as an example of how to read and interpret small bowel MR images.

Data analysis is usually started by reading the T2-weighted single-shot fast spin echo or the 2D T1-weighted gradient echo postcontrast images. The authors usually start by analyzing the late 2D postcontrast images, searching for areas of increased signal enhancement (Fig. 11). Most pathologic entities of the small bowel demonstrate thickening of the wall. The 2D postcontrast MR images offer high sensitivity for the detection of small bowel wall abnormalities and for all extraluminal changes, such as enlarged lymph nodes or abscess formations. Areas of bowel wall thickening are further characterized by analyzing the T2-weighted precontrast or dynamic contrast-enhanced images.

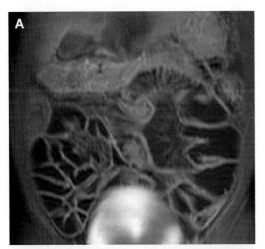

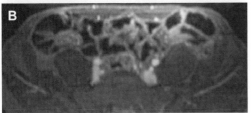

Fig. 10. Flash 2D images are acquired 3 to 5 minutes after intravenous contrast administration. These images allow the detection of subtle lesions of the small bowel wall and the surrounding tissue. They also represent the preferred data set for the detection of lymph nodes. The authors usually acquire these images in the coronal (*A*) and transverse (*B*) planes.

As mentioned previously, MR imaging is able not only to detect changes of inflammatory bowel disease but to determine the activity of specific lesions [21,30–32]. It is of note that patients who have CD can have multiple lesions at different stages of inflammation or even different types of the disease [29].

On T2-weighted images, the bowel wall itself must be analyzed. There are different mural patterns that can help to specify the type of activity. Fistulae can also be detected using these data sets, because fistulae or abscesses often appear as spiculated lesions with a fluid-equivalent signal in the center.

This is followed by assessment of the dynamic images. Normally, active inflammation has an early and strong uptake in the arterial phase, whereas the fibrostenosing type of lesion shows a delayed and more moderate uptake of contrast [21,31,33].

Finally, the TrueFisp images and the MIP images of the arterial phase need to be evaluated. Hyperemia or wall edema is usually also present in most of the changes related to CD [34–37]. It is a sensitive indicator for pathologic changes of the bowel wall. On TrueFisp imaging and the MIP reconstructions, the corkscrew arteries or the so-called "comb-sign"

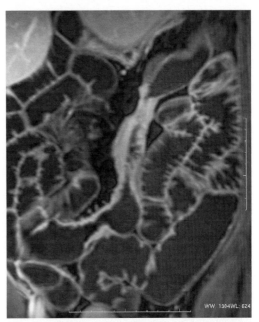

Fig. 11. Coronal fat-saturated volumetric interpolated breath-hold examination after intravenous administration of gadolinium showing skip lesions of the neo-terminal ileum with wall thickening, a laminar pattern of enhancement, deep ulceration, and structuring. (*Courtesy of* H. Bungay, MD, Oxford, United Kingdom.)

can easily be identified (Fig. 12). These are engorged vasa recta of the affected bowel segment that develop because of the prolonged or chronic hyperemia.

For 3T imaging, the work flow of image interpretation should not change. Because of the higher CNR, however, it should be easier to identify smaller lesions compared with 1.5T imaging [38]. These marked differences, especially after administration of contrast, should be helpful for improved lesion detection. In the authors' clinical experience, however, lesion characterization currently does not benefit from the higher field strength and its subsequently higher CNR, because a multitude of known patterns already allow for the adequate characterization of these lesions [11]. These patterns are well known and should not change significantly at higher field strength.

Summary

3T imaging of the small bowel: what's hot, what's not

The main challenge for 3T imaging of the small bowel has been the large field of view (FOV) covering the whole abdomen, with most of the initial problems being solved. T1-weighted imaging is ready for prime time. These sequences provide the coverage, SNR, and CNR for improving imaging

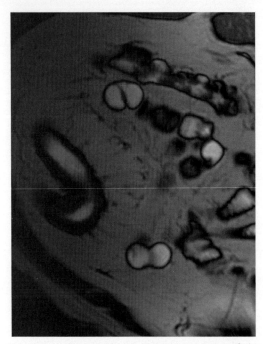

Fig. 12. Comb sign. The engorged vasa recta of the chronic inflammation are easily seen on these TrueFisp images. These are sensitive indicators for pathologic changes of an affected bowel segment.

significantly when compared with 1.5 T. This is similar to contrast-enhanced dynamic MR angiography, where these sequences have proven to be reliable and robust, clearly benefiting from the increased signal available at 3T [39,40].

Certain problems remain for T2-weighted imaging. The limitation of the SAR in relation to the FOV leads to compromises and trade-offs. These result in loss of the CNR or spatial or temporal resolution. Improved coils implementing multi-channel systems, gradient designs, and adapted sequences with modified radiofrequency (RF) waveforms or parallel imaging techniques should help to overcome these restrictions in the near future. There are already reasonable solutions for T2-weighted imaging of the abdomen, as mentioned previously [41]. Thus, using 3T technology with its inherently better SNR might improve image quality and speed. Both together should lead to a gain of diagnostic confidence in cases of small bowel pathologic findings and allow implementation of a robust sequence protocol that can be performed routinely.

References

[1] Pennazio M. Capsule endoscopy: where are we after 6 years of clinical use? Dig Liver Dis 2006; 38:867–78.

[2] May A, Ell C. Push-and-pull enteroscopy using the double-balloon technique/double-balloon enteroscopy. Dig Liver Dis 2006;38:932–8.

[3] Podolsky DK. Inflammatory bowel disease. N Engl J Med 2002;347:417–29.

[4] Singer AJ, Richman PB, Kowalska A, et al. Comparison of patient and practitioner assessments of pain from commonly performed emergency department procedures. Ann Emerg Med 1999; 33:652–8.

[5] Bender GN, Maglinte DD, Kloppel VR, et al. CT enteroclysis: a superfluous diagnostic procedure or valuable when investigating small-bowel disease? AJR Am J Roentgenol 1999;172:373–8.

[6] Prassopoulos P, Papanikolaou N, Grammatikakis J, et al. MR enteroclysis imaging of Crohn disease. Radiographics 2001;21. Spec No:S161–72.

[7] Berther R, Patak MA, Eckhardt B, et al. Mannitol as a neutral oral contrast in abdominal MDCT: a comparison of low attenuation contrast versus positive intraluminal contrast. Presented at the RSNA 92nd Scientific Assembly and Annual Meeting 2006. Chicago, 2006.

[8] Paulsen SR, Huprich JE, Fletcher JG, et al. CT enterography as a diagnostic tool in evaluating small bowel disorders: review of clinical experience with over 700 cases. Radiographics 2006; 26:641–57 [discussion: 657–62].

[9] Bender GN, Timmons JH, Williard WC, et al. Computed tomographic enteroclysis: one methodology. Invest Radiol 1996;31:43–9.

[10] Raptopoulos V, Schwartz RK, McNicholas MM, et al. Multiplanar helical CT enterography in patients with Crohn's disease. AJR Am J Roentgenol 1997;169:1545–50.

[11] Fidler J. MR imaging of the small bowel. Radiol Clin North Am 2007;45:317–31.

[12] Debatin JF, Patak MA. MRI of the small and large bowel. Eur Radiol 1999;9:1523–34.

[13] Borthne AS, Abdelnoor M, Storaas T, et al. Osmolarity: a decisive parameter of bowel agents in intestinal magnetic resonance imaging. Eur Radiol 2006;16:1331–6.

[14] Ajaj W, Goehde SC, Schneemann H, et al. Oral contrast agents for small bowel MRI: comparison of different additives to optimize bowel distension. Eur Radiol 2004;14:458–64.

[15] Schunk K, Kersjes W, Schadmand-Fischer S, et al. [A mannitol solution as an oral contrast medium in pelvic MRT]. Rofo Fortschr Geb Rontgenstr Neuen Bildgeb Verfahr 1995;163:60–6 [in German].

[16] Patak MA, Froehlich JM, von Weymarn C, et al. Non-invasive distension of the small bowel for magnetic-resonance imaging. Lancet 2001;358: 987–8.

[17] Lauenstein TC, Schneemann H, Vogt FM, et al. Optimization of oral contrast agents for MR imaging of the small bowel. Radiology 2003;228: 279–83.

[18] Laghi A, Carbone I, Catalano C, et al. Polyethylene glycol solution as an oral contrast agent for

MR imaging of the small bowel. AJR Am J Roentgenol 2001;177:1333–4.

[19] Horton KM, Eng J, Fishman EK. Normal enhancement of the small bowel: evaluation with spiral CT. J Comput Assist Tomogr 2000;24:67–71.

[20] Boudiaf M, Jaff A, Soyer P, et al. Small-bowel diseases: prospective evaluation of multi-detector row helical CT enteroclysis in 107 consecutive patients. Radiology 2004;233:338–44.

[21] Florie J, Wasser MN, Arts-Cieslik K, et al. Dynamic contrast-enhanced MRI of the bowel wall for assessment of disease activity in Crohn's disease. AJR Am J Roentgenol 2006;186:1384–92.

[22] Schindera ST, Merkle EM, Dale BM, et al. Abdominal magnetic resonance imaging at 3.0 T what is the ultimate gain in signal-to-noise ratio? Acad Radiol 2006;13:1236–43 [in German].

[23] Lee JK, Marcos HB, Semelka RC. MR imaging of the small bowel using the HASTE sequence. AJR Am J Roentgenol 1998;170:1457–63.

[24] Gourtsoyiannis N, Papanikolaou N, Grammatikakis J, et al. MR enteroclysis protocol optimization: comparison between 3D FLASH with fat saturation after intravenous gadolinium injection and true FISP sequences. Eur Radiol 2001;11:908–13.

[25] Gourtsoyiannis NC, Grammatikakis J, Papamastorakis G, et al. Imaging of small intestinal Crohn's disease: comparison between MR enteroclysis and conventional enteroclysis. Eur Radiol 2006;16:1915–25.

[26] Crohn B, Ginzburg L, Oppenheimer G. Regional ileitis: a pathologic and clinical entity. JAMA 1932;99:1323–9.

[27] Sandler RS, Golden AL. Epidemiology of Crohn's disease. J Clin Gastroenterol 1986;8:160–5.

[28] Karlinger K, Gyorke T, Mako E, et al. The epidemiology and the pathogenesis of inflammatory bowel disease. Eur J Radiol 2000;35:154–67.

[29] Maglinte DD, Gourtsoyiannis N, Rex D, et al. Classification of small bowel Crohn's subtypes based on multimodality imaging. Radiol Clin North Am 2003;41:285–303.

[30] Gourtsoyiannis N, Papanikolaou N, Grammatikakis J, et al. Assessment of Crohn's disease activity in the small bowel with MR and conventional enteroclysis: preliminary results. Eur Radiol 2004;14:1017–24.

[31] Maccioni F, Bruni A, Viscido A, et al. MR imaging in patients with Crohn disease: value of T2-versus

T1-weighted gadolinium-enhanced MR sequences with use of an oral superparamagnetic contrast agent. Radiology 2006;238:517–30.

[32] Sempere GA, Martinez Sanjuan V, Medina Chulia E, et al. MRI evaluation of inflammatory activity in Crohn's disease. AJR Am J Roentgenol 2005;184:1829–35.

[33] Low RN, Sebrechts CP, Politoske DA, et al. Crohn disease with endoscopic correlation: single-shot fast spin-echo and gadolinium-enhanced fat-suppressed spoiled gradient-echo MR imaging. Radiology 2002;222:652–60.

[34] Koh DM, Miao Y, Chinn RJ, et al. MR imaging evaluation of the activity of Crohn's disease. AJR Am J Roentgenol 2001;177:1325–32.

[35] Miao YM, Koh DM, Amin Z, et al. Ultrasound and magnetic resonance imaging assessment of active bowel segments in Crohn's disease. Clin Radiol 2002;57:913–8.

[36] Schreyer AG, Golder S, Scheibl K, et al. Dark lumen magnetic resonance enteroclysis in combination with MRI colonography for whole bowel assessment in patients with Crohn's disease: first clinical experience. Inflamm Bowel Dis 2005;11:388–94.

[37] Schreyer AG, Rath HC, Kikinis R, et al. Comparison of magnetic resonance imaging colonography with conventional colonoscopy for the assessment of intestinal inflammation in patients with inflammatory bowel disease: a feasibility study. Gut 2005;54:250–6.

[38] Upponi S, Planner A, Anderson E, et al. MR enteroclysis: a comparison of sequences at 3T. Presented at the 18th Annual Meeting and Postgraduate Course, ESAGR. Lisbon (Portugal), June 12–15, 2007.

[39] Nael K, Fenchel M, Krishnam M, et al. High-spatial-resolution whole-body MR angiography with high-acceleration parallel acquisition and 32-channel 3.0-T unit: initial experience. Radiology 2007;242:865–72.

[40] Nael K, Saleh R, Lee M, et al. High-spatial-resolution contrast-enhanced MR angiography of abdominal arteries with parallel acquisition at 3.0 T: initial experience in 32 patients. AJR Am J Roentgenol 2006;187:W77–85.

[41] van Gemert-Horsthuis K, Florie J, Hommes DW, et al. Feasibility of evaluating Crohn's disease activity at 3.0 Tesla. J Magn Reson Imaging 2006;24:340–8.

MAGNETIC RESONANCE IMAGING CLINICS

Magn Reson Imaging Clin N Am 15 (2007) 395–402

MR Colonography: 1.5T versus 3T

Thomas C. Lauenstein, MD[a],*, Bettina Saar, MD[b],
Diego R. Martin, MD, PhD[a]

- Patient preparation
- Technical considerations of MR colonography at 3T
  Signal-to-noise ratio
  Radiofrequency coils
  Susceptibility artifacts
- Sequence protocols and image quality

Fast imaging with steady-state precession
T2-weighted single-shot fast spin echo
T1-weighted three-dimensional gradient echo
- Clinical outcomes
- Summary
- References

MR colonography (MRC), a noninvasive method to evaluate colorectal disease, was first described by Luboldt and colleagues [1] in 1997. After the rectal administration of a water-based enema or gasiform distending media such as air or CO_2 [2–5], an assessment of the bowel wall can be performed either on the acquired source data or on virtual endoscopic reformations [6,7]. Other than optical colonoscopy, MRC enables a visualization of the colon even in the presence of high-grade stenoses [8,9]. Moreover, all structures adjacent to the intestine are displayed, thereby allowing the assessment of simultaneous abdominal disease [10]. Most patients prefer virtual colonography to optical colonoscopy [11,12].

Most MRC approaches during the last decade were performed at 1T [13] or 1.5T [10,14–16]. Within recent years scanners with higher field strengths have become commercially available and have been implemented clinically. First reports on MRC at 3T demonstrate the feasibility of this method [17,18]. This article focuses on the technical requirements and clinical outcomes of MRC at

1.5T and 3T and describes the advantages and limitations of MRC at both field strengths.

Patient preparation

The principles of patient preparation are similar for MRC at 1.5T and 3T. Patients who have general contraindications to MR imaging, such as cardiac pacemakers or cardioverter defibrillators, should be excluded. Patients who have hip prostheses or osteosynthetic material in the spine should not be examined, because considerable artifacts in the abdomen and pelvis may impede obtaining an image of diagnostic quality in the colon and/or rectum. Some type of bowel preparation must be performed, because examinations of unprepared bowel may result in both false-positive (stool particles simulating colorectal masses) and false-negative results (colorectal lesions masked by residual stool). To this end patients should undergo bowel cleansing and/or fecal tagging [19–21]. Furthermore, the colon must be distended to allow a reliable evaluation of the bowel wall. Otherwise,

[a] Department of Radiology, The Emory Clinic, 1365 Clifton Road, Bldg A, Suite AT-627, Atlanta, GA 30322, USA
[b] Institut für Diagnostische, Interventionelle, und Pädiatrische Radiologie der Universität Bern, Inselspital, CH-3010 Bern, Switzerland
* Corresponding author.
E-mail address: tlauens@emory.edu (T.C. Lauenstein).

doi:10.1016/j.mric.2007.06.006

nondistended colonic segments can mimic bowel wall thickening, thereby leading to possible misinterpretation of inflammation or even colorectal malignancy.

The rectal application of different agents, including water-based fluids, CO_2, or room air, has been proposed for colonic distension [3–5]. Furthermore, spasmolytic agents (eg, 20 mg of scopolamine or 1 mg of glucagon) should be administered intravenously to help obviate bowel spasms, minimize artifacts caused by bowel motion, and provide higher levels of bowel distension [22,23]. Depending on the patient's preference, positioning can be either prone or supine. For signal reception, dedicated surface array coils should be used.

Technical considerations of MR colonography at 3T

The transfer of MR imaging protocols from 1.5T to 3T for abdominal imaging harbors some pitfalls. Several issues, including image characteristics, presence of artifacts, management of specific absorption rate (SAR), and hardware-related modifications, must be addressed. Considerations that play a particularly important role for MRC at 3T are the signal-to-noise ratio, radiofrequency (RF) coils, and susceptibility artifacts.

Signal-to-noise ratio

The RF signal generated at a field strength of 3T is four times greater than that generated at 1.5T, but the signal-to-noise (SNR) is only doubled because of the simultaneous twofold increase of noise [24,25]. The increased overall SNR may allow improved spatial resolution and/or a considerable reduction in acquisition time. These advantages can be particularly important for the detection of smaller colorectal polyps (< 5 mm) or even flat adenomas, because the sensitivity and specificity for detecting these lesions at 1.5T are poor [10]. Furthermore, shorter acquisition times can be beneficial in patients who are not able to hold their breath for a longer period.

Radiofrequency coils

Only a limited variety of RF coils currently are available at 3T. The development of new surface coils will be crucial to allow greater anatomic coverage, lower SAR values, and improved implementation of parallel imaging techniques to be achieved with MRC at 3T. In particular, greater anatomic coverage in the z-axis is important because of the extension of bowel loops in craniocaudal direction. Hence, MRC ideally should encompass an anatomic coverage from the upper abdomen (including right and

left colonic flexure) down to the pelvis (including sigmoid colon and rectum).

Susceptibility artifacts

Susceptibility artifacts are increased at 3T compared with 1.5T and thus may reduce the image quality of MRC [26–28]. They arise at interfaces of materials of different susceptibility such as metal and soft tissue or gas and soft tissue. Although the administration of a liquid rectal enema is advocated for most MRC approaches, the presence of residual air within the bowel lumen cannot be avoided. Although susceptibility artifacts can be helpful in some respects (eg, for the detection of free intraperitoneal gas), they may impede an assessment of parts of the colonic wall.

Sequence protocols and image quality

A high contrast between bowel lumen and wall is mandatory for the depiction of colorectal pathologies. The contrast mechanisms depend strongly on the type of the rectal enema and the applied MR sequences. As with other abdominal MR imaging applications, it is important to collect data under breathhold conditions to avoid (respiratory) motion artifacts. Hence, acquisition times should not exceed 15 to 20 seconds, a period that is feasible for most patients. The implementation of parallel imaging has been especially helpful in decreasing acquisition times. Otherwise, data collection should be subdivided into several image blocks. After the collection of a localizer sequence, a comprehensive MRC protocol should encompass three different types of sequences (Figs. 1 and 2; Table 1), described in the following sections. Pitfalls of these sequences at 3T are discussed also, and possible optimization strategies are proposed.

Fast imaging with steady-state precession

Different vendor-specific have been used for fast imaging with steady-state precession (FISP): Balanced Fast Field Echo (Philips Medical Systems, Best, The Netherlands), fast imaging employing steady-state acquisition (FIESTA) (General Electric Medical Systems, Milwaukee, Wisconsin), and true fast imaging with steady-state precession (True-FISP) (Siemens Medical Solution, Erlangen, Germany). FISP images allow a good anatomic overview of abdominal and pelvic structures by providing a mixture of both T1 and T2 contrast. A particular advantage of this sequence is its relative insensitivity to motion, which is helpful in patients who are unable to hold their breath. FISP data should be acquired without fat suppression so mesenteric changes (eg, the presence of lymph nodes or pericolic stranding) can be appreciated better.

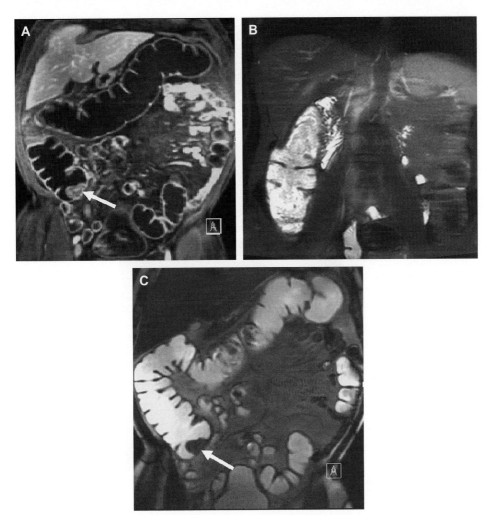

Fig. 1. MRC images obtained at 3T in coronal plane. (*A*) Contrast-enhanced T1-weighted gradient-recalled echo. The arrow indicates a 2.5-cm carcinoma in the ascending colon. (*B*) T2-weighted single-shot with fat saturation. (*C*) FISP. The arrow indicates a 2.5-cm carcinoma in the ascending colon.

Furthermore, this sequence is powerful in detecting inflammatory processes, such as the changes of Crohn's disease or ulcerative colitis [15].

FISP imaging is relatively sensitive to main B0 field inhomogeneity, resulting in banding artifacts at the margins of the field of view and at air/tissue interfaces. At 3T banding artifacts can be more evident because of increased field inhomogeneity effects (Fig. 3). A simple approach to compensate for the distortion is to split the acquisition into multiple groups along the z-axis, thereby recentering the image field to the center of the magnet and thus improving the B0 homogeneity.

Another important consideration is tissue contrast, which improves with lower TR and TE and higher flip angles. A decrease in flip angle is necessary at 3T, however, because of SAR constraints. Hence, a lower RF pulse is used, resulting in an increase of minimum TR and TE. To overcome the undesirable decrease of contrast, a lower B1 gradient can be used, and slice thickness should be increased at 3T. Overall, imaging quality of FISP-type sequences is still superior at 1.5T, because banding artifacts severely compromise the image quality at 3T.

T2-weighted single-shot fast spin echo

The differentiation between active and nonactive (ie, fibrotic) inflammatory changes of the colon is one of the clinical questions that often must be addressed when MRC is performed. To that end, the acquisition of single-shot T2-weighted sequences with fat saturation is important. Edema in or adjacent to the bowel wall as a marker for active disease can be depicted easily on the T2 fat saturated images [29,30].

On 1.5T the TR for single-shot fast spin echo (SSFSE) images usually is chosen in a way that

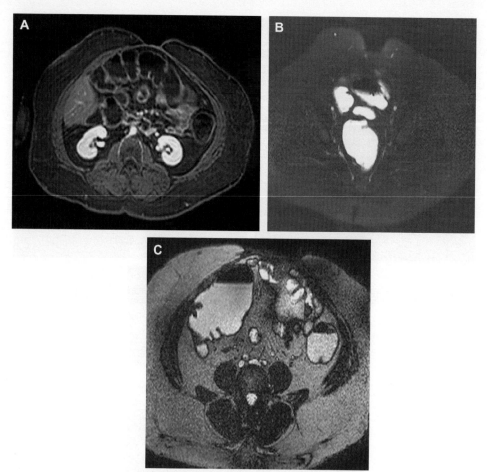

Fig. 2. MRC images obtained at 1.5T in axial plane. (*A*) Contrast-enhanced T1-weighted gradient-recalled echo. (*B*) T2-weighted single-shot with fat saturation. (*C*) FISP.

lowers acquisition times but still preserves T2 signal and typically is between 700 and 1000 milliseconds. On 3T, however, SAR limits minimum TR, which for current techniques is approximately 1500 milliseconds. Thus, SSFSE produces a single slice only every 1.5 seconds, and more than one breathhold usually is required to cover the abdomen and pelvis fully. SAR may lead to another problem: at 1.5T the SSFSE echo train is formed as a series of 180° refocusing RF pulses, but this can be difficult at 3T because of SAR constraints. Therefore, the refocusing pulses are reduced (eg, to 150°) to decrease the rate of energy deposits. Finally, there is a higher rate of T2* decay at 3T, and SSFSE techniques are more prone to blurring from T2* effect. A solution can be the use of parallel

Table 1: Comparison of sequence parameters for MR colonography at 1.5T and 3T

Parameter	2D FISP without fat suppression		2D Single-shot T2-weighted with fat suppression		3D T1-weighted gradient-recalled echo with fat suppression	
	1.5T	*3T*	*1.5T*	*3T*	*1.5T*	*3T*
TR (milliseconds)	3.7	4.7	676	1500	3.1	3.1
TE (milliseconds)	1.7	1.9	100	84	1.2	1.3
Flip angle (°)	60	45	90	90	10	10
Slice thickness (mm)	4 mm	6 mm	6–7 mm	6–7 mm	2 mm	3 mm

Abbreviations: 2D, two-dimensional; 3D, three-dimensional; FISP, fast imaging with steady-state precession.

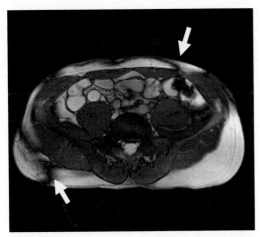

Fig. 3. FISP MRC image at 3T. Typical banding artifacts are noted in the periphery of the body (*arrows*).

imaging techniques allowing compacting the echo train length, thereby decreasing the effective echo time and thus providing sharper image resolution. Overall, the image quality of SSFSE sequences is fairly similar at 1.5T and 3T, unless dielectric artifacts compromise the images acquired at the higher field strength.

T1-weighted three-dimensional gradient echo

T1-weighted images should be collected with and without intravenous gadolinium. The three-dimensional acquisition should be performed at 20 seconds (arterial phase), 60 seconds (portal venous phase), 120 seconds (delayed contrast phase), and 180 seconds (equilibrium contrast phase). The

benefits of this sequence are related to the high spatial resolution with nearly isotropic voxel size and to information gained about tissue perfusion. Hence, polyps or carcinomas can be distinguished reliably from residual stool particles or air bubbles, which can mimic colorectal lesions (Fig. 4). Although tissue enhancement always is found in real colonic masses, pseudolesions never enhance after gadolinium administration [10,16].

The image quality (including blurring artifacts) at 3T is more influenced by changes in TE. Therefore, a maximum sampling bandwidth should be used to achieve minimum TE. Although the SNR is decreased, the advantages of persistent image quality outweigh this drawback. Overall, contrast-enhanced T1-weighted three-dimensional gradient-recalled echo sequences at 3T are superior to those at 1.5T because of the improved SNR and better efficiency of gadolinium-based contrast agents at higher field strengths.

A recent study by Rottgen and colleagues [17] directly compared the image quality of MRC at field strengths of 1.5T and 3T. Twenty patients underwent MRC at both 1.5T and 3T. For signal reception a four-element torso coil was used at both field strengths, and the same sequence types, including FISP, T2-weighted SSFSE, and T1-weighted gradient-recalled echo sequences, were collected. The image quality for each sequence was rated using a five-point scale, with higher values indicating better image quality. There were no significant differences for the T1-weighted gradient-recalled echo and T2-weighted SSFSE sequences, but the quality of FISP images was found to be superior at 1.5T. Thus, overall image quality was not increased at 3T. Table 1

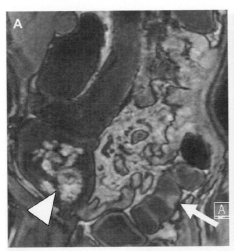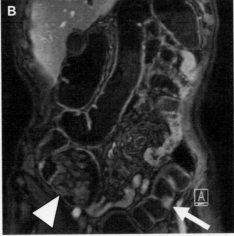

Fig. 4. T1-weighted images at 3T (*A*) before and (*B*) after intravenous gadolinium administration. A 1.2-cm polyp in the sigmoid colon shows marked contrast enhancement (*arrow*), whereas residual stool in the ascending colon already exhibits high signal on the precontrast scan and does not enhance after gadolinium administration (*arrowhead*).

displays an overview of current image parameters for all three major sequence types at 1.5T and 3T.

Clinical outcomes

Most clinical studies assessing the diagnostic impact of MRC have been conducted at 1.5T [10,14,31–34]. The largest, a recently published study Kuehle and colleagues [14], examined a screening population of 315 subjects. All participants were prepped using a fecal-tagging protocol. They ingested a tagging solution containing diatrizoic acid, barium, and locust bean gum with all main meals within 48 hours before MRC. No bowel cleansing was performed. A rectal water enema was applied for bowel distension, and data acquisition included pre- and postgadolinium T1-weighted images as well as FISP images. As a standard of reference, optical colonoscopy was performed in all patients within 4 weeks following MRC. The sensitivity of MRC for the detection of colorectal masses seemed to depend on the lesion size. Although the sensitivity for detecting polyps smaller than 5 mm was only 10.5%, the sensitivity for detecting lesions larger than 10 mm was as high as 73.9%. Most of the lesions missed on MRC were hyperplastic polyps. The sensitivity of MRC for clinically relevant adenomatous polyps larger than 5 mm, which are the main target for colorectal cancer screening, was almost 85%. Furthermore, the specificity and negative predictive values of MRC, which are particularly important for a screening method, were higher than 90%.

Hartmann and colleagues [31] performed a similar trial, using MRC to examine 100 patients who had a higher risk profile for colorectal disease. Unlike the study by Kuehle and colleagues [14], all patients underwent bowel cleansing for the MR imaging examination, and optical colonoscopy was performed on the same day. A total of 114 lesions were detected by optical colonoscopy (107 polyps, 7 carcinomas). MRC correctly identified all adenomatous lesions larger than 10 mm, and the sensitivity for the detection of polyps between 6 and 9 mm was nearly 85%. On a per-patient basis, overall sensitivity was 89%, and specificity was 96%.

In contrast to 1.5T, only preliminary data about the diagnostic accuracy of MRC at 3T are available. This lack of information results mostly from the recent implementation of MRC at 3T; more data certainly will be published within the coming years. Shin and colleagues [35] sought to establish the feasibility of MRC at 3T. They examined seven patients who had high-risk profiles for colorectal disease. Very small polyps between 2 and 6 mm were seen by means of MRC. Image quality was diagnostic in all patients, and no significant motion or parallel image artifacts were seen.

Saar and colleagues [36] presented the first clinical results of MRC at 3T. They proved the feasibility of MRC at 3T in 50 patients and compared MR imaging results with findings of subsequent colonoscopy (Fig. 5). They achieved images of diagnostic quality in more than 90% of their subjects. On a per-patient basis the sensitivity and specificity of MRC for the detection of colorectal masses were 92% and 96%, respectively. Ten of 46 polyps were not seen on MRC images, but all missed lesions were smaller than 5 mm. An overview of clinical results at 1.5T and 3T is shown in Table 2.

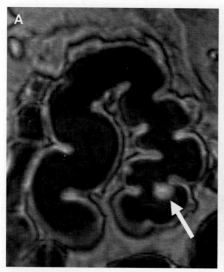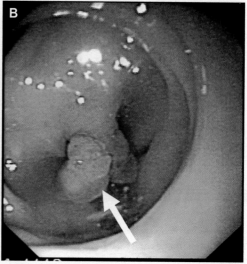

Fig. 5. (A) Pedunculated polyp (*A, B; arrows*) in the sigmoid colon. (B) Correlation of T1-weighted postcontrast MRC at 3T with subsequent finding of optical colonoscopy.

Table 2: Literature comparing the diagnostic accuracy of MR colonoscopy at 1.5T and 3T for the detection of colorectal masses

Author	Year	Field strength (T)	# Patients	Sensitivity[a] (%)	Specificity[a] (%)	Polyps[b] 6–10 mm (%)	Polyps[b] > 10 mm (%)
Ajaj et al [10]	2003	1.5	120	93	100	89	100
Hartmann et al [31]	2006	1.5	100	89	96	84	100
Kuehle et al [14]	2007	1.5	315	36	90	85	81
Saar et al [36]	2006	3	50	92	96	100	100

[a] Results on a patient basis.
[b] Sensitivity on a lesion basis for the depiction of adenomatous polyps.

Summary

MRC at 1.5T is an established method for assessing colorectal disease. Most clinical studies have shown MRC at 1.5T to have excellent diagnostic accuracy for the detection of clinically relevant adenomatous polyps larger than 5 mm. As yet the experience with MRC at 3T is limited. The feasibility of MRC at the higher field strength has been demonstrated, and the first clinical results indicate that MRC at 3T is more sensitive than MRC at 1.5T for the depiction of smaller polyps, mainly because of improvements in contrast-enhanced three-dimensional T1-weighted gradient-recalled echo. Radiologists, however, must be aware of technical pitfalls, because MRC at 3T is more prone to certain types of image artifacts, and scanning protocols must be adjusted.

References

[1] Luboldt W, Bauerfeind P, Steiner P, et al. Preliminary assessment of three-dimensional magnetic resonance imaging for various colonic disorders. Lancet 1997;349:1288–91.

[2] Luboldt W, Frohlich JM, Schneider N, et al. MR colonography: optimized enema composition. Radiology 1999;212:265–9.

[3] Bielen DJ, Bosmans HT, De Wever LL, et al. Clinical validation of high-resolution fast spin-echo MR colonography after colon distention with air. J Magn Reson Imaging 2005;22:400–5.

[4] Ajaj W, Lauenstein TC, Pelster G, et al. MR colonography: how does air compare to water for colonic distention? J Magn Reson Imaging 2004; 19:216–21.

[5] Lomas DJ, Sood RR, Graves MJ, et al. Colon carcinoma: MR imaging with CO2 enema—pilot study. Radiology 2001;219:558–62.

[6] Royster AP, Fenlon HM, Clarke PD, et al. CT colonoscopy of colorectal neoplasms: two-dimensional and three-dimensional virtual-reality techniques with colonoscopic correlation. AJR Am J Roentgenol 1997;169:1237–42.

[7] Geenen RW, Hussain SM, Cademartiri F, et al. CT and MR colonography: scanning techniques, postprocessing, and emphasis on polyp detection. Radiographics 2004;24:e18.

[8] Ajaj W, Lauenstein TC, Pelster G, et al. MR colonography in patients with incomplete conventional colonoscopy. Radiology 2005;234:452–9.

[9] Hartmann D, Bassler B, Schilling D, et al. Incomplete conventional colonoscopy: magnetic resonance colonography in the evaluation of the proximal colon. Endoscopy 2005;37:816–20.

[10] Ajaj W, Pelster G, Treichel U, et al. Dark lumen magnetic resonance colonography: comparison with conventional colonoscopy for the detection of colorectal pathology. Gut 2003;52: 1738–43.

[11] Svensson MH, Svensson E, Lasson A, et al. Patient acceptance of CT colonography and conventional colonoscopy: prospective comparative study in patients with or suspected of having colorectal disease. Radiology 2002;222: 337–45.

[12] Kinner S, Kuehle CA, Langhorst J, et al. MR colonography vs. optical colonoscopy: comparison of patients' acceptance in a screening population. Eur Radiol 2007 [Epub ahead of print].

[13] Saar B, Heverhagen JT, Obst T, et al. Magnetic resonance colonography and virtual magnetic resonance colonoscopy with the 1.0-T system: a feasibility study. Invest Radiol 2000;35: 521–6.

[14] Kuehle CA, Langhorst J, Ladd SC, et al. MR colonography without bowel cleansing–a prospectivecross-sectional study in a screening population. Gut 2007;56:1079–85.

[15] Lauenstein TC, Ajaj W, Kuehle CA, et al. Magnetic resonance colonography: comparison of contrast-enhanced three-dimensional vibe with two-dimensional FISP sequences: preliminary experience. Invest Radiol 2005;40:89–96.

[16] Lauenstein TC, Goehde SC, Debatin JF. Fecal tagging: MR colonography without colonic cleansing. Abdom Imaging 2002;27:410–7.

[17] Rottgen R, Herzog H, Bogen P, et al. MR colonoscopy at 3.0T: comparison with 1.5T in vivo and a colon model. Clin Imaging 2006;30: 248–53.

[18] Wessling J, Fischbach R, Borchert A, et al. Detection of colorectal polyps: comparison of multidetector row CT and MR colonography in a colon phantom. Radiology 2006;241:125–31.

[19] Florie J, Jensch S, Nievelstein RA, et al. MR colonography with limited bowel preparation compared with optical colonoscopy in patients at increased risk for colorectal cancer. Radiology 2007;243:122–31.

[20] Papanikolaou N, Grammatikakis J, Maris T, et al. MR colonography with fecal tagging: comparison between 2D turbo FLASH and 3D FLASH sequences. Eur Radiol 2003;13:448–52.

[21] Lauenstein T, Holtmann G, Schoenfelder D, et al. MR colonography without colonic cleansing: a new strategy to improve patient acceptance. AJR Am J Roentgenol 2001;177:823–7.

[22] Froehlich JM, Patak MA, von Weymarn C, et al. Small bowel motility assessment with magnetic resonance imaging. J Magn Reson Imaging 2005;21:370–5.

[23] Rogalla P, Lembcke A, Ruckert JC, et al. Spasmolysis at CT colonography: butyl scopolamine versus glucagon. Radiology 2005;236:184–8.

[24] Hussain SM, Wielopolski PA, Martin DR. Abdominal magnetic resonance imaging at 3.0 T: problem or a promise for the future? Top Magn Reson Imaging 2005;16:325–35.

[25] Norris DG. High field human imaging. J Magn Reson Imaging 2003;18:519–29.

[26] Merkle EM, Dale BM. Abdominal MRI at 3.0 T: the basics revisited. AJR Am J Roentgenol 2006;186:1524–32.

[27] Merkle EM, Dale BM, Paulson EK. Abdominal MR imaging at 3T. Magn Reson Imaging Clin N Am 2006;14:17–26.

[28] Lewin JS, Duerk JL, Jain VR, et al. Needle localization in MR-guided biopsy and aspiration: effects of field strength, sequence design, and magnetic field orientation. AJR Am J Roentgenol 1996;166:1337–45.

[29] Florie J, Wasser MN, Arts-Cieslik K, et al. Dynamic contrast-enhanced MRI of the bowel wall for assessment of disease activity in Crohn's disease. AJR Am J Roentgenol 2006;186:1384–92.

[30] Maccioni F, Bruni A, Viscido A, et al. MR imaging in patients with Crohn disease: value of T2- versus T1-weighted gadolinium-enhanced MR sequences with use of an oral superparamagnetic contrast agent. Radiology 2006;238:517–30.

[31] Hartmann D, Bassler B, Schilling D, et al. Colorectal polyps: detection with dark-lumen MR colonography versus conventional colonoscopy. Radiology 2006;238:143–9.

[32] Pappalardo G, Polettini E, Frattaroli FM, et al. Magnetic resonance colonography versus conventional colonoscopy for the detection of colonic endoluminal lesions. Gastroenterology 2000;119:300–4.

[33] Martin DR, Yang M, Thomasson D, et al. MR colonography: development of optimized method with ex vivo and in vivo systems. Radiology 2002;225:597–602.

[34] Saar B, Meining A, Beer A, et al. Prospective study on bright lumen magnetic resonance colonography in comparison with conventional colonoscopy. Br J Radiol 2007;80:235–41.

[35] Shin LK, Hargreaves B, Beaulieu C, et al. MR colonography at 3T using 1D- and 2D-accelerated autocalibrated parallel imaging. Presented at the Annual Meeting of the International Society for Magnetic Resonance in Medicine (ISMRM). Berlin, May 2007.

[36] Saar B, Gschossmann JM, Stoupis C, et al. Colorectal lesion characterization by using MR-colonography at 3T using dynamic scanning: an initial experience. Presented at the Annual Meeting of the European Society of Gastrointestinal and Abdominal Radiology. Heraklion, June 2006.

MAGNETIC
RESONANCE
IMAGING CLINICS

Magn Reson Imaging Clin N Am 15 (2007) 403–431

MR Imaging of Gynecologic Diseases at 3T

Lindsay Turnbull, FRCR, MD*, Susanne Booth, MRCOG

- Clinical requirements
- Current situation
- MR technical details
- Chemical shift artifact
- Fat suppression
- Susceptibility-related artifacts
- Image shading artifacts
- Imaging protocols
- Tissue contrast
- Clinical imaging
- Ovarian imaging
- Benign ovarian disease
- Benign cystic ovarian lesions
- Cystadenoma
- Cystadenofibroma
- Mature ovarian teratoma
- Endometriomas

- Pelvic inflammatory disease and tubo-ovarian collections
- Torted adnexal lesions
- Benign solid ovarian masses
- Undiagnosed adnexal mass
- Malignant ovarian tumors
  - *Types of ovarian tumor*
  - *Imaging characteristics*
  - *Staging*
  - *Residual disease*
  - *Predicting response to NAC*
- Endometrium
- Cervix
- Vulva
- Future developments
- References

Clinical requirements

MR imaging using anatomic, chemical, and functional information offers huge potential for the management of the gynecologic patient. By differentiating benign from malignant disease with very high specificity, it can aid the selection of patients requiring further treatment and determine the level of urgency. Staging accuracy, which equals that obtained at laparotomy, allows appropriate clinical expertise to be organized before surgery or the deferment of surgery until later in the treatment pathway and is a cost-effective use of resources. In the future the development of biomarkers should allow MR to predict responsiveness of inoperable tumors to treatment along with determining response during treatment using techniques to examine neovascularity, tissue viability, and chemical composition. This article compares and contrasts MR imaging of gynecologic conditions at 1.5 and 3T and to define a role for high-field imaging for these clinical conditions.

Current situation

Although considerable attention has been paid to neurologic, orthopaedic, vascular, and cardiac MR imaging, there has been less interest to date in

This work was supported by Yorkshire Cancer Research.
Centre for MR Investigations, Hull Royal Infirmary, Anlaby Road, Hull HU3 2JZ, UK
* Corresponding author.
E-mail address: l.w.turnbull@hull.ac.uk (L. Turnbull).

1064-9689/07/$ – see front matter © 2007 Elsevier Inc. All rights reserved.
mri.theclinics.com

doi:10.1016/j.mric.2007.08.001

imaging of the pelvis, particularly imaging of gynecologic conditions. Ultrasound imaging is traditionally used and although good for initial triage purposes it lacks detail, particularly in the obese patient who has excessive gaseous distension of bowel and in the presence of ascites. Ultrasound imaging lacks the ability to characterize hemorrhage or fat with accuracy, examines the pelvic side walls poorly, and provides limited anatomic detail of the internal composition of organs. More importantly it is subjective and open to operator expertise. Computed tomography provides better delineation of pelvic side wall structures but fails to provide information concerning alterations in the signal intensity or internal anatomy of pelvic organs, even following the administration of intravenous contrast agents. As a consequence MR imaging is now the modality of choice in the assessment of the female pelvis.

There is a large body of work and experience to support the use of MR imaging at field strengths of 1.5T and less, and to a lesser degree at 3T. MR imaging has been used extensively to investigate a wide range of gynecologic neoplasms, including those arising from the cervix, uterus, ovary, and vulva. Similar work performed at 3T, with its increased signal-to-noise ratio, is proving encouraging and although published data are limited, the higher spatial resolution seems to provide more clinically relevant information [1,2].

MR technical details

MR imaging offers excellent soft tissue contrast and superb multiplanar facilities unrivaled by other techniques. Although 3.0T whole-body MR systems provide approximately a factor of two increase in the signal-to-noise ratio compared with currently used 1.5T machines, important technical issues, such as chemical shift, susceptibility variations, image shading, specific absorption rate, and radiofrequency wavelength must be addressed as the field strength doubles. As expected, protocols developed for 1.5T are not immediately translatable to 3.0T.

Chemical shift artifact

The chemical shift artifact in the frequency-encoding direction shifts signal from lipid relative to water by a fixed number of pixels. At 3T water resonates at a frequency that is 420 to 440 Hz higher than lipids. The fat–water chemical shift is therefore twice the number of pixels compared with 1.5T imaging. This leads to noticeable bright/dark rims around tissue interfaces. These can be eliminated using fat-suppression techniques, although some information about the soft tissues within the pelvis

may then be lost. An alternative remedy is to double the receiver bandwidth, and although this leads to a reduction in signal-to-noise by a factor of 1.4, this is compensated for by the doubling in signal to noise ratio (SNR) resulting in an overall gain at 3T. Chemical shift artifacts in the slice select direction result in superimposition of fat from an adjacent slice on the image obscuring anatomic detail. This can be minimized by increasing the bandwidth of the radiofrequency (RF) pulses, but because the specific absorption rate is linear proportional to the RF bandwidth one disadvantage of doubling the RF bandwidth is an increasing in RF heating, which may be problematic for sequences that operate close to regulatory limits for RF heating, including some turbo spin echo/fast spin echo (TSE/FSE) sequences. In most clinical situations, however, the chemical shift artifact is not problematic and does not impinge on image interpretation.

Fat suppression

The greater separation of the resonant frequencies of water and fat at 3T, compared with 1.5T, is used to good effect in chemical shift–specific fat-suppression techniques. The diagnostic accuracy of MR imaging of the female pelvis is frequently increased by contrast enhancement, which is seen to advantage after fat suppression. Uniform fat suppression can be achieved routinely at 3T, with the exception of patients who have substantial metallic implants, such as prosthetic hip joints, which produce inhomogeneities in local B_0. New sequences based on the two-point Dixon technique are being developed by manufacturers to provide even greater reduction in the signal from fat, to limit the artifacts produced by metallic implants and minimize acquisition times thereby reducing movement artifact. These sequences typically provide separate fat and water "only" images, a feature of particular relevance to pelvic imaging.

Susceptibility-related artifacts

Local variations in the main magnetic field cause susceptibility artifacts, including image distortion and local areas of hypo- or hyperintensity. These are seen with 3T compatible implants and devices and can be reduced to levels seen at 1.5T by doubling the receiver bandwidth. Although it was originally believed that abdominal imaging would be compromised by susceptibility artifact from gas within bowel, this is not a recognized problem. Ingested items that produce susceptibility artifact are occasionally seen, including iron tablets and steel shot (Fig. 1), and in some instances necessitate re-scanning after an appropriate time interval.

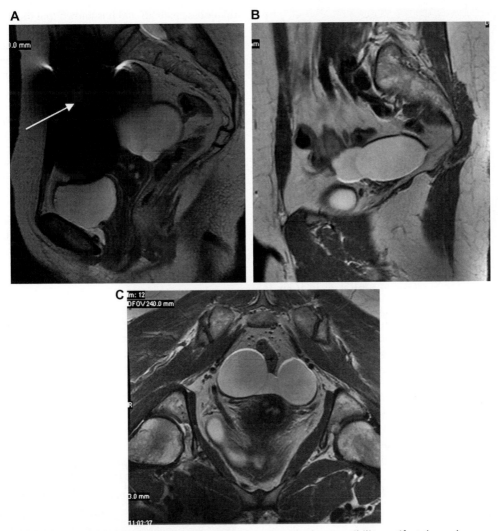

Fig. 1. Presence of steel shot ingested in food produced marked susceptibility artifact (*arrow*) on sagittal T2W-FSE-XL images obtained at 3T (*A*) requiring repeat examination after several days' delay. (*B, C*) Sagittal and oblique images.

Image shading artifacts

One of the major problems identified for pelvic imaging at 3T is image shading and uneven contrast resulting from spatial variations in the transmit B_1 field. This is particularly prominent in patients who have large intra-abdominal fluid collections either secondary to ascites or to large cystic structures. The resulting signal loss reduces or in the worst cases eliminates detail potentially resulting in a failed examination. This artifact is present in FSE/TSE images and in single-shot sequences as shown in Figs. 2 and 3. There is still debate over the cause of these artifacts, although they are believed to be caused by a combination of dielectric effect, reduced radiofrequency penetration, mismatched RF transmit values, and receiver coil issues.

The RF wavelength at the Larmor frequency for ^{1}H at 3T (26 cms) is shorter than that applied at 1.5T (52 cms) and is similar to the dimensions of the body. This smaller wavelength at higher field strengths leads to regional interference and hence marked inhomogeneities of the RF field, leading to variable cancellation of the RF excitation causing areas of shading or signal drop-off. The effect is modulated by the conductivity of the medium through which the RF wave passes. The use of high SNR surface coils may increase the conspicuity of these effects. Because we have no control over the RF wavelength at 127 Hz, B_1 receive-field correction can be applied that uses low-resolution maps from body and surface coils to partially correct signal intensity variations.

Pads filled with a medium of high electric permittivity can also significantly reduce the signal

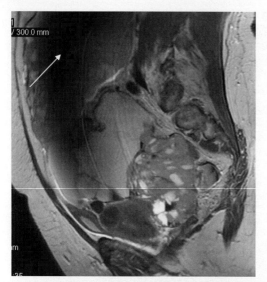

Fig. 2. T2W-FSE-XL sagittal image (FSE-XL TR 3740s, TE 91.7s; 32 cm FOV; matrix 448 × 224; 3 NEX; BW 41.7 kHz; 3 mm thickness) of significant "shading" artifact obtained at 3T in patient with gross ascites, secondary to ovarian cystadenocarcinoma, resulting in poor visualization of intra-pelvic/abdominal pathology.

inhomogeneity, although their mode of action is still debated. There are undoubtedly B_1 inhomogeneities in the transmit field that lead to spatial variations in the flip angle and the benefits of dielectric pads may be partially attributable to alteration in the geometry of the body reducing the variability of the transmit field. The imaging shading present varies according to body habitus. Smaller patients tend to produce more prominent shading artifact

than obese patients and it is known that the dielectric constant of muscle is higher than that of fat, resulting in a wavelength that is two to three times longer in fat [3]. Manufacturers are currently working on novel RF shimming techniques and multiple transmit channels to equalize the RF flip angle profile and initial results seem promising.

The image shading present is sequence dependent and choice of a sequence in which the signal is insensitive or has an acceptable dependence on flip angle [4] is recommended. Although obvious on two-dimensional T2W FSE/TSE and single shot sequences, three-dimensional (3D) T1W fast spoiled gradient echo (FSPGR) and low angle volume acquisition (LAVA) sequences are little affected by shading and when contrast enhanced provide excellent image quality. Typical examples of the information obtained are shown in Figs. 4 and 5.

Imaging protocols

Imaging protocols for gynecologic conditions must be tailored to the clinical question posed. Most examinations commence with high-resolution T2W imaging in sagittal and axial planes with additional images obtained perpendicular to the uterine long axis and in other planes according to the pathology

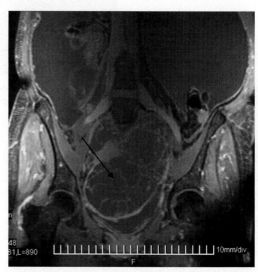

Fig. 4. Image quality substantially improved on post-contrast T1W-LAVA-DE sequence (TR 4.3s, TE 1.3s, BW 166.7 kHz, FOV 46 × 36 cm, matrix 316 × 512 Z512, thickness 3 mm, TA 1:22 minutes) obtained at 3T. Coronal image demonstrates good internal anatomy within the tumor (ovarian cystadenocarcinoma arrowed). Note lack of phase-encoding artifact in LAVA-DE images particularly with respect to large bowel and short acquisition time.

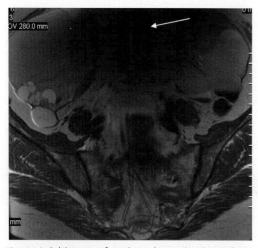

Fig. 3. Axial image of patient shown in Fig. 2 shows significant shading artifact, resulting in very poor visualization of pathology present.

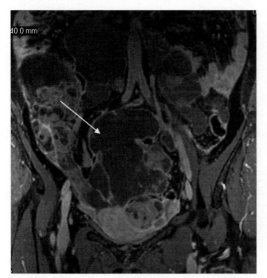

Fig. 5. Coronal image similar to that shown in *Fig. 4.*

present. T1W images are acquired pre- and postcontrast in many situations the latter is a thin-slice 3D acquisition allowing reformatting in multiple orientations. The increased SNR available at 3T provides excellent resolution even at a slice thickness of less than 1 mm, producing high-quality reformatted images as shown in *Figs. 6 and 7*. Such detail would be impossible to achieve at 1.5T and translates into improved cancer patient diagnosis and hence optimized patient management.

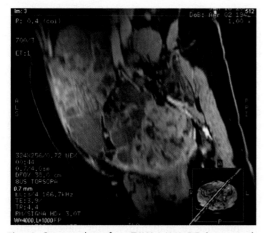

Fig. 6. Source data fromT1W LAVA-DE images obtained axial at 3T (water-only images) on patient shown in *Figs. 4 and 5*, produces reasonable quality reformatted information in an oblique plane for interrogation of cyst wall integrity, but detail reduced because of acquisition of source axial data using slice thickness of 4 mm.

In patients who have suspected recurrent tumor dynamic contrast-enhanced MR imaging (DCE-MRI) is acquired using a 4-mm slice thickness at a temporal resolution between 15 and 30 seconds, depending on the coverage required, using a T_1W volume-acquisition technique, to enable inclusion of an arterial input function if required, with tissue T_1 obtained using a multiple flip-angle gradient echo technique for subsequent pharmacokinetic modelling. This acquisition would not be feasible at 1.5T; compromises would be required in either slice thickness, overall coverage, or in the temporal resolution used.

The clinical usefulness of multiparametric quantitative MR imaging in patients who have cancer undergoing neoadjuvant chemotherapy for primary inoperable disease is now the focus of much research. To predict eventual treatment outcome early in the course of treatment a functional rather than morphologic approach is undertaken, examining parameters that reflect delivery of blood and oxygen, hypoxic status, and tissue microstructure. This approach uses a combination of data obtained from pharmacokinetic modelling of contrast-enhanced data, mapping of the apparent coefficient of water (ADC), and single voxel ^1H MR spectroscopy.

Tissue contrast

There are few studies that have directly compared the clinical usefulness of pelvic imaging at 3T with 1.5T imaging with respect to the familiarity of image quality and tissue contrast. Morakkabati-Spitz and colleagues [1] adapted a T2W TSE 1.5T protocol for 3T and to reduce the number of potential variables used the same spatial resolution, acquisition time, repetition, and echo times for both field strengths. They studied 19 patients comparing 3T images for visualization of the uterine zonal anatomy or delineation of pathologic findings, rating the findings as better, equal, or worse than 1.5T images. Scans were also evaluated for tissue contrast by comparing signal difference between muscle and bone marrow and for overall image quality by examining the presence of artifacts, visual SNR, and detail delineation, and no significant difference was found between the field strengths. They advised parameter optimization to exploit the potential of 3T systems.

Clinical imaging

There is now a substantial body of evidence to indicate the clinical usefulness of MR imaging of the female pelvis with results regularly outperforming those obtained by ultrasound and CT scanning.

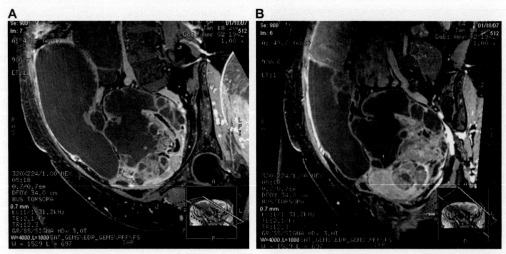

Fig. 7. Better-quality reformatted data from T1W-FSPGR images on patient shown in *Figs. 4–6* due to the use of thinner slice source images (0.7 mm), allowing excellent circumferential interrogation of cyst wall. Oblique images shown (*A*, *B*) of the extensive malignancy present within the pelvis. Images obtained at 3T.

Ovarian imaging

MR imaging studies have focused on the development of techniques to optimize the differentiation of benign from malignant ovarian masses, comparing surgical findings with preoperative MR findings to determine staging accuracy, assessing the ability of MR imaging to determine operability essential for optimization of initial management, determining response to treatment in the neoadjuvant and adjuvant settings, and examining the ability of MR imaging to detect tumor recurrence using conventional imaging and MR spectroscopy.

Benign ovarian disease

The differentiation of benign from malignant ovarian pathology may dictate the timing and necessity for surgery, the extent and type of surgery performed, and the need for a gynecologic oncologist in clinical management. Benign ovarian pathology can be divided into cystic and solid lesions.

Benign cystic ovarian lesions

Functional cysts of the ovary occur regularly throughout the menstrual cycle and are commonly diagnosed and assessed using ultrasound scanning. They are well defined, rounded or oval in shape, normally measure less than 3 cm in diameter, have smooth thin walls, have bright signal intensity contents on T2W imaging, and show no endocystic projections. On T1W imaging they have low signal intensity contents (Fig. 8). A corpus luteum has a more collapsed appearance, often slightly thickened but smooth walls, and may demonstrate hemorrhagic contents.

MR imaging is also reported to be of value in the assessment and further investigation of polycystic ovarian syndrome in obese adolescents [5]. By contrast with transabdominal ultrasound MR provided greatly improved delineation of the structural components of the ovary, including the total ovarian volume and follicle count, the mean follicular count per two-dimensional cross-sectional area, and stromal area. Although this work was performed at 1.5T improved detail would be obtained at 3T, particularly in the morbidly obese in whom imaging at 3T with even the integral body coil produces good quality information. DCE-MRI likewise has fewer limitations at 3T compared with 1.5T. Erdem and colleagues [6] have reported more rapid and intense contrast uptake with greater contrast washout in patients who have polycystic ovarian syndrome secondary to greater ovarian stromal vascularization compared with normal ovulating control subjects. Such information may aid clinical management.

Cystadenoma

Cystadenomas are larger and typically occur in an older population when it is important to exclude the presence of malignancy. They have a similar morphologic appearance to benign functional cysts and show no endocystic projections. It is important to confidently exclude the presence of endocystic projections by performing high-resolution T2W imaging and T1W imaging pre- and postcontrast enhancement. Use of a 3D volume acquisition with

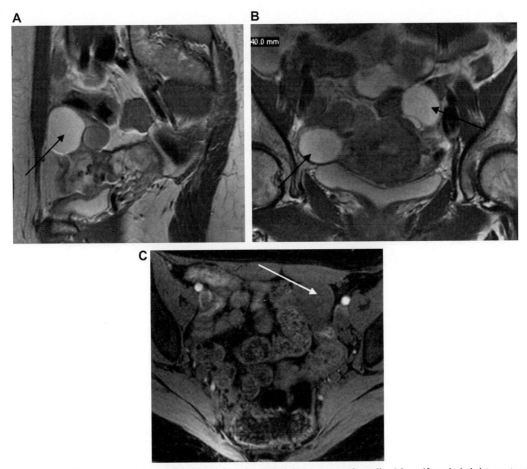

Fig. 8. Benign functional ovarian cysts (*arrows*). Well-defined thin smooth wall with uniformly bright contents on T2W-FSE sagittal (*A*) and axial (*B*) imaging and low signal intensity contents on T1W-LAVA-DE sequence (*C*), with no evidence of enhancement following IV contrast administration. Small hemorrhagic cyst noted posterior to benign functional cyst on the sagittal image. All images obtained at 3T.

a slice thickness of less than 1 mm provides excellent evaluation and permits reformatting in multiple directions to exclude pathology. The image quality obtainable at 3T is superior to 1.5T with a more confident diagnosis possible by virtue of the increase SNR, allowing thinner slices with reduced partial volume averaging effects. A typical example is shown in Fig. 9. The use of low flip-angle 3D acquisitions using the two-point Dixon technique at 3T can be acquired in approximately 90 seconds providing coverage of the entire pelvic contents. This short scan time virtually eliminates unconscious movement artifact, which despite the use of intravenous antiperistaltic agents may still degrade image quality. These sequences, depending on the manufacturer, also provide post-processed fat and T1 weighted water only images, which allow the discrimination of fat, fluid, or hemorrhagic cyst contents. Diagnosis of a benign ovarian cyst

together with normal CA125 measurement would allow conservative management of cysts if patients were asymptomatic. Although in its infancy, proton magnetic resonance spectroscopy of the pelvis may compliment and extend imaging findings. There have now been several reports of in vivo point resolved MR spectroscopy, using a TE of 136 msec, detecting elevated N-acetyl-L-aspartate signal in ovarian mucinous cystadenoma [7].

Cystadenofibroma

Cystadenofibroma typically is a multilocular cystic mass with low signal intensity peripherally distributed contents on T2W imaging, often with associated smaller cystic loculi. On T2W imaging the solid component of the tumor is of very low signal intensity and contains very high signal intensity cysts producing a "black sponge"–like appearance

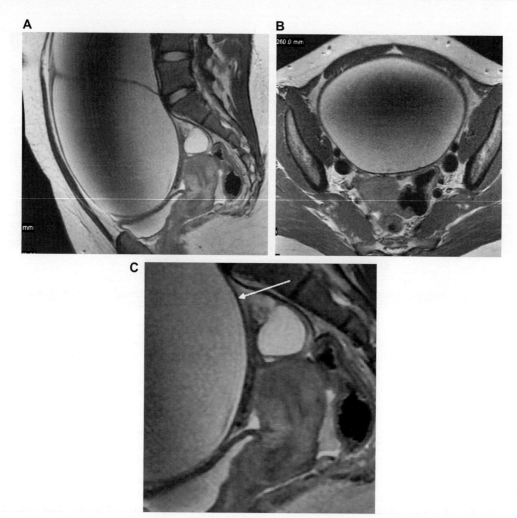

Fig. 9. Ovarian cystadenoma. Thin well-defined smooth wall on T2W-FSE-XL sagittal (*A*) and axial (*B*) images with uniformly bright signal intensity contents. Images obtained at 3T. Magnified view of cyst wall (*C*) (*arrow*) shows excellent detail and is useful to confirm findings.

[8]. This appearance is attributable to the presence of dense fibrous stromal proliferation with scattered islands of cystic glandular structures (Fig. 10). A recent report by Jung and colleagues [9], however, commented that diffuse or partial low signal thickening of the cyst wall without a definite solid component was as commonly found but that neither demonstrated the prominent contrast uptake evident with cystadenocarcinofibromas. It is important to diagnose these lesions preoperatively to avoid excessive surgery, but they can be difficult to distinguish from borderline ovarian tumors, which will be discussed later.

Mature ovarian teratoma

Germ cell tumors represent 15% to 20% of ovarian tumors and consist of teratomas, dysgerminomas, endodermal sinus tumors, choriocarcinoma, embryonal carcinoma, polyembryoma, and mixed germ cell tumors. The most common of these are teratomas that occur in three forms: mature (benign) teratomas (dermoid cyst); immature (malignant) teratomas; and monodermal or specialized teratomas, for example struma ovarii, which consists of mature thyroid tissue and ovarian stroma. Mature teratomas of the ovary appear cystic on ultrasound imaging and are typically found in the reproductive years. They contain hair, sebaceous material, teeth, and may contain differentiated tissues, including bone, cartilage, muscle, thyroid follicles, gastrointestinal, respiratory and other tissues. They are well defined, oval or rounded lesions replacing or arising from the ovary and may be bilateral. They contain predominantly bright signal intensity contents on T2W and T1W imaging attributable to fat, which

A

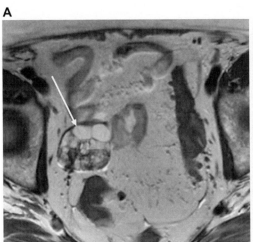

B

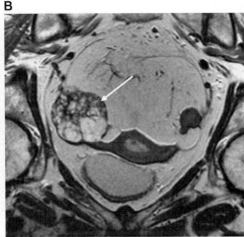

Fig. 10. Cystadenofibroma well visualized on T2W FSE-XL sequence (axial [*A*] and oblique [*B*] images). Typically the solid component of the tumor (*arrow*) is of very low signal intensity and contains very high signal intensity cysts producing a black sponge–like appearance.

often has a granular-type appearance, together with solid elements (Rokitansky's protuberance), which are typically eccentrically placed on the capsule of the lesion and contain hair and teeth. The diagnosis is clinched with fat suppression. They can be rapidly and elegantly assessed using a combination of T2W FSE/TSE and 3D dual-echo LAVA sequences as shown in Fig. 11.

Endometriomas

Endometriotic cysts arise from seeding of the peritoneal cavity with ectopic foci of endometrium, which respond to hormonal stimulation and undergo repeated hemorrhage thereby enlarging forming cysts. These most frequently occur on the ovaries (76%) but are also found on the anterior and posterior cul-de-sac (69%), posterior broad ligament (47%), uterosacral ligament (36%), uterus (11%), colon (4%), and small bowel (0.5%). Endometriomas are well-defined cysts that may show wall thickening, nodularity, and septations. They are characterized by the "shading" sign, which is the finding of reduction in signal intensity on T_2W imaging of an adnexal cyst that is hyperintense on T_1W images. Although these changes were initially described as either focal or diffuse [10–12], it is now recognized that there is commonly complete loss of signal or dependent layering of cyst contents on T_2W imaging, with a hypointense fluid level. With these criteria MR imaging at 1.5T or less has a diagnostic accuracy of 91% to 96%, a sensitivity of 90% to 92%, and a specificity of 91% to 98% [10,13,14]. Because of the excellence of these results it is unlikely that significant improvement can be

achieved at 3T, but sequence times can be reduced particularly with the use of sequences such as a 3D dual-echo LAVA (Fig. 12).

Pelvic inflammatory disease and tubo-ovarian collections

Pelvic inflammatory disease is a common and costly condition among women of reproductive years. It can lead to infertility, ectopic pregnancy, and chronic pelvic pain. Laparoscopy is routinely performed for diagnosis but this requires general anesthesia, is an invasive procedure, and may lead to complications [15]. MR imaging at 1.5T has been shown to have a powerful role in this condition and can detect tubo-ovarian abscesses, hydro- or pyosalpinges or polycystic-like ovaries with a sensitivity of 95%, a specificity of 89%, and an overall accuracy of 93% compared with comparative values of 81%, 78%, and 80% for transvaginal ultrasound [16]. Figs. 13 and 14 indicate that at least as good results should be obtainable at 3T. Actinomycosis, tuberculosis, and xanthogranulomatous inflammation are rare but specific causes of tubo-ovarian abscess that may be misdiagnosed as malignancy. Tubo-ovarian actinomycosis frequently has a predominantly solid appearance with linear, solid, enhancing tissue extending from the mass or small rim-enhancing lesions in the solid component. Tuberculous lesions typically mimic peritoneal carcinomatosis of ovary, but the lack of an obvious ovarian primary lesion aids differentiation (Fig. 15). Tubo-ovarian xanthogranulomatous inflammation demonstrates relatively nonspecific

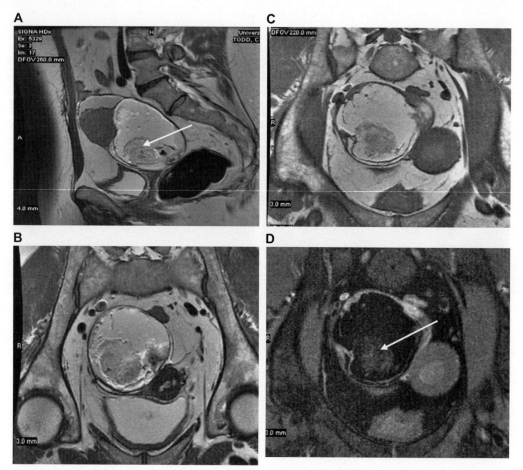

Fig. 11. Mature teratoma (dermoid cyst). Typical appearance with well-defined contours, bright but heterogeneous contents on T2W-FSE imaging, and peripherally distributed "solid" element because of Rokitansky's nodule (sagittal [*A*] and oblique [*B*], *arrow*). Presence of fatty contents seen to advantage on T1W SE (*C*) and on postcontrast T1W FSPGR image (*D*), which demonstrates signal nulling with fat-suppression pulse. Note enhancement of the Rokitansky's nodule in image *D* (*arrow*). All images obtained at 3T.

findings [17]. The increased detail obtainable at 3T should aid diagnosis of these conditions.

Torted adnexal lesions

The diagnosis of adnexal torsion can be difficult to establish, but recent reports suggest that MR imaging has an important role to play. Torsion may occur either in the presence of additional pathology or in isolation, particularly during pregnancy when 10% to 20% of all ovarian torsions occur. A torted normal ovary is enlarged, and the ovarian stroma is hyperintense on T2W imaging because of edema (Fig. 16) [18]. Torted ovarian masses frequently demonstrate irregular polypoid-type thickening of the wall, show no contrast uptake, and may be associated with edema of the adjacent pelvic

fat together with free fluid, although the latter is also a normal physiologic finding (Fig. 17).

Benign solid ovarian masses

Ovarian fibromas are benign neoplasms that arise from the connective tissue stroma of the ovary and constitute 4% of all ovarian neoplasms. On MR imaging they are typically well-encapsulated masses, which are of homogeneous low signal intensity on T1W and T2W imaging, occasionally demonstrating calcification or cystic degeneration, the latter giving rise to a whorled pattern centrally (Fig. 18). Typically they show only minimal contrast uptake. One percent of cases are associated with Meigs syndrome with the development of ascites and pleural effusions. The relative homogeneity of most of these lesions allows diagnosis, but the

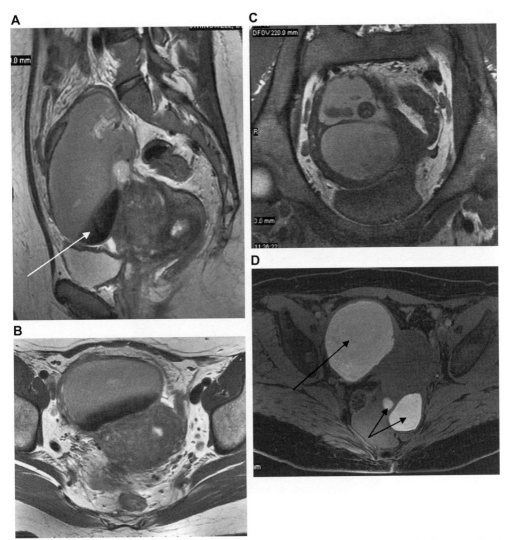

Fig. 12. Shading artifact (*arrow*) present within endometrioma on T2W-FSE image typical of longstanding hemorrhagic contents (*A, B, C*). Note presence of hypointense fluid level layering out posteriorly within the pelvic lesion. Presence of hemorrhagic contents giving rise to bright signal intensity confirmed on T1W LAVA-DE images water-only image (*D*). Note the presence of endometriosis in both ovaries (*arrows*) and the detail obtained in T1W-LAVA-DE sequence, which was acquired in only 1:22 minutes at 3T.

differential includes ovarian or broad ligament leiomyoma, lymphoma, metastasis, or a solid ovarian malignancy, such as germ cell, thecoma, or Brenner tumors. Because many of these lesions present with similar morphologic appearances, it is unlikely that 3T will aid in the differential diagnosis.

Undiagnosed adnexal mass

There are several reports examining the role of MR imaging, in comparison with CT and ultrasound scanning, for evaluating adnexal masses. These studies, predominantly performed at 1.5T, report greater specificity and accuracy for MR imaging. Sohaib and colleagues [19] quoted vales of 83.7% and 88.9%, respectively, compared with 39.5% and 63.9% for combined transabdominal and transvaginal ultrasound.

We have performed MR imaging at 3T on 191 patients who had adnexal masses, of whom 172 had ovarian disease as their primary diagnosis on histology. The remaining 19 patients had primary uterine pathology, with an incidental finding of coexisting ovarian disease (13 endometrial adenocarcinomas, 3 uterine sarcomas, and 3 benign leiomyomas). Primary ovarian malignancy was diagnosed in 77

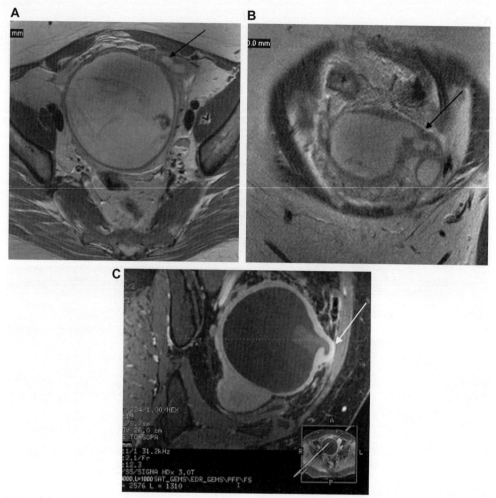

Fig. 13. Confident diagnosis of tubo-ovarian collection made using combination of (*A, B*) T2W-FSE-XL and (*B*) postcontrast T1W FSPGR imaging. Axial (*A*) and (*B*) T2W FSE images demonstrate a well-defined cystic structure with thickened walls that have a smooth inner surface, with a tubular structure arising from the supero-anterior aspect of the lesion (*arrow*). The postcontrast T1W reformatted FSPGR images (*C*) confirm the lack of endocystic projections and clearly demonstrate the presence of an associated hydrosalpinx.

patients, 20 of whom had borderline malignancies. In those patients found to have benign disease there were 3 cases of ovarian torsion, 22 benign teratomas, and a further 52 cases of benign ovarian tumors, predominantly cystadenomas and fibromas. Analysis of these data for the detection of malignant ovarian neoplasm revealed a sensitivity of 92% and a specificity of 76%. There were a total of 6 cases of misdiagnosis of benign disease in the presence of malignancy. Five of these were borderline (stage 1A) tumors believed to be either cystadenomas or cystadenofibromas on MR imaging because of the appearance of the cyst walls on T2W imaging and the lack of contrast enhancement on T1W imaging (Fig. 19). Histopathology revealed no naked eye abnormality in these cases, but changes were noted

microscopically. There was a further single case of a microscopic squamous cell cancer arising in a pre-existing mature cystic teratoma.

Malignant ovarian tumors

Types of ovarian tumor

Surface epithelial tumors are the most common type accounting for approximately 60% of all cases, with serous tumors the most common subtype. Germ cell tumors are the second largest group accounting for approximately 20% of ovarian neoplasms, with immature teratomas, dysgerminomas, and yolk sac tumors being the most frequent. Sex-cord stromal tumors account for approximately 10% of cases, and are composed of various cell types derived

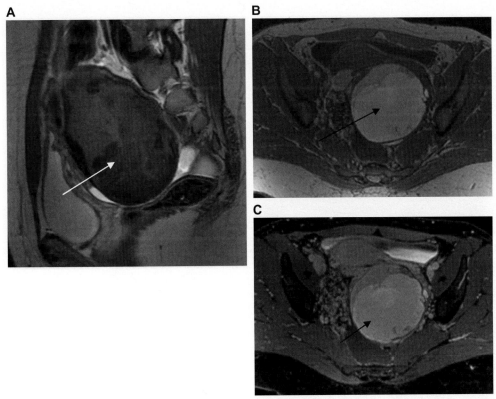

Fig. 14. Presence of low, albeit mixed, signal intensity contents on sagittal T2-weighted FSE imaging (*A*) and bright signal intensity contents on axial T1 W LAVA-DE image (*B*) with no significant enhancement on the water-only axial T1W-LAVA-DE postcontrast image (*C*) is typical of hemorrhage of variable age in to a tubo-ovarian collection (*arrows* on all images).

from gonadal stroma and sex cords. They include the most hormonally active tumors, namely granulosa cell and Sertoli Leydig tumors. Metastatic neoplasms of the ovary account for 6% to 7% of ovarian tumors and constitute an important group, because the therapy for primary ovarian malignancies is often different from that used for tumors derived from other primary sites.

Imaging characteristics

Malignant ovarian tumors often present as medium to large pelvic masses that have either a mixed solid and cystic appearance or alternatively are entirely solid. The most common surface epithelial tumors, whether serous, mucinous, endometrioid, or clear cell in type, present as an irregularly shaped mass, the cystic portions of which contain papillary ingrowths; the well differentiated show extensive papillarity and the moderate to poorly differentiated are characterized by decreasing degrees of papillarity, resulting in an increasing chaotic internal architecture. Hemorrhage into the cysts and areas of necrosis are variable findings. For typical examples

see Figs. 20–22. The solid components typically show rapid and intense contrast uptake on dynamic scanning, with variable enhancement on delayed imaging depending on the rapidity of contrast washout. In general, serous tumors tend to have uniformly bright cyst contents, whereas mucinous tumors demonstrate variable signal intensity of cyst contents. The various histologic subtypes of malignant adenocarcinomas, papillary adenocarcinomas, papillary cystadenocarcinomas, and malignant adenofibromas and cystadenofibromas are indistinguishable on MR imaging. Tumors of borderline malignant potential are fluid-filled cystic structures, many of which produce prominent papillary excrescences on the ovarian cortical surface with no evidence of invasion of the cyst wall (Fig. 23). The papillary excrescences enhance postcontrast, in comparison with the underlying low signal intensity cyst wall. This enhancement allows differentiation from cystadenomas and cystadenofibromas in most but not all cases, because in some patients microscopic changes alone exist and the lesions are indistinguishable on MR imaging. The

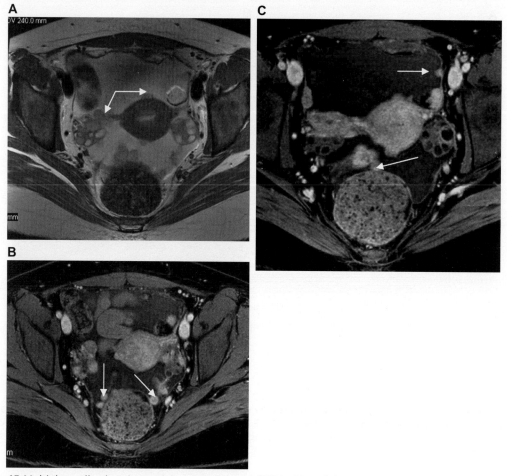

Fig. 15. Multiple small enhancing nodules present on axial T2W-FSE-XL (*A*), T1W gadolinium-enhanced LAVA-DE (water only) images (*B, C*) in patient who has intraperitoneal tuberculosis (some of which are indicated with arrows). These are indistinguishable from metastatic ovarian and other malignancies on imaging although in this patient the ovaries were clearly visualized and of normal appearance for patient's age. All images obtained at 3T.

increased detail provided by 3T imaging should detect the subtle changes present in a greater percentage of cases, however, allowing these patients to be managed appropriately. Malignant Brenner tumors often mimic ovarian fibromas and have no specific distinguishing features. Of the sex-cord stromal tumors, granulosa cell tumors are the most distinctive because of the frequent finding of hemorrhage that occurs into the cysts and may result in a hemoperitoneum, and because of estrogenic effects causing prominence of the endometrial strip and increased density of the breast parenchyma (Fig. 24). Dysgerminomas and immature teratomas are predominantly solid, with the latter often containing areas of hemorrhage or necrosis. Yolk sac tumors by contrast contain cystic elements and are indistinguishable from other mixed solid and cystic malignant ovarian tumors. Clinical presentation and age at

onset often aid the differential diagnosis, but in general this is limited to solid versus mixed solid and cystic causes. Although of interest the primary role of MR imaging is in confirming malignancy and in determining the stage at presentation, which affects clinical management and provide prognostic information.

Staging

Staging of malignancy (International Federation of Gynecology and Obstetrics [FIGO] stage 1a to 4) is crucial in determining optimal treatment. Determination of capsular integrity is potentially optimized at 3T because of the detail obtained and the ability to collect very thin slices (less than 1 mm) for reformatting circumferentially around the capsular surface. This also allows definition of potential involvement of surrounding tissues by tumor. Quyyum and

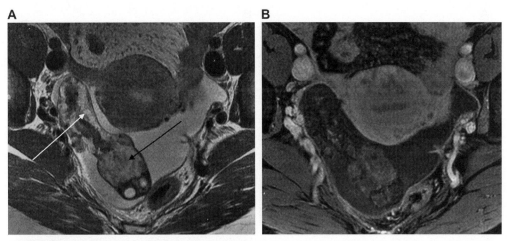

Fig. 16. Enlarged hyperintense ovary (*black arrow*) with thickened and prominent broad ligament (*white arrow*) on axial T2W-FSE imaging (*A*) due to torsion. Minimal contrast uptake seen on the postgadolinium axial T1W-FSPGR image (*B*). All images obtained at 3T.

colleagues [20] determine the relative accuracy of CT and MR imaging for detection of inoperable sites before cytoreductive surgery in a series of 137 patients who had newly diagnosed primary epithelial ovarian cancers. These were defined as tumor present at one or more of the following sites: peritoneal implants greater than 2 cm in diameter in the porta hepatis, intersegmental fissure, gall bladder fossa, subphrenic space, gastrohepatic ligament, lesser sac, or root of the small bowel mesentery; retroperitoneal lymphadenopathy greater than 2 cm in diameter above the renal hila; or hepatic or abdominal wall invasion. Results showed that CT and MR imaging at 1.5T were equally effective in predicting suboptimal debulking with sensitivity, specificity, positive predictive value (PPV), and negative predictive values (NPVs) of 76%, 99%, 94%, and 96%, respectively, suggesting that selection of patients according to imaging findings might reduce inappropriate surgery.

In other studies CT and MR performed at 1.5T have similar accuracies for the diagnosis and staging

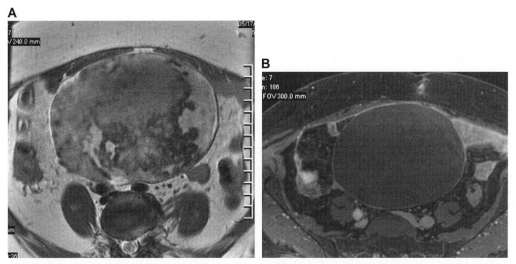

Fig. 17. Well-defined, encapsulated intraperitoneal mass, with prominent thickened internal septations on axial T2W-FSE imaging (*A*) but no enhancement evident on axial T1W FSPGR sequence (*B*), all obtained at 3T. Appearances in keeping with torted ovarian lesion. The nature of the mass may be difficult to determine in these cases because the normal internal architecture is destroyed. In this case the pathology was inadequate and a diagnosis of indeterminate cyst was made by default.

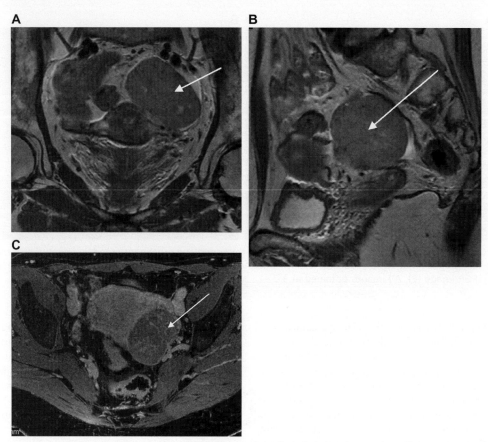

Fig. 18. Typical appearance of an ovarian fibroma (*arrow*) with well-defined smooth wall, low signal intensity contents and whorled central structure on oblique and sagittal T2W-FSE imaging (*A, B*), with minimal contrast uptake seen on axial T1W FSPGR sequence (*C*). All images obtained at 3T.

of ovarian malignancy ranging from 60% to 90% [21–27]. The overall findings indicate that MR imaging is superior to Doppler ultrasound and CT in determining malignancy, but there seems to be no difference in the accuracy of CT and MR imaging in staging the disease according to the 1999 report from the Radiology Diagnostic Oncology Group [28,29].

We have recently reviewed our own data on the staging accuracy of 3T MR imaging and have compared the results with laparotomy and histopathologic findings. Primary ovarian malignancy was diagnosed in 77 patients, 20 of whom had borderline tumors. Those patients who were suspected of having primary ovarian malignancy underwent MR imaging for preoperative assessment, using multiprojection T2W FSE imaging, postcontrast 3D LAVA-DE, and 3D T1W-FSPGR of the pelvis, with additional respiratory averaged T2W-FSE and single-shot FSE breath-held imaging of the abdomen (**Figs. 25 and 26**). All individuals underwent primary debulking surgery and subsequent histopathologic staging. Previous studies of the staging

accuracy of imaging techniques have grouped individuals into the broad categories of FIGO stages I, II, III, and IV. For the purpose of our data staging was divided into separate FIGO stages Ia to IV. The three methods of staging were compared by allotting incremental scores for FIGO stages Ia to 4 separately and the interobserver agreement between tests analyzed using quadratic weighted κ test, whereby a κ value of 0.21 to 0.40 represents a fair agreement, 0.41 to 0.60 moderate, 0.61 to 0.80 good, and 0.81 to 1.00 very good agreement. The κ value for agreement between histopathology and MR imaging was 0.866 (SE ± 0.119), which was not significantly different from the κ value for histopathology versus laparotomy at 0.926 (SE ± 0.121) indicating that MR imaging at 3T provided as reliable information as staging laparotomy. Areas of discrepancy between the MR imaging and surgical staging were seen particularly in cases in which there were microscopic metastases that could not be detected by the naked eye or with MR imaging. As MR hardware and software develop further it may be possible to improve

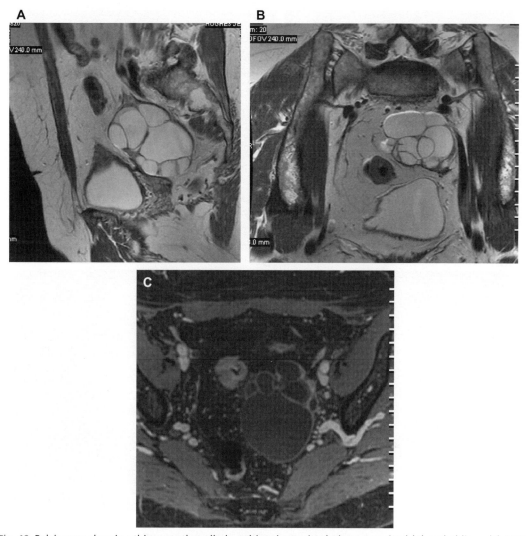

Fig. 19. Pelvic mass showing thin smooth-walled, multicystic ovarian lesion on sagittal (*A*) and oblique (*B*) T2W-FSE imaging with no enhancement evident on T1W FSPGR sequence (*C*), therefore classed as benign on imaging. Pathology subsequently showed microscopic changes consistent with borderline ovarian tumor, not seen on high-resolution imaging. All images obtained at 3T.

on these data and detect even smaller plaques of tumor in more inaccessible areas.

Because of the high proportion of borderline tumors in our final data, we performed a further analysis of the staging data for ovarian cancers alone after removing the borderline tumors. This analysis resulted in a κ value of 0.931 (SE ± 0.136) for histopathologic staging versus MR staging and a κ value of 0.958 (±0.140) for histopathologic stage versus surgical staging. Because borderline tumors are neoplasms with only microscopic features of malignancy and are notoriously difficult to diagnose preoperatively, it is justifiable to remove them from the final analysis of our data.

Residual disease

There are no reports in the literature examining the accuracy of 3T in predicting the volume of residual ovarian cancer posttreatment and only a few reports at 1.5T. Low and colleagues [30] reported on the results of 76 treated women who underwent preoperative MR imaging of the abdomen and pelvis using intravenous gadolinium-based contrast and intraluminal barium. The results were compared with surgical and histopathologic findings, serial and static CA-125, and clinical follow-up. Tumor absence was proved by normal surgical findings, clinical follow-up for at least 1 year, and normal serial CA-125 measurements. Gadolinium-enhanced images

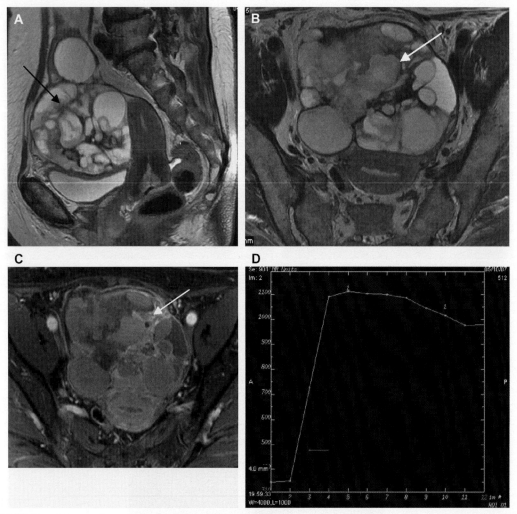

Fig. 20. Ovarian cystadenocarcinoma FIGO stage 1A. Typical appearance on sagittal (A) and oblique (B) T2W imaging with mixed solid and cystic elements, which extend to but not beyond the capsule. The lesion shows characteristic enhancement of a malignant lesion on DCE-MRI (C), with rapid and intense contrast uptake and early washout seen on the signal-intensity time curve (D) generated using FUNCTOOL software package. Postcontrast images show the extent of enhancement to good effect (D). All images obtained at 3T.

depicted residual tumor with a sensitivity of 90%, specificity of 88%, and an accuracy of 89%, compared with laparotomy results of 88%, 100%, and 89%, respectively. The positive predictive values for MR imaging, laparotomy, and serum CA-125 measurements were 98%, 100%, and 98%, respectively, and the corresponding negative predictive values were 50%, 50%, and 23%. There was a discrepancy between the MR and laparotomy findings in 14 patients. Of these MR demonstrated residual disease in 7 patients that was not found at laparotomy but was confirmed pathologically. In 6 patients laparotomy revealed small-volume residual disease not seen by MR and in a further 1 patient MR predicted small-volume residual disease, but the patient had no surgical or clinical evidence of recurrent disease at 12 months. They concluded that MR was comparable to laparotomy and superior to CA-125 measurement alone. With the improved image quality obtained at 3T at least as good results should be obtainable.

Predicting response to NAC

The efficacy of incorporating DCE imaging into the treatment planning of ovarian tumors is under investigation. Analysis of functional information derived from pharmacokinetic analysis of DCE-MRI data has revealed significant differences between eventual responders and nonresponders early in

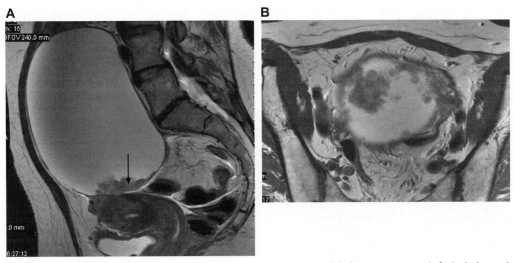

Fig. 21. Large well-defined lesion, primarily cystic in nature but with solid elements present inferiorly (*arrow*), in keeping with ovarian cystadenocarcinoma. Tumor is seen to extend to the capsular surface on both the sagittal (*A*) T2W FSE and on the oblique (*B*) T2W FSE images giving rise to irregularity and loss of clear definition of the capsule and possible early involvement of the uterine serosa. FIGO stage 1C.

the course of treatment and even at baseline for some parameters.

Endometrium

The incidence of endometrial cancer is increasing in the United Kingdom. This increase is believed to be partly because of the increasing incidence of obesity, a known risk factor for developing endometrial adenocarcinoma. Although cancers of the endometrium tend to present early, with 75% of tumors confined to the uterus, there is a group of patients in whom the usual staging and treatment procedure of total abdominal hysterectomy, bilateral salpingo-oophorectomy, and peritoneal washings is insufficient. This group has been identified by the Gynecology Oncology Group (GOG) as women who have endometrial cancer with at least one of the following: myometrial invasion greater than 50% regardless of tumor grade; extension of the tumor into the internal os or cervical stroma; adnexal or other extrauterine metastases; visibly enlarged lymph nodes; or serous, undifferentiated, clear cell or squamous histology. In these high-risk patients pelvic lymph node sampling or lymphadenectomy is required in addition to the usual surgery. In our practice patients who have cervical involvement at hysteroscopy and those who have poor prognosis pathology subtypes from uterine curetting undergo MR imaging for staging before consideration of the treatment options.

MR imaging can be helpful in staging and treatment planning for these patients. In one such study

Manfredi and colleagues [31] showed that MR imaging had a sensitivity of 87% and specificity of 91% for predicting myometrial invasion and values of 80% and 96%, respectively, for cervical invasion. Its performance for detecting lymph node involvement was less convincing, with a sensitivity of only 50% but a specificity of 95%. Extrauterine disease extension is visible on MR imaging and is thus recommended for women in whom there is a suspicion of advanced disease or in the high-risk histologic subtypes.

The use of various MR sequences for staging endometrial cancers has been investigated by several groups. Rockall and colleagues [32] assessed the diagnostic performance of T_2W and dynamic gadolinium-enhanced T_1W imaging in the preoperative assessment of myometrial and cervical invasion and to identify features that predicted nodal metastases. At 1.5T the sensitivity, specificity, PPV, and NPV for either superficial or deep myometrial invasion were 0.94, 0.50, 0.93, and 0.55 on T_2W imaging and 0.92, 0.50, 0.92, and 0.50 on T_1W imaging. For deep myometrial invasion the corresponding values were 0.84, 0.78, 0.65, and 0.91 for T_2W imaging and 0.72, 0.88, 0.72, and 0.88 on dynamic T_1W imaging. The values for cervical stromal involvement were 0.69, 0.95, 0.69, and 0.95 for T_2W imaging and 0.50, 0.96, 0.57, and 0.95 for dynamic T_1W imaging. They concluded that MRI had a high sensitivity for myometrial invasion, a high specificity for cervical invasion, and high NPV for deep myometrial and cervical invasion. Use of dynamic T_1W imaging did not improve the diagnostic performance compared with T_2W scanning. This

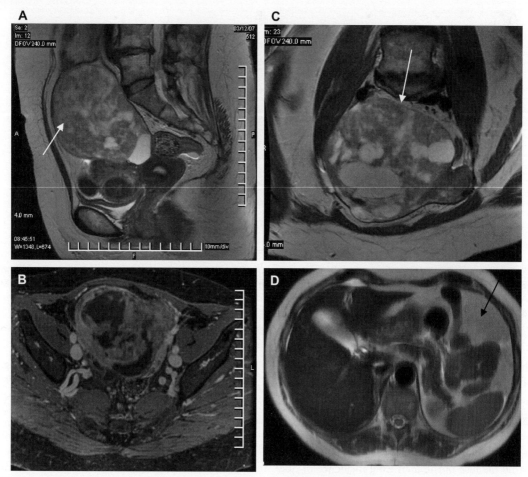

Fig. 22. Ovarian cystadenocarcinoma FIGO stage 3C by virtue of the omental disease present. Tumor appears well defined on the sagittal (*A*) and oblique (*B*) T2W-FSE images although solid elements extend to the capsular surface, which is slightly irregular and poorly visualized (*arrow*). The solid elements of the tumor are clearly seen on the T1W-FSPGR contrast-enhanced images (*C*). Omental thickening is noted on the T2W SS FSE axial images acquired during breath-holding (*D*), deep to the anterior abdominal wall as marked.

finding is in contrast to a previous report by Nasi and colleagues [33], in which the accuracy of diagnosing the depth of myometrial infiltration by MR imaging at 1.5T was improved using gadolinium-enhanced imaging compared with a T_2W sequence. They commented particularly on the improved visualization of the inner myometrium in postmenopausal women, in whom definition of the junctional zone can be problematic.

Preoperative assessment of nodal involvement by either MR or CT is known to be inaccurate. The lymph node–specific contrast agent, ferumoxtran 10, composed of ultrasmall particles of iron oxide (USPIO), has been shown to increase the sensitivity of predicting nodal metastases without loss of specificity [34]. In a group of 44 patients who had either endometrial or cervical malignancy the sensitivity, specificity, PPV, and NPV based on size criteria alone

were 27%, 94%, 60%, and 79% compared with 100%, 94%, 82%, and 100%, respectively, for USPIO-based criteria alone. Although these agents are not licensed at present, they offer the potential to greatly improve preoperative treatment planning.

There are as yet no reports of staging accuracy of endometrial cancer at 3T. Delineation of the uterine anatomy and parametrial structures is excellent, however, and the use of 3D acquisitions allows thin-slice imaging providing good quality reformatted images in all planes (Figs. 27 and 28). Initial observations are promising, but staging accuracy may still rely on the use of USPIOs for nodal assessment.

Cervix

MR imaging has proved extremely useful in the staging of cervical malignancy, which is

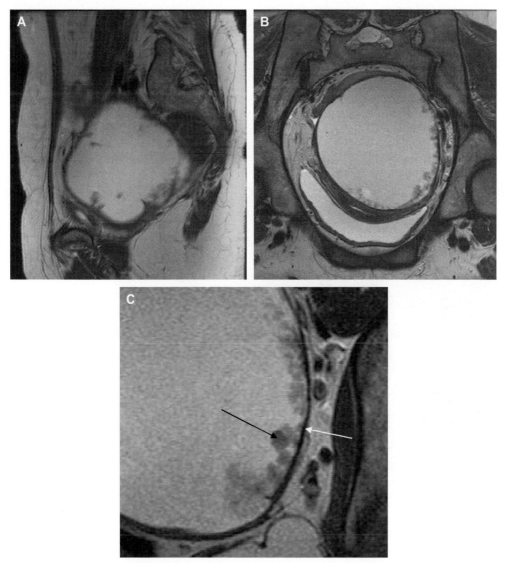

Fig. 23. Presence of small (<3 mm diameter) enhancing nodules seen deep to but separate from the capsule of the lesion on the T2W-FSE sagittal (*A*) and oblique (*B*) images, correctly diagnosed as borderline malignancy. The detail obtained at 3T (see magnified view), namely the identification of tiny endocystic projections (*black arrow*) seen separate from the capsular surface (*white arrow*), permits identification of such lesions (*C*).

traditionally staged by clinical findings and basic imaging techniques, such as chest radiograph, intravenous urogram, barium enema, cystoscopy, and sigmoidoscopy. The image quality that can be obtained with MR has allowed it to play an important role in staging, surgical and radiotherapy planning, and monitoring treatment and detecting recurrence (Figs. 29 and 30). A meta-analysis by Bipat and colleagues [35] showed that tumor detection by MR imaging had a sensitivity of 93% and an overall tumor staging accuracy of 86%. Clinical FIGO staging performed poorly giving an overall accuracy of only

47%. One of the most important features when staging early cervical disease is the presence of normal cervical stroma around the tumor. This phenomenon is best viewed on T2-weighted images in which normal cervical stroma is of low signal intensity, whereas tumor produces intermediate signal intensity. The negative predictive value for parametrial invasion is 96% [36–38], with a positive predictive value of 82% to 86% [39,40].

In addition to surface coils some groups have used endovaginal coils to improve image quality at either 0.5 or 1.5T, in particular to estimate tumor

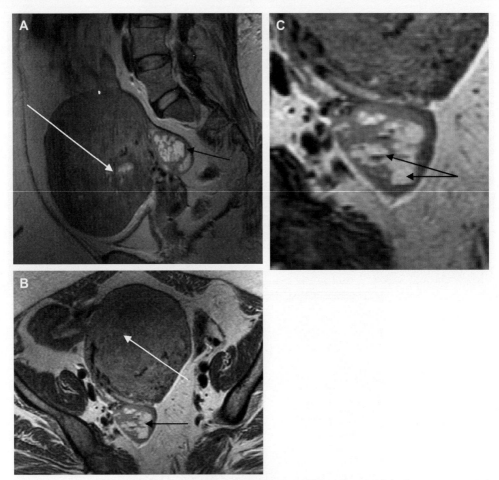

Fig. 24. Granulosa cell tumor of ovary FIGO stage 1A (*black arrow*) in patient with bulky uterus secondary to adenomyosis (*white arrow*). The ovarian lesion is composed of multiple tiny cysts, many of which contain hemorrhage. The lesion is seen on both the sagittal (*A*) and axial (*B*) T2W FSE images, but the hemorrhage is best seen layering out posteriorly on the magnified view images (*C, arrow*). The presence of hemorrhage into the cysts present, together with prominence of the endometrium and adenomyosis in a patient of 62 years (due to estrogenic stimulation), is suggestive of this particular histologic type. All images obtained at 3T.

volume because this is known to be an independent indicator of prognosis. Desouza and colleagues [41], using a combination of external phased array and endovaginal coils, reported a sensitivity and specificity of 96.9% and 59.0%, respectively, with corresponding values of 87% and 65%, respectively, for tumors less than 1 cm in diameter, with 80% and 91.3% for parametrial status and 78.6% and 72.5% for lymph node status. They commented that endovaginal imaging was particularly important for planning fertility-conserving or radical surgical treatment of early-stage cervical cancer. The same group examined the value of tumor volume measurement as a predictor of prognosis [42]. They found that only MR determination of tumor volume remained consistently and strongly associated with survival after multivariant analysis of the imaging and histopathologic parameters available before treatment ($P = .001$).

MR images have also been used to delineate the target volume and critical organs to assess the clinical usefulness of conventional, conformal, and intensity modulated (IMRT) external beam radiotherapy treatment planning of cervical cancer. Van de Bunt and colleagues [43] reported superior sparing of critical organs with IMRT with adequate coverage of the target volume. MR repeated after delivery of 30 Gy demonstrated shrinkage of the primary gross tumor volume by on average 46%. Repeated IMRT planning at this time further improved sparing of bowel and rectum in patients who had substantial tumor regression. Taylor and

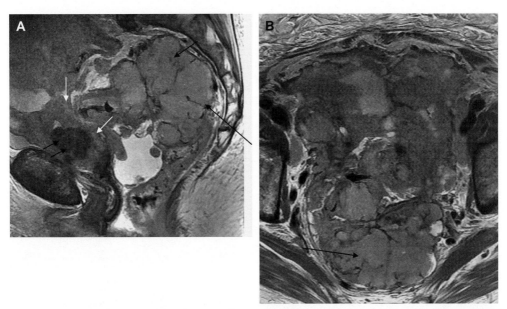

Fig. 25. Determination of involvement of surrounding structures is crucial for ovarian cancer staging. On these sagittal (*A*) and axial (*B*) T2W FSE images obtained at 3T, tumor erodes through rectosigmoid colon (*black arrow*) and diffusely involves the fundus and lower segment of the uterus (*white arrows*) which also contains a fibroid (*double black arrow*). FIGO stage 4.

colleagues [44] also demonstrated the potential to reduce the radiation dose to normal tissue by using iron oxide–enhanced MR imaging of pelvic node groups. By using a modified margin of 7 mm around the iliac vessels as a surrogate target for pelvic nodes the coverage of specific nodal groups could be increased and the volume of normal tissue irradiated reduced. Mayr and colleagues [45] have

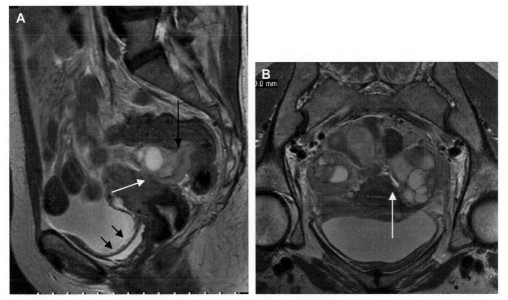

Fig. 26. Advanced ovarian cystadenocarcinoma with deposits involving the sigmoid colon (*black arrows*), peritoneal reflections of the pelvis (*double black arrows*) and uterine body (*white arrows*) in addition to bilateral ovarian masses. These are clearly seen on the sagittal (*A*) and oblique (*B*) T2-weighted FSE-XL images.

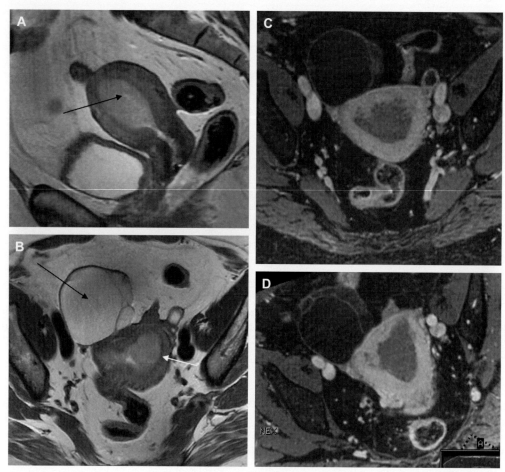

Fig. 27. Endometrial carcinoma. Typical appearance on sagittal (*A*) and axial (*B*) T2W-FSE imaging at 3T of inter- mediate signal intensity tumor (*arrow*) expanding the uterine cavity and invading the overlying low signal in- tensity junctional zone, which represents involvement of the inner myometrium. The junctional zone is marked with white arrow on image b. This extends from fundus to internal os representing FIGO stage 1B dis- ease. This is confirmed on the axial postcontrast 3D T1W FSPGR imaging (*C*), which allows good delineation of tumor margins. The 3D data set can be reformatted in any orientation desired to determine tumor extent and the integrity of the serosal aspect of the uterus (*D*). Oblique view shown in *D*. Benign ovarian cystadenoma noted incidentally (*black arrow, B*).

also used functional MR imaging as a prognostic factor in advanced cervical malignancy.

Vulva

There has been limited work performed with re- gard to vulval cancer and MR imaging. Overall im- aging in vulval cancer has a limited role in the evaluation of the primary site because this is read- ily assessed clinically. In larger tumors MR imaging is of help in evaluating the extent of disease in pa- tients who have advanced tumor involving the per- ineum, vagina, and anal canal (Fig. 31). Because groin lymphadenectomy is performed for both

diagnostic and therapeutic reasons, and groin node status is the most important single prognos- tic factor, the detection of metastases with imaging may allow better treatment planning. Lymph node metastases can be detected on MR imaging with a sensitivity of 85.7% and specificity of 82.1% [46]. Other studies have shown MR imaging to be much less accurate at detecting lymph node me- tastases with sensitivities of 40% to 50%, although highly specific at 97% to 100% [47]. New tech- niques for detecting lymph node involvement with ultra-small superparamagnetic iron oxide– enhanced MR imaging are producing encouraging results, although still only on a research basis [48].

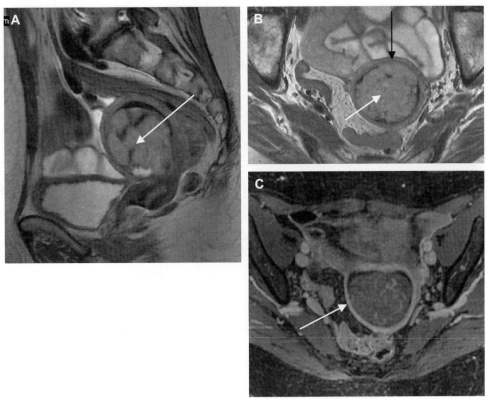

Fig. 28. Carcinosarcoma of the endometrium showing heterogeneous signal intensity structures replacing normal endometrium on both the sagittal (*A*) and axial (*B*) T2W FSE images (*white arrow*). There is loss of delineation of the endometrial/junctional zone interface on the dorsal aspect of the uterine body due to early tumor infiltration (*black arrow*). FIGO stage 1B. The tumor extent is clearly seen postcontrast on the fat-suppressed T1W FSPGR sequence (*C*) and the integrity of the serosal aspect of the uterus (*white arrow*) confirmed. All images obtained at 3T.

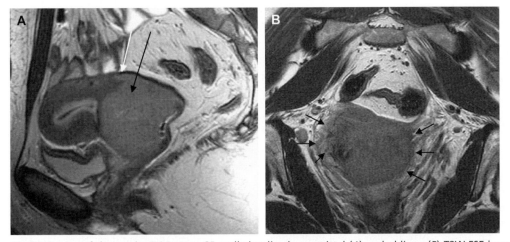

Fig. 29. Carcinoma of the cervix, FIGO stage 2B well visualized on sagittal (*A*) and oblique (*B*) T2W FSE images acquired at 3T. The intermediate signal intensity tumor mass (*black arrow, A*) is replacing the cervix, filling the endocervical canal and extending through the overlying low signal intensity stromal ring into the parametrium bilaterally (*black arrows, B*). There is possible early extension in to the lower uterine segment on the sagittal sections (*white arrow*).

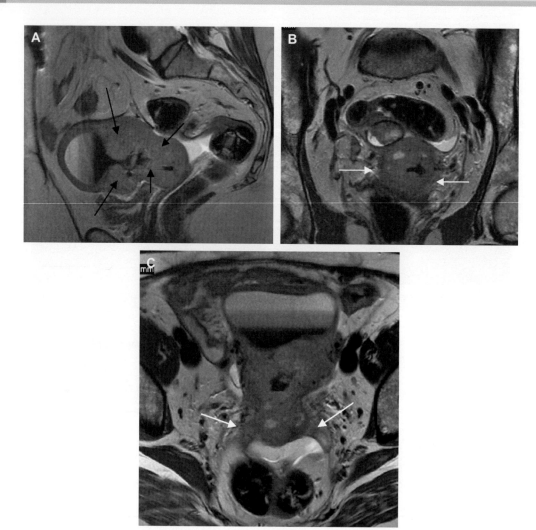

Fig. 30. T2W FSE sagittal (*A*) and oblique (*B*, *C*) images obtained at 3T of an extensive carcinoma of the cervix (*black arrows*) invading uterus. This has resulted in obstruction of the uterine cavity at the level of the internal os producing a hematocolpos (note variable age of hemorrhage, *B* and *C*). Bilateral parametrial invasion is noted with absence of the normal low signal intensity stromal ring, in keeping with FIGO stage 2B disease.

Future developments

MR imaging is an evolving tool for determination of gynecologic disease, which benefits from the move to imaging at 3T but which will be further advanced with the introduction of higher-order channel receivers and fast imaging sequences. It has major capabilities for the diagnosis, detection, and monitoring of malignancy and benefits from being noninvasive and three-dimensional allowing visualization of the extent of disease and its angiogenic properties. There are also several limitations, including the shading artifact present with ascites or very large cysts, the poor diagnostic accuracy of lymph node determination, and the inevitable failure to resolve pathology at the microscopic level.

Research continues focusing on the use of higher field strengths with improved spatial and temporal resolution data, artifact reduction, improving the understanding of the mechanism of contrast enhancement at the cellular level, and development of macromolecular and targeted contrast agents. Software is also being developed to enable functional and anatomic images to be fused in a digital imaging and communications in medicine-compliant format for input into radiotherapy planning systems. This software produces morphologically optimized enhancement data. These data are more suitable for contouring and planning radiotherapy distributions and may improve tumor control and reduce side effects by boosting the dose to the vascular part of the planning target volume.

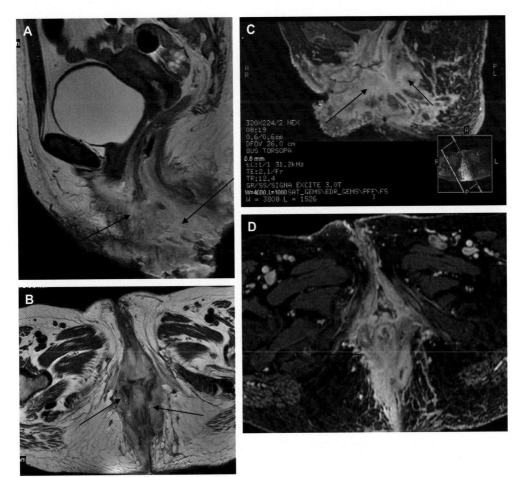

Fig. 31. Extensive squamous carcinoma of vulva (*black arrows* throughout all images) involving the labia and extending into the introitus, anal canal, and soft tissues of the buttocks. Sagittal (*A*) and axial (*B*) T2W FSE images provide useful information concerning the extent of disease present but use of 3D postcontrast T1W-FSPGR sequence, using slice thickness of 0.6 mm, allows reformatting to optimally demonstrate crucial structures such as urethra, paravaginal fat, and rectum, as shown in images *C* and *D*. All images obtained at 3T.

References

[1] Morakkabati-Spitz N, Gieske J, Kuhl C, et al. MRI of the pelvis at 3T: very high spatial resolution with sensitivity encoding and flip-angle sweep technique in clinically acceptable scan time. Eur Radiol 2006;16:634–41.

[2] Kataoka M, Kido A, Koyama T, et al. MRI of the female pelvis at 3T compared to 1.5T: evaluation on high-resolution T2-weighted and HASTE images. J Magn Reson Imaging 2007;25:527–34.

[3] Gabriel S, Corhout E. The dielectric properties of biological tissues. Phys Med Biol 1996;41:2231–49.

[4] Wang D, Heberlein KA, LaConte S, et al. Inherent insensitivity to RF inhomogeneity in flash imaging. Magn Reson Med 2004;52:927–31.

[5] Yoo RY, Sirlin CB, Gottschalk M, et al. Ovarian imaging by magnetic resonance imaging in obese adolescent girls with polycystic ovarian syndrome: a pilot study. Fertil Steril 2005;84(4):985–95.

[6] Erdem CZ, Bayar U, Erdem LO, et al. Polycystic ovary syndrome: dynamic contrast-enhanced ovarian MR imaging. Eur J Radiol 2004;51(1):48–53.

[7] Hascalik S, Celik O, Sarac K, et al. Clinical significance of N-acetyl-L-aspartate resonance in ovarian mucinous cystadenoma. Int J Gynecol Cancer 2006;16(1):423–6.

[8] Takeuchi M, Matsuzaki K, Kusaka M, et al. Ovarian cystadenofibroma—characteristic magnetic resonance findings with pathological correlation. J Comput Assist Tomogr 2003;27(6):871–3.

[9] Jung DC, Kim SH, Kim SH. MR imaging findings of ovarian cystadenofibroma and cystadenocarcinofibroma: clues for the differential diagnosis. Korean J Radiol 2006;7(3):199–204.

[10] Togashi K, Nishimura K, Kimura I, et al. Endometrial cysts: diagnosis with MR imaging. Radiology 1991;180:73–8.

[11] Nishimura K, Togashi K, Itoh K, et al. Endometrial cysts of the ovary: MR imaging. Radiology 1987;162:315–8.

[12] Woodward P, Sohaey R, Mezzetti TP. Endometriosis: radio-pathological correlation. Radiographics 2001;21:193–216.

[13] Sugimura K, Okizuka H, Imaoka I, et al. Pelvic endometriosis: detection and diagnosis with chemical shift imaging. Radiology 1993;188:435–8.

[14] Scoutt LM, McCarthy SM, Lange R, et al. MR evaluation of clinically suspected adnexal masses. J Comput Assist Tomogr 1994;18:609–18.

[15] Jacobson L, Westrom L. Objectivized diagnosis of acute pelvic inflammatory disease: diagnostic and prognostic value of routine laparoscopy. Am J Obstet Gynaecol 1969;106:1088–98.

[16] Tukeva TA, Aronen HJ, Karjalainen PT, et al. MR imaging in pelvic inflammatory disease: comparison with laparoscopy and US. Radiology 1999;210:209–16.

[17] Kim SH, Kim SH, Yang DM, et al. Unusual causes of tubo-ovarian abscess: CT and MR imaging findings. Radiographics 2004;24(6):1575–89.

[18] Ghossain MA, Hachem Y, Buy JN, et al. Adnexal torsion: magnetic resonance findings in the viable adnexa with emphasis on stromal ovarian appearance. J Magn Reson Imaging 2004;20(3):451–62.

[19] Sohaib SA, Mills TD, Sahdev A, et al. The role of magnetic resonance imaging and ultrasound in patients with adnexal masses. Clin Radiol 2005;60(3):340–8.

[20] Qayyum A, Coakley FV, Westphalen AC, et al. Role of CT and MR imaging in predicting optimal cytoreduction of newly diagnosed primary epithelial ovarian cancer. Gynaecol Oncol 2005;96(2):301–6.

[21] Forstner R, Chen M, Hricak H. Imaging of ovarian cancer. J Magn Reson Imaging 1995;5:606–13.

[22] Forstner R, Hricak H, Occhipinti KA, et al. Ovarian cancer: staging with CT and MR imaging. Radiology 1995;197:619–26.

[23] Forstner R, Hricak H, Powell CB, et al. Ovarian cancer recurrence: value of MR imaging. Radiology 1995;196(3):715–20.

[24] Kalovidouris A, Gouliamos A, Pontifex GR, et al. Computed tomography of ovarian carcinoma. Acta Radiol 1984;25:2003–8.

[25] Sanders RC, McNeil BJ, Finberg HJ, et al. A prospective study of computed tomography and ultrasound in the detection and staging of pelvic masses. Radiology 1983;146:439–42.

[26] Semelka RC, Lawrence PH, Shoemut JP, et al. Primary ovarian cancer: prospective comparison of contrast-enhanced CT and pre- and post contrast fat suppressed MR imaging, with histologic correlation. J Magn Reson Imaging 1993;3:99–106.

[27] Shiels RA, Peel KR, MacDonald HN, et al. A prospective trial of computed tomography in the staging of ovarian malignancy. Br J Obstet Gynecol 1985;92:407–12.

[28] Kurtz A, Tsimikas JV, Tempany CMC, et al. Diagnosis and staging of ovarian cancer: comparative values of Doppler and conventional US, CT, and MR Imaging correlated with surgery and histopathologic analysis—report of the Radiology Diagnostic Oncology Group. Radiology 1999;212:19–27.

[29] Tempany CMC, Zou KH, Silverman KG, et al. Staging of advanced ovarian cancer: comparison of imaging modalities—report from the Radiological Diagnostic Oncology Group. Radiology 2000;215:761–7.

[30] Low RN, Duggan B, Barone RM, et al. Treated ovarian cancer: MR imaging, laparotomy reassessment and serum CA-125 values compared with clinical outcome at 1 year. Radiology 2005;235(235):918–26.

[31] Manfredi R, Mirk P, Maresca G, et al. Local regional staging of endometrial carcinoma: role of MR imaging in surgical planning. Radiology 2004;231:372–8.

[32] Rockall AG, Meroni R, Sohaib SA, et al. Evaluation of endometrial carcinoma on magnetic resonance imaging. Int J Gynaecol Cancer 2007;17(1):188–96.

[33] Nasi F, Fiocchi F, Pecchi A, et al. MRI evaluation of myometrial invasion by endometrial carcinoma. Comparison between fast-spin-echo T2W and coronal FMPSPGR Gadolinium-dota-enhanced sequences. Radiol Med (Torino) 2005;110(3):199–210.

[34] Rockall AG, Sohaib SA, Harisinghani MG, et al. Diagnostic performance of nanoparticle-enhanced magnetic resonance imaging in the diagnosis of lymph node metastases in patients with endometrial and cervical cancer. J Clin Oncol 2005;23(12):2813–21.

[35] Bipat S, Afina SG, van der Velden J, et al. Computed tomography and magnetic resonance imaging in staging of uterine cervical carcinoma: a systematic review. Gynecol Oncol 2003;91:59–66.

[36] Janus CL, Mendelson DS, Moore S, et al. Staging of cervical carcinoma: accuracy of magnetic resonance imaging and computed tomography. Clin Imaging 1989;13:114–6.

[37] Cobby M, Browning J, Jones A, et al. Magnetic resonance imaging, computed tomography and endosonography in the local staging of carcinoma of the cervix. Br J Radiol 63(753):673–9.

[38] Sabak LL, Hricak H, Powell CB, et al. Cervical carcinoma: computed tomography and magnetic resonance imaging for preoperative staging. Obstet Gynecol 1995;86:43–50.

[39] Kaji Y, Sagimara K, Kitao M, et al. Histopathology of uterine cervical carcinoma: diagnostic comparison of endorectal surface coil and standard body coil MRI. J Comput Assist Tomogr 1994;18:783–92.

[40] Sahdev A, Sohaib A, Jacob I, et al. Performance of MRI in early cervical cancer. Presented at the ARRS 102nd Annual Meeting. 28 April–3 May 2002, Atlanta, USA [abstract]. 178;3:26.

[41] Desouza NM, Dina R, McIndoe GA, et al. Cervical cancer: value of an endovaginal coil magnetic resonance imaging technique in detecting small volume disease and assessing parametrial invasion. Gynaecological Oncology 2006;102(1): 80–5.

[42] Soutter WP, Hanoch J, D'Arcy T, et al. Pretreatment tumour volume measurement on high-resolution magnetic resonance imaging as a predictor of survival in cervical cancer. BJOG 2004;111(7):741–7.

[43] Van de Blunt L, van der Heide UA, Ketelaars M, et al. Conventional, conformal and intensity modulated radiation therapy planning of external beam radiotherapy for cervical cancer: the impact of tumour regression. Int J Radiat Oncol Biol Phys 2006;64(1):189–96.

[44] Taylor A, Rockall AG, Reznek RH, et al. Mapping pelvic lymph nodes: Guidelines for delineation in intensity modulated radiotherapy. Int J Radiat Oncol Biol Phys 2005;63(5):1604–12.

[45] Mayr NA, Yuh WT, Wang JZ, et al. Early prediction of treatment outcome: functional MR imaging and standard clinical prognostic factors in advanced cervical cancer. Int J Radiat Oncol Biol Phys 2005;63(2):S97 (Suppl 1).

[46] Singh K, Orakwue CO, Honest H, et al. Accuracy of magnetic resonance imaging of inguino-femoral lymph nodes in vulval cancer. Int J Gynecol Cancer 2006;16:1179–83.

[47] Sohaib SA, Richards PS, Ind T, et al. MR imaging of carcinoma of the vulva. AJR Am J Roentgenol 2002;178:373–7.

[48] Keller TM, Michel SCA, Frohlich J, et al. USPIO-enhanced MRI for preoperative staging of gynecological pelvic tumors: preliminary results. Eur Radiol 2004;14:937–44.

MAGNETIC
RESONANCE
IMAGING CLINICS

Magn Reson Imaging Clin N Am 15 (2007) 433–448

MR Imaging of the Prostate: 1.5T versus 3T

Daniel M. Cornfeld, MD*, Jeffrey C. Weinreb, MD

- Current role of MR imaging and magnetic resonance spectroscopic imaging in the evaluation of prostate cancer
- Evolving role of MR imaging and magnetic resonance spectroscopic imaging in the evaluation of prostate cancer
- 3T prostate imaging protocol
- Coil positioning
- Imaging protocol
- T1-weighted imaging and T2-weighted imaging
- Magnetic resonance spectroscopic imaging
- Diffusion weighted imaging
- Dynamic contrast enhancement MR imaging
- T2* mapping
- Magnetic resonance lymphography
- Summary
- References

Although it is often an indolent disease, prostate cancer is still the third leading cause of cancer death in American men [1]. Furthermore, diagnosis is invasive, and treatment can have significant morbidity.

It has been more than 2 decades since it was first suggested that MR imaging might have a role in the management of this disease [2–4], primarily for determination of extracapsular extension (ECE). Since then, there have been dramatic advances in magnetic resonance technology, and the results of numerous studies have tended to support its use. Nevertheless, there is still no consensus as to the role that MR imaging should play, and it has not achieved universal acceptance.

Within the past few years, 3T whole-body magnetic resonance scanners have become widely available for clinical use, and there is reason to believe that the increased magnetic field strength of 3T scanners provides significant benefits for prostate MR imaging. As in other areas of the body, the increased signal-to-noise ratio (SNR) at 3T should provide an opportunity for imaging the prostate with higher spatial or temporal resolution. This should lead to improvements in dynamic contrast-enhanced (DCE) imaging of the prostate. Also, it should result in improved diffusion-weighted imaging (DWI) and in vivo magnetic resonance spectroscopic imaging (MRSI) compared with 1.5T. These improvements could have important implications for assessing cancers within the gland itself.

This review presents the current data on 3T MR imaging of the prostate as well as the authors' impressions based on their experience at Yale–New Haven Hospital. Coil choice and sequence parameters as well as such advanced techniques as MRSI, DWI, and DCE are discussed.

Department of Diagnostic Radiology, Yale University School of Medicine, P.O. Box 208042, New Haven, CT 06520–8042, USA
* Corresponding author.
E-mail address: daniel.cornfeld@yale.edu (D.M. Cornfeld).

1064-9689/07/$ – see front matter © 2007 Elsevier Inc. All rights reserved.   doi:10.1016/j.mric.2007.06.004
mri.theclinics.com

Current role of MR imaging and magnetic resonance spectroscopic imaging in the evaluation of prostate cancer

Once prostate cancer is diagnosed by biopsy, it is important to determine whether the cancer has spread beyond the prostate capsule or metastasized, because prognosis and treatment options differ between organ-confined and locally advanced disease (TMN stage II versus stage III and Jewett-Whitmore stage B versus stage C). Organ-confined disease or cancer with minimal ECE may be treated with radical prostatectomy, ablation therapies, brachytherapy, or watchful waiting. Once the cancer has spread beyond the confines of the prostate gland, however, these modes of management are usually precluded and external beam radiation therapy and hormonal therapy are preferred.

Various techniques are used for staging, including digital rectal examination (DRE), prostate-specific antigen (PSA) level, biopsy Gleason score, and percentage of positive biopsies. Because of the well-documented limitations of each of these for staging, they are often used in combination; based on this information, patients are placed into low-, intermediate-, and high-risk groups for having extraprostatic disease. These methods are sometimes inaccurate, however, potentially resulting in inappropriate treatment regimens.

For an imaging test to be useful in this context, it should have high accuracy, high specificity, and low interobserver variability for determination of ECE. High accuracy and specificity ensure that patients are not excluded from a potentially curative prostatectomy secondary to a false-positive reading. Low interobserver variability ensures reproducibility of interpretation, even with less experienced readers. MR imaging has been shown to have incremental value over clinical parameters alone for prediction of ECE [5] and seminal vesicle invasion (SVI). Additionally, magnetic resonance staging can predict time to recurrence, as evidenced by rising tumor markers (eg, PSA failure) in intermediate-risk patients (as assessed by DRE, PSA, Gleason scores, and percentage of positive biopsies) [6].

On T2-weighted (T2W) images, ECE is manifest by obliteration of the retroprostatic angle, asymmetry of the neurovascular bundles, a focal irregular capsular bulge, or direct invasion into the seminal vesicles [7]. In a study of 284 patients using step histopathologic examination as a "gold standard," the most experienced reader had an accuracy of 77%, whereas the less experienced readers had accuracies of 62% to 64%. In another study, adding MRSI to T2W MR imaging increased accuracy for determination of ECE for the less experienced readers but not for the more experienced readers [8]. The number of voxels with abnormal spectra was positively correlated with the likelihood of ECE, and the combined MR imaging/MRSI findings were quite specific (>90% for both types of readers with and without spectroscopy). A more recent study of patients at low risk for ECE showed combined MR imaging/MRSI accuracy of 82% for detection of ECE. Despite the low clinical stage of the study population, 20% of the participants had surgical evidence of extraprostatic disease [9]. This is clinically useful information. In one study of 135 patients determined to be at risk for ECE based on clinical data and who were scheduled to undergo prostatectomy, MR imaging resulted in a change of the surgical plan in 28 of 36 high-risk patients [10].

The addition of DCE imaging is also reported to improve accuracy for less experienced readers [11]. T2W and fused T2W/DCE parametric maps were evaluated in 103 patients who underwent prostatectomy. Staging accuracy for the less experienced readers jumped from 79% to 87% with the addition of the DCE data. Accuracy for the advanced reader showed a trend toward improvement, but the improvement was not statistically significant. Specificity was high for T2W imaging and combined T2W imaging/DCE (>90%), but the addition of DCE improved sensitivity from 51% to 71%.

Evolving role of MR imaging and magnetic resonance spectroscopic imaging in the evaluation of prostate cancer

In response to evolving therapies for treatment of prostate cancer that are tailored for individual patients and tumors, much research is focused on using various MR imaging techniques not just for determination of ECE but for noninvasive assessment of tumor size, location, and grade [12–14]. For example, size of tumor affects radiation dose, and location of tumor is important for disease-targeted therapy. In one trial, localization of tumor by means of MR imaging altered radiotherapy treatment plans in 18% of 327 patients. The strongest predictor of PSA relapse in this group was lack of a preplanning MR imaging [15]. Other studies have shown that MR imaging has additive value to sextant biopsy and DRE in localizing peripheral zone neoplasms [16,17].

Localization of tumor is also important in cases of an elevated PSA level with a negative biopsy. The combination of MR imaging and MRSI has shown use in identifying neoplasms not detected with biopsy [18,19]. In one study, 5 of 15 localized cancers were detected using only the spectroscopic data [19]. Another study showed high specificity (88%) and negative predictive value (91%) for

MRSI in detecting neoplasm in 30 patients with an elevated PSA level and prior negative biopsy [20].

The ability of MR imaging to localize tumors within the central gland has also recently been defined. Central gland tumors can remain occult because the central gland is neither palpable nor routinely sampled by sextant biopsy. MR imaging features of central gland neoplasms include uniform low signal, ill-defined margins, lack of a capsule, and heterogenous enhancement [21,22]. Sensitivities, specificities, and accuracies for detecting tumors in the central gland are not as high as those for peripheral zone tumors. Additionally, there is a broader range of metabolites in the normal or hypertrophied central gland, which complicates using spectroscopy to differentiate central gland neoplasm from benign tissue [23]. Specifically, citrate is decreased in stromal benign prostate hyperplasia (BPH); thus, the ratios of choline plus creatine to citrate and choline to citrate may not be useful.

Finally, MR imaging has shown use in detecting recurrent neoplasm after radiation. One study showed that although interreader variability was high, the accuracy of magnetic resonance for detecting ECE and SVI before salvage prostatectomy was equivalent to the accuracy of pretreatment MR imaging [24]. Two additional studies indicate that spectroscopy is more useful than T2W imaging alone in depicting recurrent disease after external beam radiation therapy. This is because atrophic changes within the gland after radiation darken the peripheral gland on the T2W images [25,26].

In summary, MR imaging has added value to clinical data for staging prostate cancer. The addition of advanced techniques, such as spectroscopy and DCE, increase specificity, decrease interreader variability, and help inexperienced readers. MR imaging is also becoming a more accepted tool for localizing known neoplasm, localizing biopsy occult neoplasm, and detecting recurrent disease.

3T prostate imaging protocol

Before imaging, an endorectal coil (ERC) is inserted into the rectum (Medrad, Indianola, Pennsylvania) (Fig. 1). An adapter connects the ERC with an eight-element torso phased-array coil, and the two coils are used in conjunction.

At 1.5T, there is consensus that an ERC, usually in combination with a torso phased-array coil, is advantageous for prostate imaging compared with a torso coil alone [27,28]. There has been some discussion about the necessity for an ERC for prostate imaging at 3T. Some believe that the increased SNR at 3T can obviate the need for the ERC and that using only external coils would result in better patient acceptance, more uniform signal, and less compression and deformation of the gland. Examination time would be decreased, and a physician would not need to be physically present for coil placement. At this point in time, this issue has not been settled conclusively.

In one study, images of 29 patients with prostate cancer obtained by MR imaging at 1.5T using an ERC/phased-array coil were compared with images obtained by MR imaging at 3T using a phased-array coil only. Image quality was judged better using the ERC at 1.5T, but diagnostic performance was not statistically different [29]. Nevertheless, it is important to note that the 1.5T endorectal images were obtained with higher spatial resolution and more signal averaging than those obtained at 3T with the phased-array coil.

A second study compared phased-array imaging at 3T in 20 patients with combined ERC/phased-array coil imaging at 1.5T in 20 separate patients. T2W images were obtained with voxel sizes of 1.2 mm³ and 1.5 mm³. Image quality was judged equivalent at the larger pixel size only. For the higher resolution images, the 1.5T ERC coil images were superior [30].

A similar study compared image quality and staging performance at 1.5T and 3T in 22 patients with prostate cancer before prostatectomy. The 3T images obtained with an external phased-array coil were compared with 1.5T images obtained with

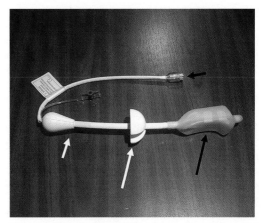

Fig. 1. The balloon-inflatable disposable ERC (Medrad, Pittsburgh, Pennsylvania). The balloon (*long black arrow*) is filled with a susceptibility-matched material, such as barium or perfluorocarbon. The curved surface of the coil is placed anterior against the prostate. The stopper (*long white arrow*) is placed against the patient's gluteal folds to prevent coil migration. The authors lay a small weight over the shaft of the coil (*short white arrow*) to prevent coil movement. The plug (*short black arrow*) attaches to the torso phased-array coil by means of an adapter.

the combined ERC/phased-array coil. Voxel size was smaller at 1.5T (1.2 mm^3 versus 1.6 mm^3). Although image quality was superior at 1.5T, staging performance was equivalent [31].

Although these early studies are useful, they do not really address the most pertinent issue: is optimal 3T prostate MR imaging better than that achievable at 1.5T, and can 3T MR imaging provide diagnostically relevant improvements compared with 1.5T? If all we are aiming for at 3T is to duplicate the results at 1.5T but without an ERC coil, MR imaging is likely to continue to play a minor role in the workup and management of prostate cancer. If prostate imaging at 3T, even if it requires an ERC, results in better and new applications, however, MR imaging may assume a pivotal role in assessment of prostate cancer.

Thus far, few published studies have attempted to address this issue. One study of 25 patients with prostate cancer showed that 3T ERC images were superior to 3T phased-array images. Motion artifacts were more prominent with the ERC, but all other imaging quality characteristics were improved. Staging accuracy was increased when using the ERC, but the capability of localizing tumor was equivalent [32].

A small study directly comparing ERC imaging at 1.5T and 3T in 10 patients showed improved image quality at 3T. Staging performance was unchanged, but the sample size was small [33]. This study was recently expanded to inlcude 46 patients with similar results [34].

The authors' experience at Yale–New Haven Hospital is that the combined ERC/phased-array coil images at 3T are better than those obtained at 1.5 T because of increased SNR and that the artifacts are no worse. The perceived improvement is nowhere near the kind of improvement one might expect from a doubling of field strength, however. This is likely attributable to two factors. First, the SNR improvement at 3T is variable, depending on the pulse sequence and the tissue imaged. In general, there is less improvement with the T2W sequences that the authors are using for prostate MR imaging. Second, the ERC has not been optimized for 3T or parallel imaging.

Thus, at the present time, the authors' impression is that optimal 3T prostate MR imaging is slightly better than at 1.5T. Nevertheless, the authors are optimistic about the development of hardware and software, which should provide significant improvement in image quality compared with 1.5T. Furthermore, they believe that the advantages of 3T for prostate imaging are likely to become most apparent for ancillary MR imaging techniques, such as MRSI, DWI, and DCE, that are still under investigation.

Coil positioning

Patients are imaged supine. Proper ERC placement involves positioning and taking steps to keep the coil from moving during the examination (see Fig. 1). When the coil moves or is in the wrong position, overall image quality is poor. The flat end of the coil is positioned flush against the posterior aspect of the prostate, centered on the prostate in the craniocaudad direction. Positioning is easily checked on the localizer images. If the coil needs to be repositioned, it should be completely deflated. If the coil is in too far, it should be removed and reinserted. Once placed, the coil does not easily move independent of the surrounding structures. A low-residue diet and preprocedure enema (self-administered the previous evening) can improve coil placement, although they are not mandatory.

To keep the coil from moving during the examination, the authors secure it to the table by placing a light weight over the coil shaft where it exits the patient. A small dielectric pad (also known as a radiofrequency [RF] cushion) or rolled towel works well. This does not rigidly fixate the coil to the table but prevents it from moving during normal respiration. Additionally, the coil comes with a round "stopper" that attaches to the shaft. Placing this stopper flush against the patient's gluteal fold keeps the coil from migrating cranially during the examination. Finally, coaching the patient to refrain from contracting his sphincter helps to reduce coil motion.

At 1.5T, the ERC is inflated with air. This is adequate for T1-weighted (T1W) and T2W imaging and is probably also adequate for DWI at 3T. The increased susceptibility gradients caused by the air–soft tissue interface at 3T significantly affects the performance of MRSI, however. Field homogeneity measurements performed on five volunteers with an ERC filled with air, barium, and liquid perfluorocarbon (PFC) showed a large posterior-anterior field gradient across the prostate when the balloon was filled with air [35]. This gradient resolved when the balloon was filled with barium or PFC. Overall field homogeneity was improved with barium and PFC versus air. The addition of higher order (nonlinear) shimming did not further increase field homogeneity. Other studies have also shown the value of using PFC when performing spectroscopy at 3T [36,37] as well as at 1.5T [38]. At the time of this writing, however, the authors still insufflate the balloon with air. This is acceptable because they are not currently performing MRSI. Although there is some distortion of the diffusion images, their diagnostic value is not significantly impaired. As the authors begin performing 3T prostate MRSI, however, they plan to use PFC instead of air.

Although barium is inexpensive and considered safe, the authors' experience is that it causes layering bright signal within the inflated balloon on the T2W images, which worsens the motion artifacts propagating through the phase direction (Fig. 2). This appearance is probably secondary to settling of the barium within solution. Additionally, on multiple occasions, the authors have had difficulty removing barium from the balloon and think that this is secondary to barium particulate obstructing the tubing. When this occurs, the authors rapidly

inject a small volume of water into the coil to dislodge the obstructing barium. Filling the balloon with water may be an acceptable substitution for susceptibility reasons but also results in high signal throughout the coil on T2W images, which propagates artifacts and can obscure portions of the prostate.

The torso phased-array coil should be placed so that there is adequate signal from the aortic bifurcation through to the pubic symphysis. This allows screening for enlarged nodes throughout the entire

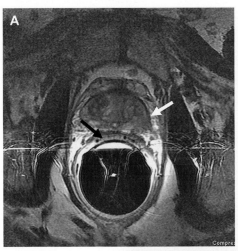

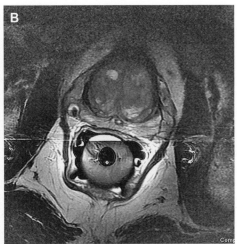

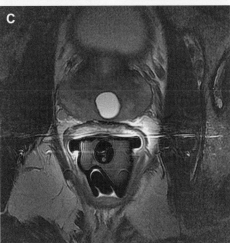

Fig. 2. (*A*) Axial T2W image through the midprostate. The ERC is filled with thick barium (the same barium you would use for a double-contrast enema). Most of the coil has no signal, which is the desired effect. There is crescentic high signal within the nondependent portion of the coil (*black arrow*), however, which is probably secondary to layering of the barium suspension. This places high signal adjacent to the prostate and worsens the appearance of phase artifacts. Neoplasm was present in the left peripheral zone (*white arrow*). (*B*) Axial T2W image through the midprostate. The ERC is filled with thin barium (the same barium you would use for a small bowel followthrough). The coil contains some signal but not much. The barium still layers, resulting in high signal against the posterior prostate. The interface between high and low signal within the coil propagates throughout the image in the phase direction. (*C*) Axial T2W image through the prostate in a patient with a utricle cyst and chronic prostatitis. The coil is incompletely distended, and is therefore more prone to motion and artifact.

pelvis. A dielectric pad is placed between the patient's abdomen and the anterior portion of the phased-array coil to mitigate the signal inhomogeneity that can plague 3T body images.

Imaging protocol

A basic prostate protocol contains axial T1W and multiplanar T2W images. MRSI, DWI, and DCE are added depending on the availability of technology and ability. The authors routinely perform DWI and DCE but do not currently have the software to perform spectroscopy at 3T.

T1-weighted imaging and T2-weighted imaging

High-resolution oblique axial and oblique coronal fast spin echo (FSE) T2W images are obtained through the prostate and seminal vesicles to evaluate for neoplasm and ECE. Some advocate also obtaining sagittal T2W images. Small field-of-view (FOV) axial FSE T1W images are acquired through the prostate to evaluate for postbiopsy hemorrhage, periprostatic nodes, and ECE. Some institutions alternatively obtain large FOV FSE T1W images through the entire pelvis to evaluate for adenopathy. Because the authors routinely give intravenous contrast, they instead perform a postcontrast T1W fat-saturated three-dimensional (3D) fast spoiled gradient echo sequence from the aortic bifurcation to the pubic symphysis as the last sequence in their examination. Sequence parameters at 1.5T and 3T are listed in Table 1.

The authors obtain the high-resolution images without parallel imaging using the body coil to transmit and the combination ERC/phased-array coil to receive. Frequency direction is anterior to posterior to prevent motion artifacts from the coil from propagating through the prostate.

The authors' experience with 3T imaging led them to increase the echo time (TE) of 100 milliseconds used at 1.5T to 140 milliseconds to accentuate the zonal anatomy of the prostate. They increase resolution by increasing the imaging matrix. Other institutions alternatively decrease the FOV (eg, from 14 cm to 12 cm). Currently, the authors' pixel resolution is 3 mm × 0.4 mm × 0.625 mm = 0.75 mm^3. Some sites have published studies with pixel resolutions of 0.35 mm^3 [39] and 0.17mm^3 [32]. To the authors' knowledge, optimal bandwidth and echo-train length have not been determined. An example of the typical image quality at 1.5T versus 3T is seen in Fig. 3.

The profile of the ERC results in high signal near the coil-prostate interface and rapid signal loss as distance from the coil increases. This makes it

Table 1: Imaging parameters for T1W and T2W sequences

	1.5 T	3 T
Axial T2W FSE	TR: 5000 TE: 102 FOV: 14 ST: 3 mm skip 0 Matrix: 256 × 192	TR: 5000 TE: 140 FOV: 14 ST: 3 mm skip 0 Matrix: 352 × 224
Coronal T2W FSE	TR: 5000 TE: 102 FOV: 14 ST: 3 mm skip 0 Matrix: 256 × 192	TR: 5000 TE: 140 FOV: 14 ST: 3 mm skip 0 Matrix: 352 × 224
Axial T1W FSE	TR: 950 TE: 9 FOV: 24 ST: 5 mm skip 1 Matrix: 256 × 160	TR: 700 TE: 7 FOV: 14 ST: 3 mm skip 0.5 Matrix: 256 × 224
Postcontrast 3D FSPGR	TR: 4 TE: 2 Flip: 12 FOV: 30–40 ST: 4 mm overlap 2 Matrix: 320 × 192 Acceleration factor: 2	TR: 4 TE: 1.6 Flip: 12 FOV: 30–40 ST: 4 mm overlap 2 Matrix: 320 × 192 Acceleration factor: 2

Abbreviations: FSPGR, fast spoiled gradient recalled; ST, slice thickness; TR, repetition time.

difficult to window the images appropriately. Postprocessing with a surface coil intensity correction (SCIC) filter corrects for this artifact. The images become grainy at the periphery but have more homogeneous signal centrally (Fig. 4). The SCIC filter is a standard filter on the authors' scanner (Signa Hdx; General Electric, Milwaukee Wisconsin). Other vendors have similar correction algorithms. The prostate group at the University of California at San Francisco (UCSF) has developed a prostate analytical coil correction (PACC) filter that tailors the surface coil correction to the exact geometry of the ERC. This produces images superior to SCIC but is not currently a commercially available product.

Magnetic resonance spectroscopic imaging

Increased magnetic field strength provides two powerful advantages for MRSI. First, the increased SNR allows smaller voxel size. MRSI voxel size at 1.5T is approximately 0.30 cm^3, and it is 0.15 cm^3 at 3T [40]. This reduces volume averaging effects

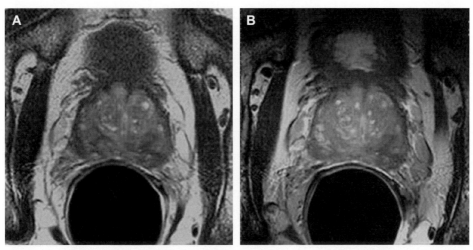

Fig. 3. Examples of T2W images at 1.5T (*A*) and 3T (*B*) using the ERC in two separate sessions in the same patient. The resolution and signal are slightly higher at 3T. (*Courtesy of* F. Coalkey, MD, San Francisco, CA.)

with periprostatic fat, postbiopsy hemorrhage, seminal vesicles, BPH nodules, and periurethral tissues.

Second, separation and height of the metabolite peaks is increased at 3T. Normal prostate tissue is characterized by a high citrate-to-choline ratio. Peripheral zone neoplasms are characterized by decreased citrate, increased choline, and decreased polyamines. At 1.5T, the choline, polyamine, and creatine peaks blend into a single peak. Criteria for identifying suspicious spectra involve measuring the ratio of choline plus creatinine to citrate, because isolating the choline peak can be difficult. At 3T, the choline peak is distinct and the ratio of choline to citrate is easier to measure (Fig. 5). The ability to identify confidently the choline peak at 3T potentially increases the specificity of MRSI.

Combined with increased spatial resolution, this also potentially improves differentiation of smaller cancers from normal tissue.

Technical challenges to MRSI at 3T include suppression of water and lipid within the prostate and surrounding tissues. One technique developed at UCSF involves a spectral spatial radiofrequency (SPRF) pulse [41]. Instead of suppressing water and lipid, this RF pulse partially excites water and completely excites metabolites from choline to citrate. The lipid frequencies are not excited. Very selective saturation (VSS) pulses refine the imaging volume to exclude periprostatic fat and the coil–soft tissue interface [42,43].

Additionally, increased J coupling of citrate at 3T causes the citrate peak to refocus at only specific

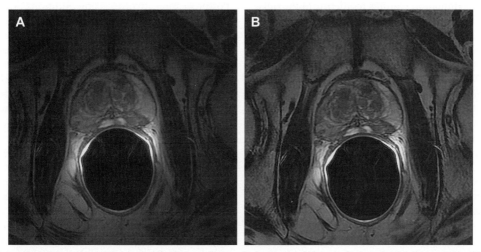

Fig. 4. Axial T2W image of the prostate before surface coil correction (*A*) and after surface coil correction (*B*). The image is more homogeneous but also more grainy after correction.

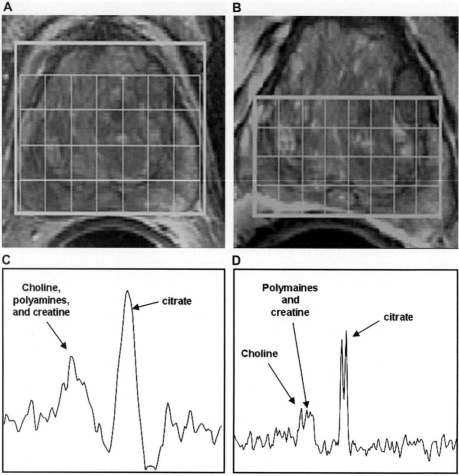

Fig. 5. Representative spectra at 1.5T and at 3T in different patients without prostate cancer. (*A, C*) Voxel prescription and sample spectra at 1.5T. The voxel size is large, and there is a single choline, polyamine, and creatine peak. (*B, D*) At 3T, the voxel size is smaller. The choline peak is seen separately from the polyamine and creatine peaks. (*Courtesy of* F. Coakley, MD, San Francisco, CA.)

TEs. This limitation requires reordering of the pulse sequence to account for the specific TE requirements [44].

Other groups have developed different solutions to these difficulties [45–49].

Use of an ERC and filling the balloon with a susceptibility neutral agent were discussed previously. Some recent work has investigated the potential of spectroscopy using only surface phased-array coils [50–53].

Although these technical challenges are the domain of physicists, chemists, and engineers, sequence prescription and postprocessing are still performed by the radiologist or technologist on site. Correct prescription involves placing the imaging volume over the prostate but excluding the seminal vesicles, rectum, and periprostatic fat; placing VSS pulses to exclude nonprostatic tissue further; and performing a linear shim in three directions.

Postprocessing involves using additional software to voxel shift, phase shift, baseline correct, and scale the spectra. These steps require additional training, time, and attention to detail. Academic sites performing prostate spectroscopy usually have a dedicated physicist or spectroscopist to monitor the acquisition and postprocessing. Thus, although MRSI at 3T is closer to everyday use, it is not yet a "push button" technique.

Diffusion weighted imaging

DWI measures the Brownian motion of free water. Diffusion is decreased in areas of increased cellularity and in areas of cellular edema secondary to the loss of ATP-dependent sodium-potassium pumps. Both conditions are believed to be present within neoplasms. The authors' experience is that increased SNR at 3T improves the quality of DWI.

The combination of increased field strength and an ERC allows for high-resolution DWI, which is an intrinsically low SNR technique.

Studies at 1.5T have shown that DWI helps to distinguish benign from malignant peripheral gland prostate tissue (Fig. 6) [14,54–56]. Although accuracy is lower for central gland tumors [57], DWI may add value to T2W images for detecting peripheral zone tumors [58,59]. Additional studies suggest that measured apparent diffusion coefficients (ADCs) predict tumor aggressiveness and response to chemotherapy [60,61].

In a recent study, 49 patients with prostate cancer and nine healthy volunteers were studied using a surface phased-array coil to generate ADC maps at 3T. There was considerable overlap between the ADC values of peripheral zone neoplasms and healthy peripheral zone tissue, but the mean ADC was significantly lower in tumors [62]. In a study of 34 patients with biopsy-proven neoplasm studied at 3T, DWI outperformed T2W imaging in identifying peripheral and central gland neoplasms [63]. Similar results at 3T have been achieved by other groups [64]. Additionally, ADC measurements from DWI are reproducible, suggesting a role for treatment monitoring [65].

The optimal diffusion gradient strength is currently unknown. Initial research used diffusion gradients with a b factor of 0 to 300 s/mm^2. Several recent abstracts have shown increased performance (measured by area under the receiver operator curve) using higher b values of 1000 to 2000 s/mm^2 [66,67].

The authors currently acquire a non–breath-hold, single-shot, echoplanar imaging (EPI)–DWI sequence using the ERC with a FOV of 18, a matrix of 160 × 200 (in-plane resolution of 1.1 mm × 0.9 mm), a slice thickness of 4 mm, and b factors

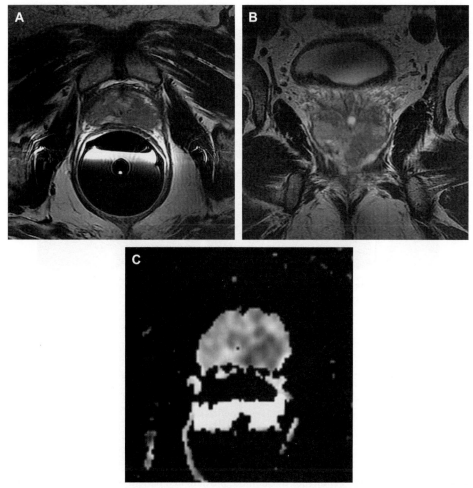

Fig. 6. Axial (*A*) and coronal (*B*) T2W images show a large neoplasm in the left midgland and apex. (*C*) Apparent diffusion coefficient (ADC) map created from DWI with b = 0 and b = 600 shows the tumor as a large area of decreased ADC.

of 0 s/mm^2 and 500 s/mm^2. Because the prostate does not contain organized directional tracts as in the brain, multidimensional acquisitions do not seem to be beneficial. Therefore, diffusion gradients are only applied in the slice direction. This minimizes image distortion. Additionally, the authors have found that setting the frequency to left/right (as opposed to anterior/posterior) for this sequence decreases distortion. The axial scan planes match the obliquity of the T2W FSE images. ADC maps are created and fused with the T2W images using commercially available software provided by the authors' vendor (Fig. 7).

Dynamic contrast enhancement MR imaging

DCE MR imaging techniques differentiate tumor from normal tissue by evaluating the kinetics of enhancement and de-enhancement. Enhancement depends on blood supply (large feeding vessels and local microvessel density) and capillary permeability. Increased blood supply and capillary permeability allow for increased enhancement. De-enhancement, or washout, depends on capillary permeability and the size of the local extravascular/extracellular space (ie, the space outside the vessels and cells). The more free space available for contrast to permeate, the longer it takes to return into the circulation. Contrast does not actually enter tumor cells. Because neoplasms parasitize large blood vessels and stimulate the growth of new ones, cause increased capillary permeability, and have decreased extravascular/extracellular space, they typically enhance and wash out more rapidly than benign tissue.

Several techniques exist for analyzing enhancement kinetics. Graphs of gadolinium concentration as a function of time can be constructed from a series of high temporal resolution images. These quantitative data can be fit to heuristic [68,69] or

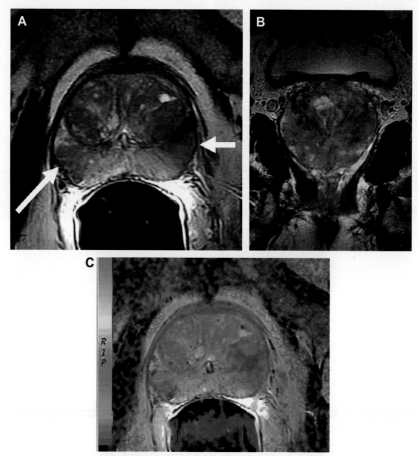

Fig. 7. Axial (*A*) and coronal (*B*) T2W images through the prostate in a patient with elevated PSA and multiple positive biopsies. Long and short white arrows in *A* show focal areas of well-defined hypointensity thought to represent peripheral zone neoplasm. (*C*) Fused ADC map and T2W image at the same level as in *A*. The regions of restricted (*blue*) diffusion correlate with the areas of neoplasm.

pharmacologic [70,71] models of tumor perfusion. The variables within these models correlate with the presence or absence of neoplasm. Qualitative data, such as peak enhancement, relative peak enhancement, maximum slope of enhancement, time to peak enhancement, and transit time, can also be calculated. A study on 36 patients with known prostate cancer suggested that relative peak enhancement was the best parameter for identifying neoplasm in the peripheral zone [72]. Simple analyses can be performed with commercially available vendor-supplied software. Fitting of the data to more rigorous heuristic or pharmacologic models requires specific software usually written by researchers within a research institution. At least one noncommercial software package is available to institutions wishing to perform these analyses [73].

To fit the enhancement curve to a pharmacologic model adequately, it is usually necessary to have three to five data points on the portion of the curve that varies the most rapidly. For prostate cancer, this requires a temporal resolution of 1 to 3 seconds. The increased SNR at 3T allows the use of high bandwidth and partial excitation imaging, which decreases imaging time. Compared with 1.5T, an identical volume can be imaged in less time but with equal SNR.

The authors' DCE protocol uses the ERC alone as a receive coil. We obtain 4-mm slices through the prostate in 2 to 4 seconds with an FOV of 14 and a matrix of 120 × 78 (in-plane resolution of 1.1 mm × 1.7 mm). Frequency direction is set anterior to posterior to decrease artifacts through the prostate. Limited coil sensitivity prevents aliasing into the gland. The authors inject gadolinium-based intravenous contrast (0.1 mmol/kg) at a rate of 2 mL/s through a peripheral intravenous line and acquire images for 5 minutes (Fig. 8).

An initial study demonstrated higher subjective image quality for DCE performed at 3T versus 1.5T [33]. A study of 20 patients with biopsy-proven prostate cancer comparing the performance of DCE MR imaging versus T2W MR imaging for localizing known prostate cancer at 3T showed increased performance using the DCE MR imaging technique. This study used a high temporal resolution technique (10 seconds), but the images were only analyzed visually [74].

Preliminary results using a pharmacologic model at 3T in 18 men with biopsy-proven prostate cancer showed that the variable associated with vascularity (known as K^{trans} and related to arterial input, macroscopic vessel density, microscopic vessel density, and capillary permeability) was higher in prostate cancer versus normal tissue. Images were acquired through the prostate every 3 seconds after contrast

administration. Combining the DCE data with the T2W images increased sensitivity (77% versus 70%) and negative predictive value (84% versus 81%) for localizing neoplasm. Specificity was not statistically different (83% versus 84%) [75].

A second study also showed a significant difference in K^{trans} between tumor and normal peripheral zone but not between tumor and benign prostatic hypertrophy. Although there remained significant overlap between K^{trans} values in tumor and normal peripheral zone tissue, within each patient, K^{trans} was greater in tumor, suggesting that focal areas of increased K^{trans} can be used to identify tumor in a heterogeneously enhancing gland [76].

An alternative approach to high temporal resolution imaging DCE MR imaging is high spatial resolution DCE MR imaging. High spatial resolution images (0.5 mm × 0.7 mm × 3 mm) can be obtained with a temporal resolution of 90 seconds. Although this temporal resolution is not high enough to fit the data to pharmacologic models, it may be sufficient to differentiate benign from malignant tissue [77]. A simple five-point time curve (precontrast plus four postcontrast points) can demonstrate qualitative enhancement and washout characteristics. In one small study, subtraction DCE images identified more and smaller neoplasms than T2W images alone [78]. Washout images (an image generated by subtracting the last postcontrast image from the first one) easily identify tissues with rapid de-enhancement (see Fig. 8). Increased SNR at 3T allows for double the pixel resolution of these postcontrast images compared with images obtained at 1.5T.

T2* mapping

A final technique, but one with limited support in the current literature, is T2* mapping. A multiecho gradient echo sequence is used to obtain images at multiple values of TE. Pixel-by-pixel signal intensities plotted as a function of TE are fit to an exponential decay to create a pixel map of T2*. In one study of eight patients with biopsy-proven prostate cancer, the T2* maps identified 17 of 18 tumors compared with 13 of 18 tumors identified by T2W imaging. Two central gland tumors were only identified on the T2* maps [79].

Magnetic resonance lymphography

Imaging with ultrasmall iron oxide particles, such as Ferumoxtran-10, is also a T2* technique. Ferumoxtran-10 is injected intravenously 24 to 36 hours before imaging and accumulates in normal lymph nodes. Normal nodes appear dark on T2* images secondary to susceptibility from the iron particles.

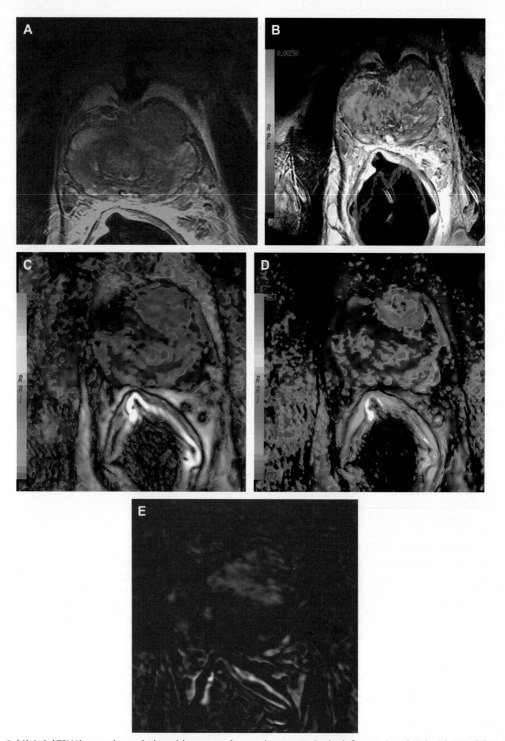

Fig. 8. (*A*) Axial T2W image through the midprostate shows a large mass in the left anterior gland with ECE. (*B*) Fused T2W/ADC map shows restricted diffusion within the tumor. (*C*) Fused T1W/perfusion map. The perfusion parameter displayed is relative signal enhancement, which is the ratio of peak signal intensity to baseline signal intensity. (*D*) Fused T1W/perfusion map. The perfusion parameter displayed is the maximum slope of increase. The parameters displayed in *C* and *D* are qualitative, and the maps were generated with commercial software obtained through the authors' vendor. More advanced parametric maps of quantitative parameters, such as K^{trans}, require conversion of signal intensity to gadolinium concentration and more advanced curve-fitting algorithms. (*E*) Subtraction images formed by subtracting the last DCE image from the peak enhancement image. The neoplasm is clearly displayed.

Nodes infiltrated with tumor do not accumulate the iron particles and remain bright on these images. Pathologic nodes as small as 5 mm can be detected with standard sequences at 1.5T [80]. Initial studies using Ferumoxtran-10 at 3T showed improved image quality at higher spatial resolution compared with images obtained at 1.5T [81]. Diagnostic performance was not evaluated. Ultrasmall iron oxide particles are not currently approved for use in the United States.

Summary

Many new techniques in prostate MR imaging are under development and refinement. Most of these techniques should benefit from the increased SNR and other features at 3T. Conventional T2W imaging can be obtained at increased spatial resolution. DWI benefits from increased signal to noise. The ability to image at increased bandwith and partial excitations without sacrificing SNR allows DCE MR imaging to be performed at higher temporal resolution. Alternatively, DCE can be performed at higher spatial resolution. MRSI benefits twofold at 3T. Voxel size is reduced by half, and there is increased separation of the choline and creatine peaks. Because volume measured by the number of voxels with abnormal spectra is correlated with the likelihood of extracapsular spread, 3T spectroscopy may also increase the accuracy of localized staging. Additionally, better identification of the choline peak increases the specificity of spectroscopy. This is especially useful in irradiated glands, where citrate is normally decreased and choline is the only peak to indicate residual or recurrent disease.

With time, more of the benefits and limitations of 3T prostate imaging should be learned. The authors anticipate that future studies of prostate imaging at 3T are likely to demonstrate increased detection and localization of smaller tumors, which can facilitate individualized therapy and perhaps identify patients in whom watchful waiting may be appropriate.

References

[1] American Cancer Society. Cancer facts and figures 2007. Publication no. 500807. Atlanta (GA): American Cancer Society; 2006.

[2] Hricak H, Williams RD, Spring DB, et al. Anatomy and pathology of the male pelvis by magnetic resonance imaging. AJR Am J Roentgenol 1983;141(6):1101–10.

[3] Hricak H, Williams RD. Magnetic resonance imaging and its application in urology. Urology 1984;23(5):442–54.

[4] Buonocore E, Hesemann C, Pavlicek W, et al. Clinical and in vitro magnetic resonance imaging of prostatic carcinoma. AJR Am J Roentgenol 1984;143(6). 1267–72.

[5] Wang L, Mullerad M, Chen H, et al. Prostate cancer: incremental value of endorectal MR imaging findings for prediction of extracapsular extension. Radiology 2004;232:133–9.

[6] D'Amico A, Whittington R, Malkowicz B, et al. Endorectal magnetic resonance imaging as a predictor of biochemical outcome after radical prostatectomy in men with clinically localized prostate cancer. J Urol 2000;164(3 Pt 1): 759–63.

[7] Yu K, Hricak H, Alagappan R, et al. Detection of extracapsular extension of prostate carcinoma with endorectal and phased-array coil MR imaging: multivariate feature analysis. Radiology 1997;202:697–702.

[8] Yu K, Scheidler J, Hricak H, et al. Prostate cancer: prediction of extracapsular extension with endorectal MR imaging and three-dimensional proton MR spectroscopic imaging. Radiology 1999;213: 481–8.

[9] Zhang J, Dave A, Ricketts J, et al. Endorectal MR imaging and proton spectroscopy for preoperative evaluation of clinical T1c prostate cancer. Proceedings of the International Society of Magnetic Resonance in Medicine 2007;15:801.

[10] Hricak H, Wang L, Wei D, et al. The role of preoperative endorectal magnetic resonance imaging in the decision regarding whether to preserve or resect neurovascular bundles during radical retropubic prostatectomy. Cancer 2004; 100(21):2655–63.

[11] Futterer J, Engelbrecht M, Huisman H, et al. Staging prostate cancer with dynamic contrast-enhanced endorectal MR imaging prior to radical prostatectomy: experienced versus less experienced readers. Radiology 2005;237:541–9.

[12] Scheidler J, Hricak H, Vigneron S, et al. Prostate cancer: localization with three dimensional proton MR spectroscopic imaging—clinicopathologic study. Radiology 1999;213:473–80.

[13] Futterer J, Heijmink S, Scheenen T, et al. Prostate cancer localization with dynamic contrast-enhanced MR imaging and proton MR spectroscopic imaging. Radiology 2006;241:449–58.

[14] Reinsberg S, Payne G, Riches S, et al. Combined use of diffusion-weighted MRI and H MR spectroscopy to increase accuracy in prostate cancer detection. AJR Am J Roentgenol 2007;188:91–8.

[15] Clarke D, Banks S, Wiederhorn R, et al. The role of endorectal coil MRI in patient selection and treatment planning for prostate seed implants. Int J Radiat Oncol Biol Phys 2002; 52(4):903–10.

[16] Mullerad M, Hricak H, Kuriowa K, et al. Comparison of endorectal magnetic resonance imaging, guided prostate biopsy and digital rectal examination in the preoperative anatomical

localization of prostate cancer. J Urol 2005;174: 2158–63.

[17] Wefer A, Hricak H, Vigneron D, et al. Sextant localization of prostate cancer: comparison of sextant biopsy, magnetic resonance imaging and magnetic resonance spectroscopy imaging with step section histology. J Urol 2000;164:400–4.

[18] Costouros N, Coakley F, Westphalen A, et al. Diagnosis of prostate cancer in patients with an elevated prostate-specific antigen level: role of endorectal MRI and MR spectroscopic imaging. Am J Roentgenol 2007;188:812–6.

[19] Ansellem-Ouazana S, Younes P, Conquy S, et al. Negative prostatic biopsies in patients with a high risk of prostate cancer. Is the combination of endorectal MRI and magnetic resonance spectroscopy imaging a useful tool? A preliminary study. Eur Urol 2005;47:582–6.

[20] Taouli B, Chin D, Stifelman M, et al. Role of 3D 1H MR spectroscopy for prospective detection of prostate cancer in men with prior negative biopsies. Proceedings of the International Society of Magnetic Resonance in Medicine 2007;15:3670.

[21] Akin O, Sala E, Moskowitz C, et al. Transition zone prostate cancers: features, detection, localization, and staging at endorectal MR imaging. Radiology 2006;239:784–92.

[22] Li H, Sugimura K, Kaji Y, et al. Conventional MRI capabilities in the diagnosis of prostate cancer in the transition zone. AJR Am J Roentgenol 2006; 186:729–42.

[23] Zakian K, Eberhardt S, Hricak H, et al. Transition zone prostate cancer: metabolic characteristics at H MR spectroscopic imaging—initial results. Radiology 2003;229:241–7.

[24] Sala E, Eberhardt S, Akin O, et al. Endorectal MR imaging before salvage prostatectomy: tumor localization and staging. Radiology 2006;238: 176–83.

[25] Coakley F, Teh H, Quayyum A, et al. Endorectal MR imaging and MR spectroscopic imaging for locally recurrent prostate cancer after external beam radiation therapy: preliminary experience. Radiology 2004;233:441–8.

[26] Pucar D, Shukla-Dave A, Hricak H, et al. Prostate cancer: correlation of MRI imaging and MR spectroscopy with pathologic findings after radiation therapy—initial experience. Radiology 2005;236: 545–53.

[27] Hricak H, White S, Vigneron D, et al. Carcinoma of the prostate gland with pelvic phased array coils versus integrated endorectal-pelvic phased array-coils. Radiology 1994;193:703–9.

[28] Engelbrecht M, Jager G, Laheij R, et al. Local staging of prostate cancer using magnetic resonance imaging: a meta-analysis. Eur Radiol 2002;12(9):2294–302.

[29] Torricelli P, Cinquantini F, Ligabue G, et al. Comparative evaluation between external phased array coil at 3T and endorectal coil at 1.5T. J Comput Assist Tomogr 2006;30(3): 355–61.

[30] Sosna J, Pedrosa I, DeWolf W, et al. MR imaging of the prostate at 3 tesla: comparison of an external phased-array coil to imaging with an endorectal coil at 1.5 tesla. Acad Radiol 2004;11: 857–62.

[31] Beyersdorff D, Taymoorian K, Knosel T, et al. MRI of prostate cancer at 1.5 and 3T: comparison of image quality in tumor detection and staging. AJR Am J Roentgenol 2005;185:1214–20.

[32] Heijmink S, Futterer J, Takahashi S, et al. A comparison of image quality and prostate cancer localization and staging performance between body array coil and endorectal coil MR imaging at 3T. Proceedings of the International Society of Magnetic Resonance in Medicine 2006;14:170.

[33] Futterer J, Scheenen T, Huisman H, et al. Initial experience of 3 tesla endorectal coil magnetic resonance imaging and H-spectroscopic imaging of the prostate. Invest Yadiol 2004;39:671–80.

[34] Heijmink S, Futterer J, Hambrock T, et al. Prostate cancer: body-array versus endorectal coil MR imaging at 3T-comparison of image quality, localization, and staging performance. Radiology 2007;244:184–95.

[35] Rosen Y, Bloch B, Lenkinski R, et al. 3T MR of the prostate: reducing susceptibility gradients by inflating the endorectal coil with a barium sulfate suspension. Magn Reson Med 2007;57: 898–904.

[36] Choi H, Ma J. Use of perfluorocarbon (PFC) in magnetic resonance spectroscopy (MRS) of the prostate: a method to improve the linewidth and quality of the spectra. Proceedings of the 90th Annual Meeting of RSNA, Chicago, November 28–December 3, 2004. p. 270.

[37] Prando A, Kurhanewicz J, Borges A, et al. Prostatic biopsy directed with endorectal MR spectroscopic imaging findings in patients with elevated prostate specific antigen levels and prior negative biopsy findings: early experience. Radiology 2005;236:903–10.

[38] Hamilton G, Middelton M, Choi S, et al. Improved MR spectral analysis for a PFC-filled endo-rectal prostate surface coil compared to an air-filled coil. Proceedings of the International Society of Magnetic Resonance in Medicine 2007;15:1400.

[39] Bloch B, Rofsky N, Baroni R, et al. 3 Tesla magnetic resonance imaging of the prostate with combined pelvic phased-array and endorectal coils: initial experience. Acad Radiol 2004;11: 863–7.

[40] Chen A, Xu D, Sotto C, et al. High resolution MRSI and DTI of prostate cancer at 3T. Proceedings of the International Society of Magnetic Resonance in Medicine 2007;15:2887.

[41] Schricker A, Pauly J, Kurhanewicz J, et al. Dual-band spectral-spatial RF pulses for prostate MR

spectroscopic imaging. Magn Reson Med 2001; 46:1079–89.

[42] Le Roux P, Gilles R, McKinnon G, et al. Optimized outer volume suppression for single-shot fast spin-echo cardiac imaging. J Magn Reson Imaging 1998;8:1022–32.

[43] Tran T, Vigneron D, Sailasuta N, et al. Very selective suppression pulses for clinical MRSI studies of brain and prostate cancer. Magn Reson Med 2000;43:23–33.

[44] Chen A, Cunningham C, Xu D, et al. 3 Tesla high resolution 3D MR spectroscopic imaging of the prostate with a MLEV-PRESS sequence. Proceedings of the International Society of Magnetic Resonance in Medicine 2005;13:261.

[45] Kim D, Margolis S, Daniel B, et al. Magnetic resonance spectroscopic imaging of the human prostate using spiral based J-resolved technique at 3 tesla main magnetic field. Proceedings of the 90th Annual Meeting of RSNA, Chicago, November 28–December 3, 2004.

[46] Kaji Y, Kuroda K, Matsuoka Y, et al. Rigorous shimming in Prostate CSI Study at 3T. Proceedings of the 90th Annual Meeting of RSNA, Chicago, November 28–December 3, 2004.

[47] Lange T, Trabesinger A, Schulte R, et al. Prostate spectroscopy at 3 tesla using two dimensional S-Press. Magn Reson Med 2006;56:1220–8.

[48] Klomp D, Scheenen T, Hambrock T, et al. A new method for optimum MRSI of prostate at 3T using adiabatic RF pulses and internal water referencing. Proceedings of the International Society of Magnetic Resonance in Medicine 2007;15:2885.

[49] Schuster C, Scheenen T, Dreher W, et al. Fast 3D proton MR spectroscopic imaging of the human prostate in vivo at 3 tesla using "spectroscopic missing pulse—SSFP". Proceedings of the International Society of Magnetic Resonance in Medicine 2007;15:1243.

[50] Yasushi K, Kuroda K, Maeda T, et al. Anatomical and metabolic assessment of prostate using a 3-tesla MR scanner with a custom-made external transceive coil: Healthy Volunteer Study. J Magn Reson Imaging 2007;25:517–26.

[51] Scheenen T, Roell S, Heijmink S, et al. 3D H-MR spectroscopic imaging of the human prostate at 3T without an endorectal coil: a step towards MR screening of prostate cancer. Proceedings of the 91st Annual Meeting of RSNA, Chicago, November 27–December 2, 2005.

[52] Guer O, Traeber F, Morakkabati-Spitz N, et al. 1H-MR spectroscopy of the prostate using a phase-array surface coil at 3T. Proceedings of the 92nd Annual Meeting of RSNA, Chicago, November 26–December 1, 2006.

[53] Mancino S, Squillaci E, Manenti G, et al. Dynamic contrast-enhanced MRI and MR spectroscopy at 3 tesla of prostate cancer with pelvic phased array coil. Proceedings of the 92nd Annual Meeting of RSNA, Chicago, November 26–December 1, 2006.

[54] Issa B. In vivo measurement of the apparent diffusion coefficient in normal and malignant prostatic tissues using echo-planar imaging. J Magn Reson Imaging 2002;16:196–200.

[55] Gibbs P, Toser D, Liney G, et al. Comparison of qualitative T2 mapping and diffusion-weighted imaging in the normal and pathologic prostate. Magn Reson Med 2001;46:1054–8.

[56] Hosseinzadeh K, Schwartz S. Endorectal diffusion-weighted imaging in prostate cancer to differentiate malignant and benign peripheral zone tissue. J Magn Reson Imaging 2004;20:645–61.

[57] Tanimoto A, Nakashima J, Shinoda K, et al. The clinical value of ADC maps in the detection of prostate cancer. Proceedings of the International Society of Magnetic Resonance in Medicine 2007;15:3661.

[58] Haider M, van der Kwast T, Tanguay J, et al. Combined T2 and diffusion weighted MRI for localization of prostate cancer. Proceedings of the International Society of Magnetic Resonance in Medicine 2007;15:3663.

[59] Chen Y, Pu Y, Liang P, et al. Prostate cancer detection in patients with intermediate prostate specific antigen levels using high resolution diffusion tensor imaging prior to transrectal ultrasound guided biopsy. Proceedings of the International Society of Magnetic Resonance in Medicine 2007;15:3658.

[60] deSouza N, Riches S, vanAs N, et al. Potential value of diffusion weighted imaging as an indicator of tumor aggressiveness in prostate cancer. Proceedings of the International Society of Magnetic Resonance in Medicine 2007;15:3659.

[61] Yoshizako T, Uchida N, Wada A, et al. The ADC value in hormone refractory prostate cancers on diffusion-weighted MR images for predicting effect of chemotherapy. Proceedings of the International Society of Magnetic Resonance in Medicine 2007;15:3662.

[62] Pickles M, Gibbs P, Sreenivas M, et al. Diffusion-weighted imaging of normal and malignant prostate tissue at 3T. J Magn Reson Imaging 2006;23:130–4.

[63] Miao H, Fukatsu H, Ishigaki T. Prostate cancer detection with 3-T MRI: comparison of diffusion-weighted and T2-weighted imaging. Proceedings of the International Society of Magnetic Resonance in Medicine 2007;61:297–302.

[64] Bourne R, Stanwell P, Ramadan S, et al. ADC of prostate tissue in vivo at 3T. Proceedings of the International Society of Magnetic Resonance in Medicine 2006;14:2248.

[65] Gibbs P, Pickles D, Sreenivas M, et al. Repeatability of diffusion imaging of the prostate at 3T. Proceedings of the International Society of Magnetic Resonance in Medicine 2005;13:268.

[66] Namiki T, Koyama K, Tanaka H, et al. Effect of diffusion-weighted imaging with very high

b-factors (2000, 3000) for detection of prostate cancer. Proceedings of the 91st Annual Meeting of RSNA, Chicago, November 27–December 2, 2005.

[67] Sano M, Ichikaa T, Tsukamoto T, et al. Detection of prostatic cancer: usefulness of high b-value diffusion-weighted MR imaging. Proceedings of the 91st Annual Meeting of RSNA, Chicago, November 27–December 2, 2005.

[68] Huisman H, Engelbrecht M, Barentsz J. Accurate estimation of pharmacokinetic contrast-enhanced dynamic MRI parameters of the prostate. J Magn Reson Imaging 2001;13:607–14.

[69] Moate P, Dougherty L, Schnall M, et al. A modified logistic model to describe gadolinium kinetics in breast tumors. Magn Reson Imaging 2004; 22:467–73.

[70] Tofts P. Modeling tracer kinetics in dynamic Gd-DTPA MR imaging. J Magn Reson Imaging 1997;7:91–101.

[71] Tofts P, Brix G, Buckley D, et al. Estimating kinetic parameters from dynamic contrast-enhanced T1-weighted MRI of a diffusible tracer: standardized quantities and symbols. J Magn Reson Imaging 1999;10:223–32.

[72] Englebrecht M, Huisman H, Laheij R, et al. Discrimination of prostate cancer from normal peripheral zone and central gland tissue by using dynamic contrast-enhanced MR imaging. Radiology 2003;229:248–54.

[73] d'Arcy J, Collins D, Padhani A, et al. Informatics in radiology (infoRAD): magnetic resonance imaging workbench: analysis and visualization of dynamic contrast-enhanced MR imaging data. Radiographics 2006;26:621–32.

[74] Kim C, Park B, Kim B. Localization of prostate cancer using 3T MRI: comparison of T2 weighted and dynamic contrast enhanced imaging. J Comput Assist Tomogr 2006;30(1):7–11.

[75] Gariib A, Jung E, Tomasson D, et al. T2 and dynamic contrast enhanced MR (DEC-MRI) imaging of prostate cancer at 3T. Proceedings of the International Society of Magnetic Resonance in Medicine 2005;13:2121.

[76] Lowry M, Turnbull L. Analysis of prostate DCE-MRI at 3T using a measured arterial input function. Proceedings of the International Society of Magnetic Resonance in Medicine 2006; 14:110.

[77] Eyal E, Block B, Furman-Haran E, et al. Pattern and model based analysis of dynamic contrast enhanced prostate MRI data. Proceedings of the International Society of Magnetic Resonance in Medicine 2007;15:523.

[78] Yu J, Chung J, Kim J, et al. Prostate cancer: added value of subtraction dynamic imaging in 3T magnetic resonance imaging with a phased-array body coil. Proceedings of the International Society of Magnetic Resonance in Medicine 2007;15: 2886.

[79] Hambrock T, Huisman H, Takahashi S, et al. T2* mapping versus T2-weighted MR imaging in localization of prostate cancer at 3 tesla. Proceedings of the 92nd Annual Meeting of RSNA, Chicago, November 26–December 1, 2006.

[80] Harisinghani M, Barentsz J, Hahn P, et al. Non-invasive detection of clinically occult lymph-node metastases in prostate cancer. N Engl J Med 2003;348(25):2491–9 Erratum in: N Engl J Med 2003 Sep 4;349(10):1010.

[81] Heesakkers R, Futterer J, Hovels A, et al. Prostate cancer evaluated with Ferumoxtran-10-enhanced T2*-weighted MR imaging at 1.5 and 3T: early experience. Radiology 2006;239:481–7.

MAGNETIC
RESONANCE
IMAGING CLINICS

Magn Reson Imaging Clin N Am 15 (2007) 449–465

Perspectives on Body MR Imaging at Ultrahigh Field

Elizabeth M. Hecht, MD[a,*], Ray F. Lee, PhD[b],
Bachir Taouli, MD[c], Daniel K. Sodickson, MD, PhD[b,d]

- ■ Radiofrequency coils
- ■ Radiofrequency homogeneity
- ■ Specific absorption rate
- ■ Main magnetic field homogeneity
- ■ Alteration of tissue contrast
  - *Arterial spin labeling*
  - *T2-weighted imaging*
  - *T2*-weighted imaging*
  - *Iron oxide contrast agents*
- ■ Chemical shift
- ■ Safety
  - *Acoustic noise*
  - *Medical devices*
- ■ Potential applications of MR imaging beyond 3T

- ■ Biochemical processes and molecular imaging
  - *Sodium (^{23}Na) MR imaging*
  - *Phosphorus (^{31}P) MR imaging*
  - *Proton (^{1}H) MR spectroscopy*
- ■ Susceptibility-sensitive T2* imaging for iron and calcium
  - *Iron-containing contrast agents*
  - *Blood oxygenation level-dependent imaging*
  - *Susceptibility weighted imaging*
- ■ Vascular imaging and characterization
- ■ Summary
- ■ References

Three Tesla (T) imaging is clearly beneficial for clinical neuroimaging, but the benefits of 3T for body imaging are as yet unclear. Beyond the brain, the opportunities and theoretical rewards of 3T are generally harder to achieve. Even if and when investigators are successful in realizing the maximum benefit of 3T in body imaging, will this lead to significant clinical benefit over 1.5T imaging? Unfortunately, the maximal theoretical benefits are not as yet achievable because there are competing effects that come into play. Nonetheless, it is the potential

for higher signal to noise ratio (SNR), greater spectral separation, and faster imaging that drives us to explore even higher field imaging. Do investigators wait until they have solved all the problems of body imaging at 3T before moving forward to working at 7T or higher? Currently, there are a handful of whole body 7T magnets available in the United States, and only slightly more worldwide. All the potential advantages that can be foreseen for clinical body imaging at 3T would logically be even greater at 7T, but so too are the challenges.

[a] Department of Radiology, New York University School of Medicine, 560 First Avenue, New York, NY 10016, USA
[b] Department of Radiology, New York University School of Medicine, 660 First Avenue, New York, NY 10016, USA
[c] Department of Radiology, New York University School of Medicine, 530 First Avenue, MRI, New York, NY 10016, USA
[d] Center for Biomedical Imaging, New York University Medical Center, 650 First Avenue, Suite 600-A, New York, NY 10016, USA
* Corresponding author.
E-mail address: hechte01@med.nyu.edu (E.M. Hecht).

1064-9689/07/$ – see front matter. Published by Elsevier Inc.
mri.theclinics.com

doi:10.1016/j.mric.2007.07.001

To achieve diagnostic image quality at 3T in the body, peripheral vasculature, and breast comparable to that of 1.5T imaging, relatively straightforward adjustments in sequence parameters are required. However, to truly maximize the benefits of 3T and improve imaging quality, new and innovative magnet, radiofrequency (RF) coil, and sequence design are required. To date, there have been few studies that have systematically compared body imaging at 1.5T and 3T. In fact, it is difficult to make such a direct comparison, as the sequence parameters and coils for 1.5T and 3T are necessarily different and, on a practical level, many institutions many not have a 1.5T and 3T magnet readily available. Currently, the paradigm for 3T body imaging is no different from that for 1.5T imaging. In most imaging centers, 1.5T body imaging protocols are modified to work more effectively at 3T and mimic the image quality of 1.5T with some expected improvement in signal to noise, fat saturation, image resolution, and acquisition time. As investigators consider approaching the challenge of even higher field imaging, should the same paradigm be followed and should they continue to work around the same problems encountered thus far at 3.0T, or should other ways of answering the clinical questions more effectively and more comprehensively be explored?

The most immediate problems of imaging at ultrahigh field strength beyond 3T are not unfamiliar, as many of them are already pressing issues at 3T: issues such as RF coils, B_1 homogeneity, specific absorption rate (SAR), safety, B_0 field homogeneity, alterations in tissue contrast, and chemical shift. In this article, these issues will be reviewed briefly in terms of how they may affect image quality at higher field strengths beyond 3T. The authors propose various approaches to overcoming the challenges and discuss potential applications of high field MR imaging as it applies to specific abdominal, pelvic, peripheral vascular, and breast imaging protocols.

Radiofrequency coils

Currently, there are only a few coils available for ultrahigh field MR imaging of the abdomen and breast. No commercial coils are available for vascular imaging, as far as the authors are aware. While theoretically, SNR increases linearly with increasing magnetic field strength, specialized coils are required to achieve such potential. Radiofrequency (B_1) homogeneity is essential to optimizing image quality. With increasing field strength, however, the interactions between coils and biologic tissue become significant. Maintaining RF (B_1) field homogeneity becomes a considerable engineering challenge requiring innovations in coil design.

At field strengths lesser than or equal to 3T, the body coil is embedded in the bore of the magnet and used for RF transmission, generally with a receive-only surface coil array for data acquisition. At ultrahigh field strength, constructing a large volume body coil for transmission is problematic because tuning becomes extremely difficult and long RF coil circuits begin to radiate a significant portion of their energy. This leads to energy and signal loss in the coil and transference of heat and electrical noise to the subject and magnet bore environment [1]. In addition, the tuning capacitance is inversely proportional to the resonance frequency, leading to impractical tuning capacitance at high field strengths. Alternatively, a coil array may be used for signal transmission and reception, but B_1 inhomogeneity is a problem. Multichannel coil arrays capable of parallel imaging become ever more crucial for high field coil design because high parallel acceleration factors will be needed at high field strength to cope with issues of SAR and to improve spatial and temporal resolution.

There are several coil designs that are currently being implemented for high field brain imaging, including birdcage, transverse electromagnetic (TEM), and microstrip coils. In a recent study, the performance of these different coils was compared at 7T [2]. The birdcage coil was found to have higher average and maximal local SAR levels when compared with TEM and microstrip coils, and B_1 field homogeneity of the loaded TEM coils was better than those of the birdcage and microstrip coils. Loaded TEM coils also demonstrated the least radiation loss. The B_1 field homogeneity of the microstrip coil was slightly better than the birdcage, although the microstrip was the most inhomogeneous when unloaded.

For human body imaging, there are a few coils that have been recently described, including an actively detunable TEM volume coil [3], an eight channel flexible TEM/stripline transceiver array [4], and a Flourine/Hydrogen ($^{19}F/^1H$) dual resonant elliptic body coil (Fig. 1) [5], all of which show great promise and are currently being implemented in the research setting for anatomic and spectroscopic imaging. B_1 shimming is a challenge at 7T, but finetuning of the transmit arrays can compensate for interactions between electromagnetic fields and the human body. To our knowledge, only one coil has been described for breast imaging at 7T: a linearly polarized solenoid coil (Figs. 2 and 3) [6].

Finally, endoluminal coils may or may not be necessary at high field strength. Ideally, imaging could be performed without endoluminal coils, but they may still play a role in body MR imaging, given the challenges of RF and B_0 homogeneity over a large field of view at ultrahigh field strength.

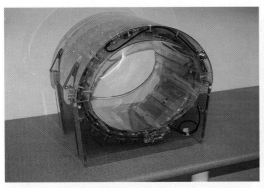 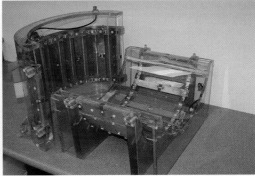

Fig. 1. Images of a $^{19}F/^{1}H$ dual resonant elliptic body coil designed specifically to image the pancreas.

Radiofrequency homogeneity

RF homogeneity is difficult to achieve and maintain as field strength increases. To create and manipulate MR signal, an RF pulse must resonate at the precessional frequency—or Larmor frequency—of the nucleus within the main magnetic field (B_0). The Larmor frequency is proportional to the magnetic field strength and gyromagnetic ratio (γ) of the nucleus being imaged. For hydrogen nuclei (ie, protons), the Larmor frequency is approximately 64 MHz at 1.5T, 128 MHz at 3T, and 298 MHz at 7T. Meanwhile, wavelength decreases with increasing frequency: 64 MHz corresponds to approximately 4.7-m wavelength in free space; 298 MHz corresponds to approximately 1 m; however, the effective wavelength is further reduced by almost an order of magnitude by the high electrical permittivity of human tissue. At increasing field strength, the interaction between the body and the coil becomes more pronounced, in part because the size of the body becomes comparable to the operating RF wavelength. Even at 3T investigators begin to notice unwanted RF behavior within the body that is typically manifested as regions of signal loss (ie, "dark spots") or, less commonly, signal brightening

(ie, "hot spots"). The RF or B_1 field distribution also becomes more unpredictable with increasing field strength because it is increasingly affected by the interaction of the coil with the body, rather than being determined by the coil design alone.

The field shaping effects of the body are commonly grouped under the general term "dielectric effects." At sufficiently high frequency, several complex electrodynamic influences are actually at work: constructive and destructive interferences, caused by wave propagation effects at the shortened wavelengths, associated with high internal permittivities; shielding effects of RF eddy currents, induced by the coil fields in electrically conductive tissues; and distortion of electromagnetic fields at tissue boundaries. Unfortunately, the net effect of all of these influences depends upon the detailed geometry and composition of the patient's body: that is, body habitus or the presence or absence of ascites or amniotic fluid. Furthermore, variations in image intensity may reflect spatial variations in RF fields associated either with spin excitation or signal detection, or with both together. Excitation field variations result in nonuniformities of flip angle across the image, which can in turn result in spatial variations of contrast.

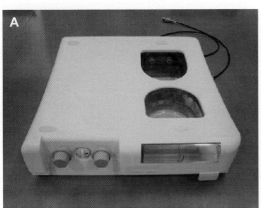 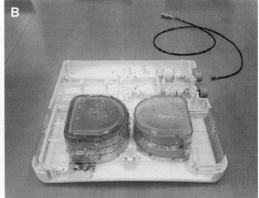

Fig. 2. (*A*) Top and (*B*) bottom of the linearly polarized solenoid coil for dedicated breast imaging at 7T.

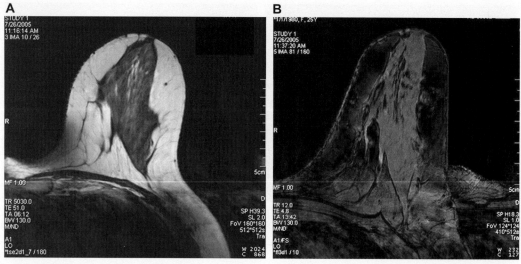

Fig. 3. Axial high resolution T1-weighted images of the left breast at 7T (*A*) without and (*B*) with frequency selective fat suppression. Note the homogenous fat suppression achieved at ultrahigh field strength caused by increased spectral separation.

As investigators move to higher field strength they need to address these issues, which represent a nontrivial difficulty, particularly for abdominal and pelvic imaging where the structures in contact with the coils can be large when compared with the RF wavelength (Fig. 4). At 3T, dielectric pads are currently used to improve signal in problem areas, such as the left lobe of the liver or in the pelvis, but results with dielectric pads may be variable at higher field strengths. Postprocessing filters have been introduced on some systems, which equalize the signal throughout an image, but this does not address the source of the problem and it does not regain lost SNR. Use of composite excitation pulses for robust preservation of transmit homogeneity have recently been described [7] and such approaches are promising for high field applications.

Improvements in coil design represent an important solution to the problem of RF inhomogeneities. If the coils can be automatically adjusted to compensate for tissue-coil interactions, then high field MR examinations can be tailored to the patient. In a preliminary study by Vaughan and colleagues [8], 9.4T imaging of the human brain was achieved and image quality was successfully optimized by using interactive multichannel RF field magnitude and phase shimming to adjust and compensate for inhomogeneity as it was encountered.

Additional control of field homogeneity may be achieved using newly described techniques for transmit parallel imaging [9,10]. These techniques excite entirely distinct patterns in each element of a transmit coil array by driving each coil with a distinct current waveform (rather than merely with

a distinct amplitude and phase, as in the case of RF shimming). Suitably optimized waveforms may be designed to accelerate complex RF pulses, but also to improve signal homogeneity and to reduce SAR [10,11].

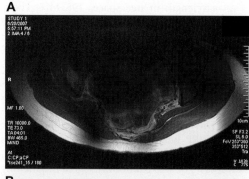

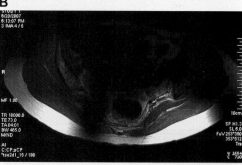

Fig. 4. Axial T2-weighted images through the pelvis in a young female volunteer at 7T demonstrating (*A*) "dielectric effects" in the pelvis with (*B*) no significant improvement demonstrated, despite placing a dielectric pad over the patient.

Specific absorption rate

The deposition of RF energy in tissue grows with increasing field strength and frequency. The traditional rule of thumb states that SAR grows as the square of the frequency, though in practice the growth is probably somewhat slower at high frequencies. In addition to baseline SAR increases, the local distribution of SAR becomes increasingly heterogeneous and subject specific, for reasons similar to those driving B_1 inhomogeneities at high field strength. Limiting SAR becomes technically challenging at high field, particularly in body and vascular imaging as many RF-intensive pulse sequences are used. Multiacquisition techniques that use ultrashort acquisition times (TR), such as time resolved imaging, are especially SAR intensive. Acceleration of data reception using parallel imaging may be used to reduce the SAR for individual data sets (by reducing the number of RF excitations required to generate any given image data set). However, multiple sequential acquisitions will approach SAR limits fairly rapidly unless very high acceleration factors are used, or unless entirely different SAR reducing techniques become available.

In general, imaging parameters will be significantly constrained by the SAR limits imposed by the US Food and Drug Administration (FDA) and implemented by manufacturers. Straightforward adjustments, such as decreasing slices per TR, decreasing flip angle, lengthening TR, increasing inter echo spacing, and prolonging the RF pulse duration can reduce SAR; however, adjusting these parameters leads to reduced coverage, alteration of tissue contrast, and diminished SNR. Therefore, new pulse sequences and coil designs are required to optimize image quality at ultrahigh field strength.

There are several new SAR-reduced sequence designs that have been successfully implemented at 3T and will also be beneficial at ultrahigh field. Variable-rate selective excitation (VERSE) uses a time varying gradient which modifies the shape of the RF pulse to reduce RF power without affecting other parameters, such as flip angle, slice profile, or acquisition time [12]. Variable flip angle sequences have also been introduced into clinical practice at 3T. These techniques use the desired image contrast and relaxation-time-dependent signal evolution to determine the optimal flip angle variation, permitting the use of longer echo train lengths and effective echo time (TE) without reaching SAR limits. Such techniques include hyperechoes [13], smooth transitions between pseudo steady states [14], and 3D T2-weighted turbo spin echo with high sampling efficiency [15].

Unfortunately, these techniques alone may not be sufficient at ultrahigh field strength. Combinations with parallel imaging may rectify the situation somewhat by reducing the number of RF pulses per unit time, albeit at some cost in SNR. It is currently believed that some of the greatest promise for SAR reduction lies in parallel transmission techniques, which can arrange for cancellation among transmit coil array elements of the electric fields responsible for energy deposition [10].

Main magnetic field homogeneity

Ultrahigh field magnets require appropriate shielding and insulation to maintain homogeneity and safety, and on a practical level this increases the cost of ultrahigh field scanners. Susceptibility effects represent both an advantage and a disadvantage of high field imaging. Generally, T2* shortening associated with magnetic susceptibility differences are major impediments in abdominal and pelvic imaging because of the interfaces between bowel gas, air in the lungs, and soft tissue, not to mention the common presence of surgical clips, sutures, metallic implants, and stents. These effects, combined with issues of respiratory and bowel motion, make imaging in the body much more challenging as field strength increases. On the other hand, the increase in susceptibility effects can be used to an advantage for functional imaging using blood oxygenation level-dependent (BOLD) effects, or for detection of pathology using ultrasmall paramagnetic iron oxide (USPIO) particles as contrast agents. The detection of iron, calcium and gas related to pneumobilia, infection, or bowel perforation should be improved at ultrahigh field strength. Bowel antiperistalsis agents and fluid, rather than air-based luminal contrast agents, will likely be required to improve image quality.

Alteration of tissue contrast

With increasing field strength, T1 relaxation times of tissues lengthen and tend to converge, while to a lesser extent, T2 relaxation times shorten. De Bazelaire and colleagues [16] demonstrated the differences in tissue relaxation times of abdominal and pelvic organs at 3T, compared with 1.5T in human volunteers, confirming the overall lengthening of T1 and shortening of T2 relaxation times. The degree of alteration of T1 and T2 is variable depending upon the organ of interest. To date, only limited data are available regarding relaxation times in the human body at 7T [17]. There is preliminary data on the relaxation times of human cartilage, demonstrating an approximately 35% increase in the T1 values of cartilage at 7T as compared with 3T, but shortening of T2 values was not demonstrated. A recent study of the human brain at various magnetic field strengths demonstrated a three-fold increase in T1 values for most brain tissue at 7T as compared with 0.2T [18]. In this same study, T1 values of arterial blood were measured and found to lengthen with increasing field strength—a fact consistent with prior in vitro data and potentially beneficial for arterial spin labeling (ASL) perfusion imaging [18].

Thus far, experiences at 3T reveal that image quality is not greatly impaired by T1 lengthening because minor adjustments of TR, TE, and flip angle can usually compensate for these effects. Nevertheless, lengthening of TR adversely affects acquisition times and higher bandwidths are required, compromising the gains in SNR expected at higher field strengths. Parallel imaging may be used to reduce TR and SAR, but again this occurs at the expense of SNR (at least when compared with unaccelerated acquisitions using the same coil arrays). At higher field strengths, alterations in T1 values and the convergence of T1 values will greatly impact sequence selection and design. The routine short TR, short TE, high flip angle sequences used in perfusion, and vascular imaging become less effective [19]. Magnetization-prepared sequences and inversion recovery T1-weighted sequences used in neuroimaging at 3T to accentuate differences in gray and white matter may also be beneficial for body imaging, to bring out subtle T1 differences at ultrahigh field strength that may not be appreciated using conventional spoiled gradient echo sequences. However, these sequences take longer to acquire, which is problematic for body imaging as it is preferable to acquire data with suspended respiration. Restore pulses that transfer transverse magnetization back to the longitudinal direction before the next RF excitation may also be used to improve tissue contrast and shorten TRs. Restore pulses may be implemented on both T1- and T2-weighted fast spin echo sequences, and in conjunction with variable flip angle methods.

Despite the challenge of bringing out contrast between tissues at ultrahigh field strength, phantom studies show that there is minimal decrease in T1 relaxivity of gadolinium chelates at 3T when compared with 1.5T [20]. This could potentially lead to greater contrast between enhancing and nonenhancing tissue at ultrahigh field strength and increase lesion conspicuity [21], which would be particularly beneficial for dynamic contrast enhanced T1-weighted spoiled gradient sequences used for perfusion imaging and angiography. In addition, T2 relaxivity of gadolinium chelates is also increased at 3T [20], such that lower concentrations of contrast material can and should be used to prevent loss of signal from T2* effects when dynamic susceptibility weighted contrast enhanced perfusion imaging is performed [22]. It remains to be seen, however, if this will lead to improvement in lesion detection, more accurate or confident diagnosis, or improved patient outcome in clinical practice. Similar considerations should be kept in mind for 7T applications.

Arterial spin labeling

ASL is a technique used to measure blood flow that requires no exogenous contrast agents. Selective inversion pulses are used to magnetically label protons in blood. Signal changes result from flowing blood and these alterations in signal can be quantified to determine blood flow to tissue. Hence, there is direct correlation between contrast and perfusion without confounding issues of permeability. The magnetic "tagging" of blood is dependent on T1. T1 must be long enough to permit detection of tissue perfusion, but short enough to allow dynamic changes to be monitored [23]. Because ASL sequences are inherently signal poor, combining them with high field strength, with its potential for higher SNR, is an attractive idea. However, subtle changes in perfusion may be harder to detect because of increasing susceptibility at high field strength. Nonetheless, the longer T1 recovery expected at high fields is advantageous for ASL imaging because blood remains magnetically "tagged" for longer periods of time, potentially leading to more sensitive measurements of flow. ASL techniques are now being implemented in cardiac and neuroimaging and are currently being explored for renal imaging [24]. ASL techniques can be challenging for abdominal applications because they require subtraction of data sets and their quality may be degraded by motion of the adjacent bowel and by respiratory motion. In general, however, there is tremendous interest in gaining insight into the hemodynamics within tissue, with the hope that this will help distinguish normal from neoplasm, or inflammatory or infectious tissue. An understanding of tissue perfusion using techniques such as ASL will potentially lead to improvements in the designing, administering, and monitoring of chemotherapeutic agents in patients with malignancy.

T2-weighted imaging

T2-weighted imaging with rapid acquisition relaxation enhancement- type sequences becomes especially problematic at higher field strengths because of dielectric effects and excessive RF power deposition. One way of reducing SAR is to use a lower flip angle, but this will compromise signal and contrast to noise. Alternatively, the RF pulse amplitude can be reduced (leading to longer RF pulses and longer echo trains) at the expense of TR and tissue blurring. T2-blurring is a more severe problem at high field strength because of the shorter T2 relaxation times. Parallel imaging combined with variable flip angle sequences or VERSE type pulses are potentially more favorable alternatives to reduce SAR, because they will not significantly compromise acquisition time or image contrast.

T2*-weighted imaging

BOLD is another technique that detects blood flow without the use of exogenous contrast agents. Local susceptibility effects induced by iron within the heme of deoxyhemoglobin may be detected and used as an endogenous contrast agent. Alterations in the ratio of oxy (diamagnetic) to deoxyhemoglobin (paramagnetic) may be appreciated on magnetic resonance, reflecting subtle microvascular differences in oxygen demand and regional oxygenation. The BOLD effect is currently being used for functional brain imaging but is also being explored for applications in the abdomen, pelvis and extremities, normal liver, kidney (including transplanted kidneys) [25–30], endometrium [31], and in calf skeletal muscle assessing ischemia, response to stimuli, and medication [32–35]. At ultrahigh field strength, the increase in susceptibility effects will likely improve sensitivity to the iron particles in hemoglobin, but in the abdomen and pelvis confounding T2* effects from adjacent structures may complicate measurement of oxygenation.

Iron oxide contrast agents

Detection of iron contrast agents improves at higher field strength because of increased susceptibility effects. Therefore, sensitivity to contrast agents, such as USPIOs, will increase at ultrahigh field strength. Exploring other similar types of paramagnetic contrast agents may be warranted for detection of pathology or possibly delivering and monitoring chemotherapeutic agents. USPIOs are used for detection of metastatic lymphadenopathy in a variety of neoplastic processes of neck, chest, abdomen, and pelvis. In addition to imaging of malignancy, several other applications for USPIO contrast agents are also under exploration, including imaging of diffuse and focal liver disease, atherosclerotic plaque, renal disease, and infection [36]. In vivo use of magnetically labeled therapeutic agents, including human stem cells [37], may benefit from higher field imaging, which may allow for improved tracking of the delivery of therapeutic agents, as well as improved monitoring of therapeutic effects.

Chemical shift

Chemical shift artifact of the first kind refers to misregistration of spatial information caused by difference in the resonant frequency of water and fat. This artifact is only appreciated in the frequency encoding (readout) direction, and is a result of erroneous mapping of the signal from lipid relative to that of fluid or water [38]. Typically, chemical shift is manifested by high and low signal bands along a lipid-water interface perpendicular to the frequency-encoding direction [38]. This difference in frequency directly relates to the main magnetic field. At 1.5T the frequency difference between fat and water is 220 Hz; at 3T it is 440 Hz, and at 7T it is about 1000 Hz. At a fixed bandwidth, the pixel width of the band-like artifact widens as field strength increases (eg, a two-pixel band at 3T grows to about five pixels at 7T, which can limit visualization of pathology, particularly around the organ edges). To reduce the artifact, the bandwidth must be increased, compromising some degree of SNR gain from the high field strength. Investigators make this adjustment at 3T and will likely also have to do so at even higher field strength. Alternatively, frequency selective fat suppression or water excitation are expected to improve as spectral separation increases with increasing field strength, and these can be used to compensate for chemical shift effects (Fig. 5) [39].

Chemical shift artifact of the second kind refers to the "India ink" artifact related to intravoxel phase cancellation, caused by differences in the resonant frequency of water and fat present in the same voxel of tissue. Chemical shift imaging is useful in body imaging and used for detection of fat within tissue. At high field the precessional frequencies of fat and

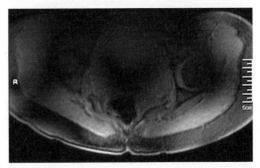

Fig. 5. Axial T1 3D frequency selective fat suppressed spoiled gradient echo image through the pelvis of a young female volunteer. Note the "dielectric effects" leading to signal loss in the center of the pelvis. Nonetheless, there is homogenous fat suppression. Homogenous fat suppression is easily achieved at 7T without significant adjustment of parameters or shimming because of the increase in spectral separation between water and fat resonances (Siemens Medical Solutions, Erlangen, Germany).

water protons increase and the time intervals, between when fat and water spins are in and out of phase with each other, get shorter and shorter. Increasing TE to encompass multiple cycles of relative spin precession can introduce undesirable T2* effects. On the other hand, short TEs associated with a single cycle are difficult to achieve and dependent on the strength and slew rate of the gradients. At ultrahigh field strength alternative means of detecting fat in the body—means such as spectroscopy, for example—may be required. Spectroscopy may be able not only to detect small amounts of fat but also to permit quantification, thus yielding more information than conventional in- and out-of-phase imaging.

Safety

Is there an upper limit as to how high a magnetic field may be used for human imaging? This of course depends largely upon issues of patient safety, such as RF-induced tissue heating and, to a lesser extent, technical issues of constructing and maintaining high-field magnets (Fig. 6). In terms of human safety, the FDA has categorized clinical MR systems with a static magnetic field of less than or equal to 8T as posing "non-significant risk" for patients over 1 month old (current FDA guidelines can be found at www.fda.gov). However, there are higher field magnets (up to 9.4T) that have been investigated and have shown the feasibility of human imaging thus far without ill effects [8]. For animals,

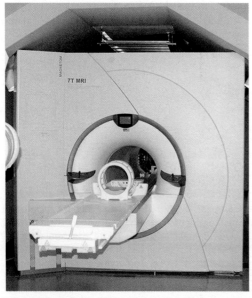

Fig. 6. 7T long bore whole MR imaging system at New York University (*Courtesy of* Siemens Medical Solutions, Erlangen, Germany; with permission).

horizontal magnet systems are available beyond 11T.

Tissue heating is a significant safety concern and potential constraint of imaging at ultrahigh field strength. Higher RF energy is deposited in tissue as the operating frequency is increased (ie, with increasing field strength). The specific limits on SAR are no more than 4 W/kg averaged over the entire body for a duration greater than or equal to 15 minutes, and no more than 8 W/kg in any gram of tissue in the head or torso for a duration of greater than or equal to 5 minutes [40].

Additional safety concerns at ultrahigh field include the side effects of motion through large magnetic fields, electrical stimulation, projectiles, uncertain effects of long-term field exposure, acoustic noise, and heating or motion of implanted devices. Side effects related to exposure to a high field magnet have been reported to include vertigo, difficulty in balancing after leaving the magnet, nausea, headache, sleepiness, numbness and tingling, muscle twitches, visual stimulation (faint flashes of light also referred to as magnetic phosphenes), and metallic tastes [8,19]. Usually these effects are transient and are precipitated when a patient is moving into the magnetic field. Alteration in the appearance of the electrocardiogram—specifically augmentation of T waves—may be seen as a result of magnetohydrodynamic effects.

Few studies have investigated the long-term effects of strong static magnetic fields. Thus far, there is no data to support the notion that exposure to a strong static magnetic field alone has carcinogenic effects. That said, some potential effects have been suggested on intracellular ion control (specifically Ca^{2+}), orientation of some cell types, and gene expression [41]. Given the move toward ultrahigh field human imaging, continued investigation is warranted. Some studies have suggested a concern for teratogenic effects in early pregnancy, based only on animal models [42–44]. Generally, MR imaging is avoided in the first trimester.

Acoustic noise

Acoustic noise level will increase at ultrahigh field strength, as the forces experienced by changing gradient currents are proportional to field strength. Noise is related to the vibration of the gradient coils. Sequences that require large gradient switching amplitudes may lead to ambient noise that can exceed national industrial exposure guidelines [45]. Unfortunately, this can cause permanent injury if appropriate measures are not taken, and there are FDA guidelines to limit exposure. Routine safety measures, such as ear plugs and headphones, are usually sufficient to reduce ambient noise to acceptable levels, but additional work is ongoing which aims to reduce noise at its source. Parallel imaging can also decrease the rate of gradient coil switching by allowing reduced k-space sampling.

Medical devices

Currently, most mechanical devices considered safe at 1.5T are also considered safe at 3T. In a study of 109 implants and medical devices (including 32 aneurysm clips) on a 3T system, only four (4%) were considered potentially unsafe. In fact, it is likely that the vast majority of devices that are considered safe at 1.5T will be safe at even higher fields; however, there may be variation depending on field strength and design of the bore. Systematic testing of medical devices is needed in order to accurately determine which devices, if any, are contraindicated.

In addition to the issue of safety, image artifacts related to implanted devices are likely to increase with increasing field strength. If a patient's particular internal hardware impairs diagnosis at ultrahigh field strength because of excessive artifact, then lower field strength would be preferable. Ideally, this should be determined before a patient is scheduled, to reduce the stress and anxiety of an indeterminate exam and rescheduling.

Potential applications of MR imaging beyond 3T

Despite the technical difficulties of imaging at higher field strengths, there is a great potential for exploring more innovative MR techniques that not only reveal anatomy and morphology, but give insight into organ function and the pathophysiology of disease processes. Conventionally used sequences at lower field strengths may not only be challenging to reproduce at higher field, they are likely to be inadequate. To improve diagnostic MR capability, more biologic-oriented approaches enabled by ultrahigh field strength should be seriously considered. The following section briefly speculates on new opportunities that emerge at ultrahigh field strength, at a physiologic, cellular, and molecular level.

Biochemical processes and molecular imaging

Hydrogen is the most abundant element in the human body and, therefore, it is the primary element used for MR imaging. However, isotopes of other elements, such as Sodium (^{23}Na), Phosphorus (^{31}P), Carbon (^{13}C), Fluorine (^{19}F), and Oxygen (^{17}O) are suitable for MR investigation and may even be preferable for certain indications. Experience with imaging of human subjects using alternative nuclei such as these is somewhat lacking in the literature because of several challenges, including the low abundance of nuclei other than hydrogen within the human body, the need for specially-tuned coils, the lower sensitivity of nuclear magnetic resonance to these nuclei, and thus the need for ultrahigh field strength magnets (Table 1).

While animal experiments have been performed, there is only preliminary data on human subjects using sodium and phosphorus for body MR imaging. These studies permit some insight into the potential of such endeavors, but the availability of ultrahigh field whole body magnets will undoubtedly promote further investigation in this field. The goal of imaging with alternative nuclei, in general, is to gain insight into function and physiology rather than focus on morphology.

Currently the nuclei of interest that have begun to emerge for body applications, and might especially benefit from ultrahigh field strengths, include ^{23}Na and ^{31}P. The applications range from functional assessment of normal physiology to investigation of pathologic processes, such as ischemia, infection, transplant rejection, fibrosis and neoplasm.

Sodium (^{23}Na) MR imaging

Renal imaging with ^{23}Na is one of the most promising applications. Renal physiology and sodium concentration are intertwined and directly related to the function of the kidney and, therefore, sodium imaging may provide a quantitative and regionally specific measure of renal function; alterations in sodium concentration may be an early sign of renal impairment. The feasibility of human body imaging with sodium was demonstrated in the 1980s [46,47]. More recently, data is emerging in rat models and human subjects that may prove useful in a clinic setting.

In a study by Maril and colleagues [48], sodium MR imaging was performed in a 4.7T magnet in normal, diuretic, and obstructed rat kidneys in vivo. Normal kidneys demonstrated an increase in sodium signal intensity from the edge of the cortex through the outer and inner medulla that was further quantified, based on reference in vivo and ex vivo measurement of cortical and medullary T1 and T2 relaxation times. In rats exposed to a diuretic, there were quantifiable alterations in the sodium gradient from cortex to medulla over time, with an initial increase in sodium signal in the inner medulla and, to a lesser degree, in the renal cortex; over time the gradient almost cancelled with the expected increase in sodium urine concentration. In acutely obstructed kidneys (induced by ligation), renal enlargement was depicted on proton MR imaging and

Table 1: Relative abundance of nuclei in the human body, resonance frequency, and sensitivity at various field strengths

Nucleus	Abundance in the body	Gyromagnetic ratio (γ) (MHz/T)	Resonance frequency at 1.5T (MHz)	1.5T Sensitivity compared with ^{1}H	Resonance frequency at 3T (MHz)	3T Sensitivity compared with ^{1}H at 1.5T	Resonance frequency at 7T (MHz)	7T Sensitivity compared with ^{1}H at 1.5T
^{1}H	88 M	42.58	63.9	100%[b]	127.7[a]	200%	298.0	467%
^{13}C	~50 mM	10.68	16.1	1.6%	32.1	3.2%	74.9	7.4%
^{31}P	75 mM	17.25	25.9	6.6%	51.7	13.3%	120.7[a]	30.9%[b]
^{23}Na	80 mM	11.27	16.9	9.3%	33.8	18.5%	78.8	43.2%[b]
^{17}O	16 mM	-5.77	8.7	2.9%	17.3	5.8%	40.4	13.6%
^{19}F	4 µM	40.08	60.1	83.4%	120.2[a]	167%	280.4	389%

These are relative sensitivities and are not corrected for abundance

[a] Note the proximity in resonance frequencies of ^{1}H and ^{19}F at 3T to ^{31}P at 7T, suggesting that a coil tunable to the frequencies of ^{1}H and ^{19}F imaging at 3T could potentially also be used for ^{31}P imaging at 7T.

[b] Note the relative sensitivity of ^{31}P and ^{23}Na at 7T are approaching that of ^{1}H at 1.5T, suggesting feasibility of higher resolution imaging and spectroscopy with ^{31}P and ^{23}Na at 7T.

diminished parenchymal thickness and perihilar atrophy was observed on histology. On sodium MR imaging, there was an approximately two-fold decrease in the cortico-outer medullary sodium gradient, as compared with normal kidney, along with reduction of the gradient from the outer medulla to the papillary tip. Despite these changes, serum creatinine did not change, likely because of compensatory changes in the contralateral kidney, emphasizing the regionally specific role of imaging. In two cases of spontaneously obstructed kidneys there were no morphologic changes; the sodium gradient was maintained compatible with retained function, but there was distortion in the distribution of the sodium because of the hydronephrosis. In another study by the same group, there was a 21% reduction in the cortico-outer medullary sodium gradient and a 40% decrease in the inner medulla to cortex sodium ratio gradient in rates with acute tubular necrosis (ATN) [49]. At pathology, only focal ATN was demonstrated, suggesting a high sensitivity to the disease process even in its early stages.

More recently, Maril and colleagues [50] investigated the feasibility of sodium MR imaging of the human kidney at 3T in six normal volunteers. Sodium distribution was assessed before and following water deprivation for 12 hours. A sodium gradient was observed with increasing concentration of sodium from cortex to medulla, with a medulla to cortex ratio of approximately 2.4, which increased with water deprivation to 2.7, based on regions of interest-based analysis. Based on pixel by pixel analysis, the slope of signal to noise curve along the corticomedullary axis revealed an increase of 25% from cortex to medulla. The authors note the requirement of short TEs for sodium MR imaging as a consequence of the ultrashort T2 times of a significant (approximately 60%) component of the ^{23}Na population.

In another preliminary study of renal sodium MR imaging and BOLD imaging of human kidneys at 3T, a normal healthy volunteer was compared with five patients, including two with chronic renal failure and three with transplanted kidneys, two of whom were in chronic renal failure [51]. Normally functioning kidneys demonstrated a corticomedullary gradient of sodium concentration, while the gradient was lacking in many regions of the chronic failure kidneys. BOLD imaging revealed that a preserved corticomedullary sodium gradient correlated well with the presence of relative medullary hypoxia, whereas in chronic renal failure there was no corticomedullary differentiation with decreased oxygenation in the cortex and loss of relative hypoxia in the medulla.

Taken together these studies suggest the role of in vivo sodium imaging for the direct regional assessment of renal function. With the increased sensitivity offered by 7T, it appears that implementation of such imaging strategies can be achieved in clinically reasonable scan times with adequate spatial resolution and contrast to noise ratio.

Sodium MR imaging may also have oncologic applications beyond those established for brain tumors. Sodium is considered a sensitive indicator of cellular integrity and cellular metabolism [52]. Tissue sodium concentration is determined by the combination of intracellular and extracellular volume fractions and can be increased by changes in either compartment. Intracellular pH, intracellular sodium concentrations, increased Na^+/H^+ transporter activity, and Na^+/potassium (K^+) adenosine triphosphatase (Na^+/K^+-ATPase) activity have all been linked to tumor malignancy [52]. In a recent study of patients with breast lesions using sodium and proton MR imaging at 1.5T, sodium concentrations were consistently found to be elevated in proven histologic malignant breast lesions, when compared with glandular tissue, adipose tissue, and benign lesions [52].

Myocardial viability has also been assessed using sodium MR imaging in animal models. Viable myocytes contain lower concentrations of intracellular sodium when compared with extracellular, because of active outward transport of sodium by Na^+/K^+-ATPase [53]. In ischemia, intracellular sodium concentrations rise. If reperfusion occurs in a timely fashion intracellular concentrations return to baseline; if not, concentrations remain high [53]. This could conceivably also be used for assessing ischemia and viability in other muscles as well.

Phosphorus (^{31}P) MR imaging

Studies of ^{31}P offer more challenges than sodium MR imaging, primarily because of the even shorter T2 relaxation times requiring the use of ultrashort TEs. While regional variations in sodium concentration are of interest (as in the study of renal function), investigations of phosphorus focus on the relative balance of key phosphate-containing metabolites and, therefore, spectroscopic approaches are warranted (note that in principle spectroscopic imaging would allow regional depiction of various metabolite concentrations). Phosphorus (^{31}P) spectroscopy can detect relative concentrations of high energy phosphate metabolites, including adenosine triphosphate (ATP), inorganic phosphate (Pi), phosphocreatine (PCr), phosphomonoesters (PME), and phosphodiesters (PDE), alterations in the concentrations of which have been associated with ischemia, enzyme deficiencies, and tumors [54]. As with spectroscopy in general, higher field strength will lead to increased peak amplitude and spectral separation, potentially improving delineation of various metabolites. Practically, one might expect rapid progress in ^{31}P imaging for two reasons: first, proximity of the resonance frequencies of ^{1}H and ^{19}F at 3T to ^{31}P at 7T suggests that a coil tunable to the frequencies of ^{1}H and ^{19}F imaging at 3T could potentially also be used for ^{31}P imaging at 7.0T. Second, the relative sensitivities of ^{31}P and ^{23}Na at 7T are approaching that of ^{1}H at 1.5T, suggesting feasibility of higher resolution imaging and spectroscopy with ^{31}P and ^{23}Na at 7T (see Table 1). Consequently, applications of phosphorus MR imaging already contemplated at lower field strength might be expected to improve at 7T. These include spectroscopic studies of muscle activity and function [55], studies of pH, liver [56,57] and renal function including transplanted organs [54,58,59], and oncology such as breast [60] and cervical cancer [61]. In the liver, the phosphorylated metabolites mentioned above are of interest, but while PCr is a dominant peak seen in musculoskeletal imaging, it is not typically seen in the liver because of its low contribution to hepatic metabolism [56].

In an earlier study of cirrhosis involving 85 patients, Menon and colleagues [57] found that there were significant differences in metabolite ratios when compared with healthy controls, with elevation of PME ratios and a reduction in PDE (thought to be an indicator of cell membrane integrity) ratios. Progressive and significant increases in PME and ATP were associated with increasing functional impairment of the liver, and there were some notable differences between spectra of cirrhotic livers of different etiologies with diminished Pi ratio in alcoholic cirrhosis and primary sclerosing cholangitis. In a more recent study by Dezortova and colleagues [56], levels of PDE and ATP were significantly lower in cirrhosis when compared with control livers, and this correlated well with the Child Pugh score. This study went on to further attempt to determine if spectroscopy could differentiate between various etiologies of cirrhosis and found that alcoholic etiology was associated with lower Pi, but no difference in cholestatic liver disease. The multicomponent nature of PME and PDE peaks make discerning subtle differences in metabolite concentrations difficult at lower field strengths. At higher field strengths better delineation of the individual peaks and perhaps resolution of additional peaks could elucidate the biochemic signature of various disease processes.

Proton (^{1}H) MR spectroscopy

Spectroscopy of ^{1}H will also benefit from ultrahigh field strength for similar reasons. However, many of the detracting issues present at low field strength will also need to be addressed at high field. In fact, high field strength will accentuate many of the artifacts, including patient motion and susceptibility-induced field disturbances; higher order and local shimming techniques are likely to prove critical. However, the potential benefits of high signal to noise and increased spectral resolution are appealing for many of the applications currently being explored at 1.5 and 3T, such as oncology using spectroscopy to distinguish between benign and malignant processes, assessment of tumor grade and response to therapy, or assessment of diffuse liver diseases, such as fatty infiltration and cirrhosis.

Detecting the presence or absence of fat within the liver is important for many disease processes. MR imaging at 1.5 and 3T is very sensitive to detecting both fat and iron and, at first thought, ultrahigh field strength may not seem that beneficial. However, one of the deficiencies of MR imaging thus far is the inability to quantify liver fat content, let alone detect very subtle shifts in either perfusion or metabolism that may precede or be associated with their accumulation. Unfortunately, in- and out-of-phase gradient recalled echo (GRE) sequences, that are commonly used to detect fat at lower field strength, will be challenging to implement at ultrahigh field strength because of the much reduced echo time differences required (out-of-phase and in-phase TEs at 1.5T are 2.2 ms and 4.4 ms; whereas at 7T the corresponding TE values would be 0.5 ms and 1.0 ms, approximately). Proton spectroscopy may be a viable alterative to conventional imaging approaches. Magnetic resonance spectroscopy (MRS) shows promise for not only detecting fat but also quantifying it, which may be useful in diagnosis and monitoring of response to therapy with superior accuracy as compared with GRE [62,63]. A recent study has demonstrated the feasibility of both breathhold liver MR imaging and ^{1}H MRS at 7.0T, although B_0 shimming was problematic in two out of four patients and further optimization is required [64].

Susceptibility-sensitive T2* imaging for iron and calcium

Sensitivity to iron and calcium will be increased at ultrahigh field strength because of the increase in magnetic susceptibility effects, and thus more pronounced T2* shortening. This has several interesting implications for oncologic imaging, metabolic, infectious, and vascular disorders using iron-containing contrast agents, as well as suggesting the use of techniques such as BOLD and susceptibility weighted imaging (SWI) to examine endogenous contrast mechanisms.

Iron-containing contrast agents

Iron-containing contrast agents such as superparamagnetic iron oxide (SPIO) and USPIO particles, have a diverse range of applications. These particles are specifically taken up by the monocyte-macrophage system and can be markers of inflammation and malignancy. In the liver, these agents are taken up by Kupffer cells, which are macrophages exclusively located in the liver. Normal uptake of these agents leads to a homogenous decrease in liver signal on GRE (T2*-weighted) imaging. Tumors (whether benign or malignant) and other lesions will remain relatively hyperintense, increasing lesion conspicuity. One of the more exciting oncologic applications using iron oxide particles is the detection and assessment of metastatic lymph node disease, with promising results for gastrointenstinal, bladder, prostate, cervical, endometrial, and breast cancer. In fact, one study comparing the use of USPIOs for assessment of prostate cancer nodal metastases at 1.5T versus 3T, found that there was superior fat and soft tissue to vessel contrast and improved delineation of lymph node borders [65] at 3T. Further benefits, such as detection of smaller metastatic lesions and pathologic lymph nodes, are anticipated at ultrahigh field strength because of increased sensitivity to the iron based contrast agent. However, undesirable blooming effects arising from such increased sensitivity may require mitigation with the use of shorter TE for imaging.

Other oncologic applications of USPIOs relate to molecular and cellular imaging. Future MR contrast agents are needed for selective labeling and visualization of targeted macromolecules or targeted cells, and for specific assessment of biologic processes in an effort to administer and monitor specific therapeutic agents [36,66]. USPIOs may prove useful for such purposes and these applications are being explored [36]. Ultrahigh field strength may offer not only the sensitivity but also the resolution required to image cellular and biochemic processes with anatomic detail.

The study of macrophage activity using USPIOs has several additional implications for inflammatory processes, such as atherosclerosis, transplant rejection, and infection [36]. Studies suggest that macrophages are a marker of unstable atherosclerotic plaques more vulnerable to rupture, and animal experiments demonstrate that USPIOs are taken up in atherosclerotic plaques [36,67,68]. One pitfall to this technique is the potential presence of calcium, which can confound characterization such that other techniques, such as Gd-chelate enhanced imaging, may also be needed. Still, ultrahigh fields may improve sensitivity to detection of vulnerable plaque and offer higher spatial resolution.

Blood oxygenation level-dependent imaging

Unlike imaging with SPIOs and USPIOs, the techniques of BOLD and SWI exploit the endogenous contrast provided by iron containing molecules (SWI and BOLD) and calcium (SWI), and are expected to become increasingly sensitive techniques with increasing field strength. BOLD has been used primarily for functional brain mapping in neuroimaging, but may offer a way of imaging tissue oxygenation, which has implications for measuring hypoxia in cancer or other disease processes, such as limb ischemia, specifically exploiting the balance of oxy- and deoxyhemoglobin and paramagnetic properties of deoxyhemoglobin. Use of inhaled Carbogen (95% O_2, 5% CO_2) during imaging can also help amplify the BOLD effect and measure tissue vascular responsiveness. A brief introduction to the applications of BOLD at lower field strengths provides a basis for speculating about ultrahigh field strength applications.

Data on BOLD imaging of abdominal and pelvic tumors are limited, but response to chemoembolization for hepatocellular carcinoma, using BOLD to measure hypoxia, shows promise in one study of a rabbit model [69]. BOLD imaging has also been used to quantify baseline R_2^* ($R_2^* = 1/T_2^*$) and Carbogen-induced changes in R_2^*, in rodent models with prolactinomas and fibrosarcomas, to predict the efficacy of radiotherapy [70].

BOLD MR imaging of the kidney has been explored for a number of applications, based on the hypothesis that failure to maintain medullary oxygenation leads to renal dysfunction [71]. Applications include study of normal renal physiology, diabetes, obstruction, arterial stenosis, the effects of administration of pharmaceuticals, and renal transplants. In a study of renal transplant, R_2^* measurements in the medullary regions of transplant kidneys in acute rejection were significantly lower than those of normal kidneys and kidneys with ATN [29], suggesting a promising nononcologic clinical application.

Another potential clinical use of BOLD is for functional imaging of ischemia and hyperemia in the evaluation of peripheral arterial occlusive diseases. While conventional MR imaging does an excellent job at noninvasively monitoring vascular anatomic changes that result from atherosclerosis, it cannot offer information regarding the presence or absence of tissue injury or identify tissue at risk of limb-threatening ischemia. BOLD imaging may provide insight into metabolic changes in exercise or induced ischemia [72]. In a study by Ledermann and colleagues [32], BOLD imaging of the calves was performed in healthy volunteers during ischemia and relative hyperemia, and compared with other techniques used in practice to indirectly measure tissue perfusion and oxygenation, including Laser Doppler flowmetry and transcutaneous oxygen pressure (TcPO$_2$) respectively, and demonstrated good correlation, suggesting that BOLD may be a promising diagnostic tool for assessing both muscle perfusion and oxygenation.

The benefits of BOLD at 3T have recently been demonstrated in human volunteers, with improved baseline contrast on R$_2$* maps without degradation by susceptibility effects, although the TE should be modified to compensate for the expected increase in susceptibility effects at even higher field strength [73]. While BOLD MR imaging suffers from low signal, the higher signal to noise and increased sensitivity to the BOLD effect at ultrahigh field strength may enable this physiologic imaging approach.

Susceptibility weighted imaging

SWI, exploiting both the magnitude and phase sensitivities of GRE imaging to magnetic susceptibility effects, offers overall increased sensitivity to magnetic field disturbances that might arise from accumulation of iron (including blood products) or calcium [74]. Although SWI is already sensitive at 1.5T and 3T, and primarily used in neuroimaging applications, capabilities are predicted to increase at ultrahigh field strength and that may benefit both body and neuroimaging. One intriguing application is in breast imaging to detect microcalcifications that are associated with malignancy. Despite the advantages of dynamic contrast enhanced MR imaging over conventional mammography, MR imaging does not depict the subtle microcalcifications that are easily seen on conventional mammography. Currently, work is underway at the authors' institution to explore the use of SWI in breast cancer imaging at 3T, and look to ultrahigh field strength for future work because of its increased sensitivity to microcalcification and promise of higher resolution imaging [75]. Other potential applications might include detection of subtle signs of hemorrhage or blood products within the body, or characterization of atherosclerotic plaque.

Vascular imaging and characterization

One potential advantage of ultrahigh field strength would be to further explore and implement vascular imaging techniques that use mechanisms of endogenous contrast, rather than depend on exogenous contrast agents, such as gadolinium chelates. At the same time, it is appealing to supplement anatomic vascular imaging with plaque characterization and functional information regarding tissue perfusion, hypoxia, and ischemia as discussed above. Noncontrast enhanced techniques, such as time-of-flight (TOF) magnetic resonance angiography (MRA) and ASL perfusion techniques, would benefit from the high signal to noise and lengthening of T1 expected at ultrahigh field strength. TOF benefits, for example, from the T1 lengthening because it will accentuate the contrast of in-flowing blood with better suppression of background signal. Preliminary results comparing intracranial TOF MRA at 7T versus 3T demonstrates improved visualization of small peripheral vessels, although there was a modest amount of increased ghosting along the phase encoding direction in some data [76]. There are potential pitfalls at ultrahigh field strength. The T1 of the blood pool is also longer, so saturation effects will be more pronounced, particularly with 3D techniques, and acquisition time may be prolonged secondary to SAR considerations. However, parallel imaging could compensate for both these problems, although at the expense of SNR; this may, however, not be significant given the baseline high SNR at ultrahigh magnetic field strength. Modulating the RF pulse, as discussed previously, could reduce SAR. Gadolinium contrast enhanced imaging, although feasible [77], will be more challenging because of the modified T1, T2* effects, SAR, and artifacts. Ultrahigh field strength can also benefit noninvasive methods of measuring tissue perfusion, such as ASL, which again benefits not only from increased SNR but also from the longer blood T1 values, offering prolonged "tag" or "label" persistence.

Summary

One of the major motivations for exploring ultrahigh field strength is the quest for higher signal to noise. Unfortunately, the theoretical gains are somewhat diminished by competing factors, which typically require parameter adjustments that reduce SNR. If signal was the only goal however, why not just scan for longer periods of time by increasing the number of signal averages? It is clear that imaging at ultrahigh field strength is more challenging for not only technical reasons, such as B$_1$ inhomogeneity, SAR, B$_0$ field inhomogeneity, changes in tissue contrast, and chemical shift effects, but also for practical reasons. Patients are likely to experience more side effects, exam time may be lengthened, and medical devices or implants considered MR safe at 1.5T may be deemed incompatible at higher field strengths or may markedly degrade the image quality and reduce diagnostic quality. Therefore, it should be clear that the benefits of ultra high field imaging must outweigh the risks and negative aspects. If we merely attempt to recreate the diagnostic imaging quality of 1.5T and 3T, then ultrahigh field imaging will likely disappoint.

Addressing a clinical question, using the same routine anatomic protocols optimized for 1.5T and currently being optimized for 3T may not be possible at ultrahigh field strength. Therefore, perhaps these same clinical questions may be answered in another more comprehensive way, using approaches that become increasingly feasible at ultrahigh field. However, lower field magnet systems (1.5T or 3T) may remain preferable for a subset of patients and for many routine clinical applications, while ultrahigh field imaging may be reserved for specific clinical questions that require functional or metabolic characterization in addition to anatomic imaging. If we aim to maximize the opportunities and advantages of ultrahigh field imaging, such as imaging with alternative nuclei, susceptibility weighted imaging, and spectroscopy, in the context of a particular clinical problem in an effort to obtain not only basic anatomic information but additional functional or physiologic information, then there appears to be a strong future opportunity for ultrahigh field MR in body imaging.

References

[1] Vaughan JT, Adriany G, Garwood M, et al. Detunable transverse electromagnetic (TEM) volume coil for high-field NMR. Magn Reson Med 2002;47(5):990–1000.

[2] Wang C, Shen GX. B1 field, SAR, and SNR comparisons for birdcage, TEM, and microstrip coils at 7T. J Magn Reson Imaging 2006;24(2):439–43.

[3] Vaughan JT, Adriany G, Snyder CJ, et al. Efficient high-frequency body coil for high-field MRI. Magn Reson Med 2004;52(4):851–9.

[4] Snyder CJ, DelaBarre L, Van de Moortele PF, et al. Stripline/TEM transceiver array for 7T body imaging [164]. In: Berlin (Germany): Proc Intl Soc Mag Reson; 2007. p. 164.

[5] Lee RF, Stefanescu C, Xue R, et al. A 19F/1H dual resonant elliptic body coil that is double tuned by ellipticity. In: Proc Intl Soc Mag Reson 15. 2007. Berlin (Germany): 2007.

[6] Lee RF, Moy L, Brown R, et al. 7T high resolution breast MRI. In: Proc Int Soc Mag Reson Med 15; 2007. Berlin (Germany): 2007.

[7] Collins CM, Wang Z, Mao W, et al. Array-optimized composite pulse for excellent whole-brain homogeneity in high-field MRI. Magn Reson Med 2007;57(3):470–4.

[8] Vaughan T, DelaBarre L, Snyder C, et al. 9.4T human MRI: preliminary results. Magn Reson Med 2006;56(6):1274–82.

[9] Katscher U, Bornert P, Leussler C, et al. Transmit SENSE. Magn Reson Med 2003;49(1):144–50.

[10] Zhu Y. Parallel excitation with an array of transmit coils. Magn Reson Med 2004;51(4):775–84.

[11] Zhang Z, Yip CY, Grissom W, et al. Reduction of transmitter B1 inhomogeneity with transmit SENSE slice-select pulses. Magn Reson Med 2007;57(5):842–7.

[12] Hargreaves BA, Cunningham CH, Nishimura DG, et al. Variable-rate selective excitation for rapid MRI sequences. Magn Reson Med 2004;52(3):590–7.

[13] Hennig J, Scheffler K. Hyperechoes. Magn Reson Med 2001;46(1):6–12.

[14] Hennig J, Weigel M, Scheffler K. Multiecho sequences with variable refocusing flip angles: optimization of signal behavior using smooth transitions between pseudo steady states (TRAPS). Magn Reson Med 2003;49(3):527–35.

[15] Lichy MP, Wietek BM, Mugler JP 3rd, et al. Magnetic resonance imaging of the body trunk using a single-slab, 3-dimensional, T2-weighted turbo-spin-echo sequence with high sampling efficiency (SPACE) for high spatial resolution imaging: initial clinical experiences. Invest Radiol 2005;40(12):754–60.

[16] de Bazelaire CM, Duhamel GD, Rofsky NM, et al. MR imaging relaxation times of abdominal and pelvic tissues measured in vivo at 3.0 T: preliminary results. Radiology 2004;230(3):652–9.

[17] Regatte RR, Schweitzer ME. Ultra-high-field MRI of the musculoskeletal system at 7.0T. J Magn Reson Imaging 2007;25(2):262–9.

[18] Rooney WD, Johnson G, Li X, et al. Magnetic field and tissue dependencies of human brain longitudinal 1H2O relaxation in vivo. Magn Reson Med 2007;57(2):308–18.

[19] Hu X, Norris DG. Advances in high-field magnetic resonance imaging. Annu Rev Biomed Eng 2004;6:157–84.

[20] Rohrer M, Bauer H, Mintorovitch J, et al. Comparison of magnetic properties of MRI contrast media solutions at different magnetic field strengths. Invest Radiol 2005;40(11):715–24.

[21] Trattnig S, Ba-Ssalamah A, Noebauer-Huhmann IM, et al. MR contrast agent at high-field MRI (3 Tesla). Top Magn Reson Imaging 2003;14(5):365–75.

[22] Trattnig S, Pinker K, Ba-Ssalamah A, et al. The optimal use of contrast agents at high field MRI. Eur Radiol 2006;16(6):1280–7.

[23] Detre JA, Zhang W, Roberts DA, et al. Tissue specific perfusion imaging using arterial spin labeling. NMR Biomed 1994;7(1–2):75–82.

[24] de Bazelaire C, Rofsky NM, Duhamel G, et al. Arterial spin labeling blood flow magnetic resonance imaging for the characterization of metastatic renal cell carcinoma(1). Acad Radiol 2005;12(3):347–57.

[25] Djamali A, Sadowski EA, Samaniego-Picota M, et al. Noninvasive assessment of early kidney allograft dysfunction by blood oxygen level-dependent magnetic resonance imaging. Transplantation 2006;82(5):621–8.

[26] Djamali A, Sadowski EA, Muehrer RJ, et al. BOLD-MRI assessment of intrarenal oxygenation and oxidative stress in patients with chronic kidney allograft dysfunction. Am J Physiol Renal Physiol 2007;292(2):F513–22.

[27] Thoeny HC, Zumstein D, Simon-Zoula S, et al. Functional evaluation of transplanted kidneys with diffusion-weighted and BOLD MR imaging: initial experience. Radiology 2006;241(3): 812–21.

[28] Tumkur SM, Vu AT, Li LP, et al. Evaluation of intra-renal oxygenation during water diuresis: a time-resolved study using BOLD MRI. Kidney Int 2006;70(1):139–43.

[29] Sadowski EA, Fain SB, Alford SK, et al. Assessment of acute renal transplant rejection with blood oxygen level-dependent MR imaging: initial experience. Radiology 2005;236(3): 911–9.

[30] Hofmann L, Simon-Zoula S, Nowak A, et al. BOLD-MRI for the assessment of renal oxygenation in humans: acute effect of nephrotoxic xenobiotics. Kidney Int 2006;70(1):144–50.

[31] Kido A, Koyama T, Kataoka M, et al. Physiological change of the human uterine myometrium during menstrual cycle: evaluation using BOLD MRI imaging. In: 2005. Miami (FL): 2005. p. 539.

[32] Ledermann HP, Heidecker HG, Schulte AC, et al. Calf muscles imaged at BOLD MR: correlation with TcPO2 and flowmetry measurements during ischemia and reactive hyperemia–initial experience. Radiology 2006;241(2):477–84.

[33] Ledermann HP, Schulte AC, Heidecker HG, et al. Blood oxygenation level-dependent magnetic resonance imaging of the skeletal muscle in patients with peripheral arterial occlusive disease. Circulation 2006;113(25):2929–35.

[34] Bulte DP, Alfonsi J, Bells S, et al. Vasomodulation of skeletal muscle BOLD signal. J Magn Reson Imaging 2006;24(4):886–90.

[35] Noseworthy MD, Bulte DP, Alfonsi J. BOLD magnetic resonance imaging of skeletal muscle. Semin Musculoskelet Radiol 2003;7(4):307–15.

[36] Corot C, Petry KG, Trivedi R, et al. Macrophage imaging in central nervous system and in carotid atherosclerotic plaque using ultrasmall superparamagnetic iron oxide in magnetic resonance imaging. Invest Radiol 2004;39(10):619–25.

[37] Bos C, Delmas Y, Desmouliere A, et al. In vivo MR imaging of intravascularly injected magnetically labeled mesenchymal stem cells in rat kidney and liver. Radiology 2004;233(3): 781–9.

[38] Hood MN, Ho VB, Smirniotopoulos JG, et al. Chemical shift: the artifact and clinical tool revisited. Radiographics 1999;19(2):357–71.

[39] Merkle EM, Dale BM, Paulson EK. Abdominal MR imaging at 3T. Magn Reson Imaging Clin N Am 2006;14(1):17–26.

[40] Guidance of industry and FDA Staff: criteria for significant risk investigation of MR diagnostic devices. Available at: http://www.fda.gov/cdrh/ode/guidance/793.html. 2003. Accessed July 14, 2003.

[41] Miyakoshi J. Effects of static magnetic fields at the cellular level. Prog Biophys Mol Biol 2005; 87(2–3):213–23.

[42] Yip YP, Capriotti C, Talagala SL, et al. Effects of MR exposure at 1.5 T on early embryonic development of the chick. J Magn Reson Imaging 1994;4(5):742–8.

[43] Heinrichs WL, Fong P, Flannery M, et al. Midgestational exposure of pregnant BALB/c mice to magnetic resonance imaging conditions. Magn Reson Imaging 1988;6(3):305–13.

[44] Tyndall DA, Sulik KK. Effects of magnetic resonance imaging on eye development in the C57BL/6J mouse. Teratology 1991;43(3): 263–75.

[45] Foster JR, Hall DA, Summerfield AQ, et al. Sound-level measurements and calculations of safe noise dosage during EPI at 3 T. J Magn Reson Imaging 2000;12(1):157–63.

[46] Granot J. Sodium imaging of human body organs and extremities in vivo. Radiology 1988; 167(2):547–50.

[47] Ra JB, Hilal SK, Oh CH, et al. In vivo magnetic resonance imaging of sodium in the human body. Magn Reson Med 1988;7(1):11–22.

[48] Maril N, Margalit R, Mispelter J, et al. Functional sodium magnetic resonance imaging of the intact rat kidney. Kidney Int 2004;65(3): 927–35.

[49] Maril N, Margalit R, Rosen S, et al. Detection of evolving acute tubular necrosis with renal 23Na MRI: studies in rats. Kidney Int 2006;69(4): 765–8.

[50] Maril N, Rosen Y, Reynolds GH, et al. Sodium MRI of the human kidney at 3 Tesla. Magn Reson Med 2006;56(6):1229–34.

[51] Rosen Y, Bondonyi-Kovacs G, Hindman N, et al. BOLD and sodium MRI of the human kidney: preliminary experience with patients [abstract 2733]. In: Proc Intl Soc Mag Reson Med. Berlin (Germany): 2007. p. 2733.

[52] Ouwerkerk R, Jacobs MA, Macura KJ, et al. Elevated tissue sodium concentration in malignant breast lesions detected with non-invasive (23)Na MRI. Breast Cancer Res Treat 2007.

[53] Kim RJ, Lima JA, Chen EL, et al. Fast 23Na magnetic resonance imaging of acute reperfused myocardial infarction. Potential to assess myocardial viability. Circulation 1997;95(7): 1877–85.

[54] Grist TM, Charles HC, Sostman HD. 1990 ARRS Executive Council Award. Renal transplant rejection: diagnosis with 31P MR spectroscopy. AJR Am J Roentgenol 1991;156(1):105–12.

[55] Boesch C. Musculoskeletal spectroscopy. J Magn Reson Imaging 2007;25(2):321–38.

[56] Dezortova M, Taimr P, Skoch A, et al. Etiology and functional status of liver cirrhosis by 31P MR spectroscopy. World J Gastroenterol 2005; 11(44):6926–31.

[57] Menon DK, Sargentoni J, Taylor-Robinson SD, et al. Effect of functional grade and etiology on in vivo hepatic phosphorus-31 magnetic resonance spectroscopy in cirrhosis: biochemical basis of spectral appearances. Hepatology 1995; 21(2):417–27.

[58] Taylor-Robinson SD, Sargentoni J, Bell JD, et al. In vivo and in vitro hepatic phosphorus-31 magnetic resonance spectroscopy and electron microscopy in chronic ductopenic rejection of human liver allografts. Gut 1998;42(5):735–43.

[59] Chu WC, Lam WW, Lee KH, et al. Phosphorus-31 MR spectroscopy in pediatric liver transplant recipients: a noninvasive assessment of graft status with correlation with liver function tests and liver biopsy. AJR Am J Roentgenol 2005;184(5): 1624–9.

[60] Twelves CJ, Porter DA, Lowry M, et al. Phosphorus-31 metabolism of post-menopausal breast cancer studied in vivo by magnetic resonance spectroscopy. Br J Cancer 1994;69(6):1151–6.

[61] Morimoto T, Obata T, Ohno T, et al. Phosphorous-31 magnetic resonance spectroscopy of cervical cancer using transvaginal surface coil. Magn Reson Med Sci 2005;4(4):197–201.

[62] Ruel M, Lepanto L, Bilodeau M. Noninvasive quantification of liver triglycerides in steatosis patients using MR methods. In: Proc Intl Soc Mag Reson Med. Berlin (Germany): 2007. p. 3547.

[63] Chang JS, Taouli B, Salibi N, et al. Opposed-phase MRI for fat quantification in fat-water phantoms with 1H MR spectroscopy to resolve ambiguity of fat or water dominance. AJR Am J Roentgenol 2006;187(1):W103–6.

[64] Snyder AL, Snyder CJ, DelaBarre L, et al. Preliminary experience with liver MRI and 1H MRS at 7 Tesla [729]. In: Proc Intl Soc Mag Reson Med. Berlin (Germany): 2007. p. 729.

[65] Heesakkers RA, Futterer JJ, Hovels AM, et al. Prostate cancer evaluated with ferumoxtran-10-enhanced T2*-weighted MR Imaging at 1.5 and 3.0 T: early experience. Radiology 2006;239(2): 481–7.

[66] Sosnovik DE, Weissleder R. Emerging concepts in molecular MRI. Curr Opin Biotechnol 2007; 18(1):4–10.

[67] Kooi ME, Cappendijk VC, Cleutjens KB, et al. Accumulation of ultrasmall superparamagnetic particles of iron oxide in human atherosclerotic plaques can be detected by in vivo magnetic resonance imaging. Circulation 2003;107(19): 2453–8.

[68] Ruehm SG, Corot C, Vogt P, et al. Magnetic resonance imaging of atherosclerotic plaque with ultrasmall superparamagnetic particles of iron oxide in hyperlipidemic rabbits. Circulation 2001;103(3):415–22.

[69] Rhee TK, Larson AC, Prasad PV, et al. Feasibility of blood oxygenation level-dependent MR imaging to monitor hepatic transcatheter arterial embolization in rabbits. J Vasc Interv Radiol 2005; 16(11):1523–8.

[70] Rodrigues LM, Howe FA, Griffiths JR, et al. Tumor R2* is a prognostic indicator of acute radiotherapeutic response in rodent tumors. J Magn Reson Imaging 2004;19(4):482–8.

[71] Prasad PV. Evaluation of intra-renal oxygenation by BOLD MRI. Nephron Clin Pract 2006;103(2): c58–65.

[72] Forster BB. Is functional MR imaging of skeletal muscle the ultimate tool for assessment of peripheral arterial occlusive disease? Radiology 2006;241(2):329–30.

[73] Li LP, Vu AT, Li BS, et al. Evaluation of intrarenal oxygenation by BOLD MRI at 3.0 T. J Magn Reson Imaging 2004;20(5):901–4.

[74] Haacke EM, Xu Y, Cheng YC, et al. Susceptibility weighted imaging (SWI). Magn Reson Med 2004;52(3):612–8.

[75] McGorty KA, Fazio W, Kim D, et al. Susceptibility weighted imaging (SWI) sequence for breast calcification at 3T. In: Proc Soc Mag Reson Tech. Berlin (Germany): 2007.

[76] von Morze C, Xu D, Purcell DD, et al. Intracranial Time-of-Flight R Angiography at 7T with Comparison to 3T [681]. In: Proc Intl Soc Mag Reson Med. Berlin (Germany): 2007. p. 681.

[77] Ludman CN, Morgan PS, Peters A, et al. Contrast enhanced MR angiography at 7 Tesla: challenging the limits of spatial resolution [abstract 2492]. In: Proc Intl Soc Mag Reson Med. Berlin (Germany): 2007. p. 2492.

ELSEVIER
SAUNDERS

MAGNETIC
RESONANCE
IMAGING CLINICS

Magn Reson Imaging Clin N Am 15 (2007) 467–471

Index

Note: Page numbers of article titles are in **boldface** type.

Moving?

Make sure your subscription moves with you!

To notify us of your new address, find your **Clinics Account Number** (located on your mailing label above your name), and contact customer service at:

E-mail: elspcs@elsevier.com

800-654-2452 (subscribers in the U.S. & Canada)
407-345-4000 (subscribers outside of the U.S. & Canada)

Fax number: 407-363-9661

Elsevier Periodicals Customer Service
6277 Sea Harbor Drive
Orlando, FL 32887-4800

*To ensure uninterrupted delivery of your subscription, please notify us at least 4 weeks in advance of move.